W9-BUV-775

Advances in Health Care Organization Theory

Stephen S. Mick
Mindy E. Wyttenbach
Editors

Advances in Health Care Organization Theory

JOSSEY-BASS
A Wiley Imprint
989 Market Street
San Francisco, CA 94103-1741

www.josseybass.com

Jossey-Bass books and products are available through most bookstores. To contact
Jossey-Bass directly call our Customer Care Department within the U.S. at
800-956-7739, outside the U.S. at 317-572-3986 or fax 317-572-4002.

Jossey-Bass also publishes its books in a variety of electronic formats.
Some content that appears in print may not be available in electronic books.

Library of Congress Cataloging-in-Publication Data
Advances in health care theory / Stephen S. Mick, Mindy E. Wyttenbach,
  editors.—1st ed.
    p. ; cm.
  Includes bibliographical references and index.
    ISBN 0-7879-5764-X (alk. paper)
  1. Medical care. 2. Health facilities. 3. Organization—Research.
  [DNLM: 1. Delivery of Health Care—organization &
administration—United States. 2. Community Networks—organization &
administration—United States. 3. Health Facilities—organization &
administration—United States. 4. Health Planning—organization &
administration—United States. W 84 AA1 A235 2003] I. Mick, Stephen S.
II. Wyttenbach, Mindy E., 1975-
  RA427.A446 2003
  362.1—dc21   2002155024

FIRST EDITION
HB Printing   10 9 8 7 6 5 4 3 2 1

Contents

Figures and Tables

. . . .

Figures

Tables

Acknowledgments

· ·

The faculty, students, and staff of the Department of Health Administration at Virginia Commonwealth University deserve all the
praise that I can muster for having tolerated my lapses in departmental administration and instruction while working on this edited
volume. Thank you all for your patience. Thanks, too, are due to
Andy Pasternack, our editor, for his encouragement and support
throughout this effort. Finally, great appreciation is extended to
Myron Fottler and Arnold Kaluzny, and to Kaluzny's doctoral sem-
inar, for careful and thoughtful reviews of the entire manuscript.

STEPHEN S. MICK

Thank you to my family for their support throughout the duration
of this project. I am also grateful to my coeditor for guiding me
through the ins and outs of my first editorial endeavor. Finally, I
would like to acknowledge Dr. Steve Mosher, who introduced me
to the field of health administration in the early 1990s. I truly appreciate his dedication to teaching young professionals and the invalu-
able advice that he has provided me over the years.

MINDY E. WYTTENBACH

The Editors

. . . .

Stephen S. Mick is the Arthur Graham Glasgow Professor in the Department of Health Administration at Virginia Commonwealth University. He is also the departmental chair. He received his B.A. degree in psychology (1965) from Stanford University and his M.Phil. (1972) and Ph.D. degrees in sociology (1973) from Yale University. Mick taught sociology at Middlebury College; he also taught public health and health care organization and management at Yale University, Oklahoma University, the University of Washington, Johns Hopkins University, and the University of Michigan.

Mindy E. Wyttenbach is a candidate in the doctoral program in Health Services Organization and Research at Virginia Commonwealth University. She received her B.A. degree in health care administration (1997) from Mary Baldwin College and her M.H.S. degree in health finance and management (1999) from the Johns Hopkins University Bloomberg School of Public Health.

The Contributors

. . . .

Jeffrey A. Alexander is the Richard Carl Jelinek Professor of Health Management and Policy at the University of Michigan, School of Public Health.

Jane Banaszak-Holl is an assistant professor in the Department of Health Management and Policy, University of Michigan.

James W. Begun is professor and director of the M.H.A. Program in the Department of Healthcare Management at the University of Minnesota.

Lawton R. Burns is the James Joo-Jin Kim Professor of Health Care Systems and Management and director of the Wharton Center for Health Management and Economics at the University of Pennsylvania.

Thomas A. D'Aunno is the Novartis Professor of Healthcare Management and professor of organizational behavior, INSEAD, France.

Kevin J. Dooley is a professor of management and industrial engineering at Arizona State University.

Heather Elms is an assistant professor in the Department of Management at Warrington College of Business Administration at the University of Florida, Gainesville.

David Grazman is the associate director of H∗Works at the Health Care Advisory Board Company in Washington, D. C.

John R. Kimberly is the Henry Bower Professor in the Department of Management and the Department of Health Care Systems at the Wharton School, University of Pennsylvania. He is also Visiting Professor at INSEAD in Fontainebleau, France, and Executive Director of the Wharton/INSEAD Alliance.

Roice D. Luke is a professor in the Department of Health Administration at Virginia Commonwealth University.

Etienne Minvielle is Charge de Recherche at the CNRS and a Chief Researcher at the Center for Health Economics and Administrative Research (INSERM-CNRS, Paris, France).

Thomas G. Rundall is the Henry J. Kaiser Professor of Organized Health Systems in the Division of Health Policy and Management at the University of California, Berkeley.

W. Richard Scott is Professor Emeritus in the Department of Sociology at Stanford University.

Stephen M. Shortell is the Blue Cross of California Distinguished Professor of Health Policy and Management and a professor of organizational behavior in the Division of Health Policy and Management at the University of California, Berkeley, and the Haas School of Business. He is also the Dean of the School of Public Health at Berkeley.

Stephen L. Walston is the director of graduate programs and an associate professor in the Department of Health Administration at Indiana University.

Kenneth R. White is associate professor and director of graduate programs in the Department of Health Administration at Virginia Commonwealth University.

Douglas R. Wholey is professor and chair of Public Health Administration at the University of Minnesota, School of Public Health.

James L. Zazzali is an assistant professor in the Department of Health Administration, Virginia Commonwealth University

Brenda Zimmerman is an associate professor of strategy and organization at McGill University.

Advances in Health Care Organization Theory

Themes, Discovery, and Rediscovery

Stephen S. Mick and Mindy E. Wyttenbach

T he original essays in this book are written to help advance the field of organization theory, particularly in the area of health care. In the spirit of its predecessor volume's focus on health care organization theory in the 1980s (Mick, 1990), this book continues the task of demonstrating the contribution that analysts of health care organizations can make to an understanding of what has happened in the health care sector, focusing this time on the 1990s. The chapters in this book may also presage what might happen in the current decade of the new millennium.

Both senior authors and new colleagues join together in the present volume to construct new or revised visions of how, and with what results, organization theory has provided an understanding of health care during the last decade of the previous century. Simultaneously, where we have found theory to be lacking, we have attempted to pose new and more useful paradigms.

Environmental Changes in Health Care

Characteristics of the health care environment of the 1990s caused many of us to be puzzled by what we saw. Some of what perplexed us were extensions of changes that began in the 1980s. These characteristics included the addition of nonlocal and multilayered authority structures to, and sometimes their replacement of, conventional physician-administrator-governing board structures; the convergence of hospital structures, goals, and performance regardless of profit status, or of religious or secular status; the addition of diversified services only remotely related to the provision of health care; the widespread implementation of quality improvement processes whose results are still yet to be determined; the rapid adoption of integrated delivery structures or systems (IDSs) and the almost as rapid retreat from these models; and the rapacious purchasing by hospitals of physician practices followed by the stunning financial failures of these acquisitions.

These events have occurred in a financial environment experiencing dizzying growth that, for a brief moment in the mid-1990s, appeared to have been mastered by the apparent impact of growth in managed care. But this was just a brief respite: total expenditures for health care were $647 billion in 1990 and approximately $1.3 trillion in 2000, with per capita expenditures increasing from $2,738 to $4,637 during that period. The percentage of the gross national product spent on health care was about 11.5 in 1990; it rose to about 13.2 in 2000 (Heffler and others, 2001). What were the major lines of movement and experimentation that occurred in the preceding decade?

Events and Actions in the 1990s

The environment during the 1990s within the health care sector in the United States was turbulent and fueled by uncertainties in spite of the fact that this was a period of economic prosperity for the nation. The unemployment rate during this decade was at an all-time low, and medical technology advancements were occurring and diffusing at an astonishing rate. The human genome project, pharmaceutical innovations to treat conditions such as AIDS, and the refinement of minimally invasive surgical techniques during this decade each contributed to shaping the health care delivery system that exists today.

During the 1990s, health care spending increased rapidly despite the presence of managed care in the United States. By 1995, managed care plans had become the dominant form of health insurance and enrolled 73 percent of all Americans who were covered by employer-based health benefits (Jenson, Morrisey, Gaffney, and Liston, 1997). Nevertheless, health care spending in the United States reached $1.2 trillion by 1999. Expenditures for prescription drugs more than doubled inside of ten years and in 1999 reached $100 billion (Mays, Hurley, and Grossman, 2001). By the year 2000, the number of uninsured individuals in the United States reached 44 million, or 14 percent of the U.S. population, and the over-eighty-five segment of the nation's population had increased by 35 percent from 3.1 million in 1990 to 4.2 million in 1999 (U.S. Census Bureau, 2000).

Hospital downsizing and consolidations occurred frequently during this decade, and community hospitals across the country shed 72,000 beds inside of the ten-year period as a large portion of traditionally inpatient business shifted to the outpatient sector. By the end of the decade, urgent care centers, surgi-centers, and ambulatory care clinics were operating successfully in markets across the country and had become accepted as efficient and effective alternatives to the more expensive acute care hospital setting (Heffler and others, 2001).

The presence of these trends and issues within the health care environment during the 1990s, along with many others, set the stage for countless advances in health services management, research, policy development, and theoretical analysis.

Regulatory Activity

The political environment within the 1990s was also intense, and at the beginning of the decade public support for national health care reform was at a forty-year high. At the same time, universal health insurance coverage was a priority on the agenda of policymakers at the national, state, and local levels. Thus, soon after taking office, the Clinton administration drafted the Health Security Act of 1992, which may have been the most publicized attempt at federal health care reform in recent history. Although this legislation was never passed, governmental policymakers, nongovernmental activists, business groups, trade unions, and physician organizations worked tirelessly to develop alternative reform policies and programs aimed at providing health insurance coverage for all U.S. citizens (Skocpol, 1995).

In spite of the defeat of the Health Security Act, in 1993 President Clinton signed the Family and Medical Leave Act. This was the first piece of legislation signed into law under the Clinton administration, and it had a significant impact on the health care sector in the United States. After its implementation, the act allowed working Americans to enjoy a new sense of job and health insurance coverage security in the event of a personal or family member illness. Additionally, the implementation and success of this act provided Americans with a sense of renewed confidence in the government's role in the health care sector.

In response to an increased focus on the Internet as a tool for the transmission of medical information and the diffusion of complex information systems within health care, the president signed into law the Health Insurance Portability and Accountability Act (HIPAA) in 1996. This piece of legislation, which focused on the privacy, confidentiality, and security of medical information required consumer control over personal health information. For the first time in history, lawmakers had called for the establishment of accountability guidelines for medical record use and release, security of health-related data, and public responsibility for privacy protections within the U.S. health care sector (Lumpkin, 2000). The specifications of this act would require substantial changes for managed care organizations, hospitals, physician practices, and health information technology vendors. Because its implementation was designed to occur in stages, most beyond the year 2000, the true impacts of this legislation are not yet known (Chesney, 2001).

Aside from this, President Clinton signed the Balanced Budget Act (BBA) into law in August 1997 and the Balanced Budget Refinement Act (BBRA) in 1999, both of which prompted some of the most significant changes to the Medicare and Medicaid programs since their development. These acts introduced potentially stringent cost controls for hospitals, home health agencies, and safety-net providers throughout the country. Industry experts predict that hospital profit margins could decrease by 48 percent by 2002 as a result of the BBA, which will have profound implications for the operations and financial viability of these organizations (HCIA, 2001). Furthermore, between 1997 and 1999, Medicare funding for freestanding home health agencies was reduced by 35 percent (Heffler and others, 2001). For safety-net providers, the BBA threatened subsidies that have long supported indigent care provided by these organizations, such as disproportionate share and indirect medical education payments (Dickler and Shaw, 2000; Zuckerman, Bazzoli, Davidoff, and LoSasso, 2001).

Another policy change during this decade that had a significant impact on the health care industry in the United States was the Children's Health Insurance Program (CHIP) of 1997 or Title XXI of the Social Security Act. This state and federal partnership program, which was developed to expand child health assistance to uninsured and low-income children, allocated $24 billion over a five-year period to assist states in expanding health insurance coverage to children. Federal policymakers shortly after implementation argued that the CHIP program, which was implemented quickly by states, was the most noteworthy attempt to improve access to health care for children since the inception of the Medicaid program (U.S. Health Care Financing Administration, 2001a). In spite of several limitations, many argued that this act was a step in the right direction regarding the provision of health services to children of low- to moderate-income parents (Starr, 2000).

As a result of consumer discontent with the restrictions imposed by managed care organizations during the 1990s, U.S. lawmakers formulated the Patient Bill of Rights in 1998. If signed into law, this piece of legislation would have been the first act to permit the federal government to dictate relationships between consumers, providers, and managed care organizations. Unfortunately, although aiming to support consumers, the passage of this bill was prohibited by political gridlock. While the Senate supported a version of this bill that allows consumers to sue their health plans without limitation, the House proposed that restrictions be placed on the size of such lawsuits to reduce their frequency and contain costs. By the end of the 1990s, Congress was still debating the final stipulations of this legislation, furthering the uncertain environment for health care consumers and managed care organizations into the next century.

Organizational and Financing Trends

During this period of intense health care regulatory activity, several organizational and financing trends became visible within the health care industry in the 1990s. Some of the most widespread trends included the adoption and implementation of the resource-based relative value scale (RBRVS) methodology of Medicare Part B physician payment; the rise and fall of physician practice management companies (PPMCs); a shift toward vertical and horizontal health system integration, and ultimately de-integration; a major increase in health insurance premiums; a surge to enroll Medicaid and Medicare beneficiaries into managed care programs; and an overall managed care backlash by consumers, providers, and other stakeholders in the health care industry.

One of the most significant changes to physician reimbursement policy that occurred during the 1990s was the development of the RBRVS. This new payment system for physician services under the Medicare program was established in 1992. The aim of this provider payment methodology was to recognize objective measures for the work of physicians and to create reimbursement equity for physician services across all specialties. Due to its success in eliminating irregularities within the Medicare physician fee schedule, nearly 50 percent of private health plans surveyed in 1995 reported some use of the RBRVS system (Harris-Shapiro and Greenstein, 1999). By 1998, this system was widely used by third party payers, state Medicaid agencies, and Blue Cross/Blue Shield plans across the country to determine physician reimbursement levels and capitation rates (American Academy of Pediatrics, 1998).

In the early 1990s, managed care and capitation were believed by many experts to be the next wave in health care financing and delivery. However, as physicians increasingly experienced the impact of these trends in the forms of declining reimbursements, increased administrative burden, and a general loss of control of their professional destinies, many realized that they lacked the capital, cash, and managerial expertise to survive. Thus in response, many linked with PPMCs to assist with practice asset management and managed care contracting (Hill, 1998). Although the $11 billion PPMC industry was expected to achieve a great success, within a short period of time, many physicians became discontented with the loss of control and high management fees associated with these entities. For many, PPMCs added costly and redundant layers of overhead to physician practices that did not add significant value. Ultimately, many PPMCs were unsuccessful in their attempts to manage practice costs and enhance physician revenues, and many physicians separated voluntarily from these entities (Badertscher, 1998). Subsequently, several PPMCs, such as MedPartners, went bankrupt.

The consequences of this financial failure were felt by physicians across the nation when PPMC stock value was lost and numerous physician groups within the country were left without a vehicle for contracting with managed care organizations (Hill, 1998; Lesser and Ginsburg, 2000). Health care analysts soon concluded that PPMCs had grown too quickly (Ginsburg, 2000).

In response to such misfortune, many physicians joined unions in an effort to regain the professional autonomy that they held prior to entering into PPMC affiliations (Bohlmann, 2000). In a short period of time, physician unionization emerged as trend of its own within the U.S. health care system.

By the middle of the 1990s, health care sector leaders had become enthusiastic about the prospect of the potential of integrated health care delivery systems as cost containment vehicles to provide a continuum of care to consumers. However, by the end of the decade, this organizational experimentation, like many others, had fallen to the wayside. Health care organizations across the country moved quickly away from integrated organizational models that just a few years before were believed to be the future of health care delivery within the United States. Reasons cited in the literature and the popular press for such deintegration included the large of amount of capital necessary for successful integration, administration and information technology complications, cultural differences between staff members within separate organizations aiming to integrate, and the generally high transaction costs associated with the integration process (Ginsburg, 2000), a prediction made by some observers at the beginning of the 1990s (for example, Mick, 1990).

At the same time that PPMCs and integrated delivery systems were becoming less prevalent within the United States, consumer spending on health insurance premiums was increasing. As a result of changes in employer policies regarding the provision of health insurance benefits for employees, the percentage of the total premium paid by workers for family coverage increased from 28 percent to 34 percent from 1990 to 1995. Furthermore, from 1999 to 2000, premiums increased by 8.3 percent, which reflected the highest one-year premium increase during a seven-year period (Gabel, Ginsburg, Pickreign, and Reschovsky, 2001).

Aside from these overall themes, during the 1990s enrollment patterns and health insurance product offerings changed. In spite of a projection that health maintenance organizations (HMOs) would grow within the United States during this period, and a brief movement from employers toward restrictive managed care models,

HMO enrollment grew very little (Ginsburg, 2000). Coupled with the overarching rise in consumerism that occurred during this period, consumer desires for increased choice resulted in an enrollment shift from more tightly controlled HMOs to less restrictive preferred provider organizations (PPOs) and point of service (POS) plans (Heffler and others, 2001). In 1993, POS plans covered only 9 percent of American workers, yet by 1995 this had reached 20 percent (Jenson, Morrisey, Gaffney, and Liston, 1997). This shift occurred as consumers lost the freedom to choose their provider under restrictive managed care arrangements (Marquis and Long, 1999).

Another notable change within managed care was the enrollment of Medicare and Medicaid beneficiaries in managed care plans in an effort to enhance care quality and contain costs. From 1991 to 1996, Medicaid managed care enrollment increased from 9.5 percent of total beneficiaries to 40 percent (Holahan, Zuckerman, Evans, and Rangarajan, 1998). Furthermore, by 1996, 13.3 million Medicaid recipients were enrolled in some form of managed care, and total Medicare managed care enrollment increased from 3.1 million at the end of 1995 to 6.3 million in 1999 (U.S. Health Care Financing Administration, 2001b; (Lipson, 1997). Along with this growth, however, there was a strong sense in some quarters that managed care, left unregulated, would fail in its multiple, sometimes conflicting, objectives of cost containment, improved access to care, and enhanced health care service quality.

Aside from a desire for provider choice, consumers began at an increasing rate to demand information about the health services that they received. In response to this demand and the increasing level of competition in the managed care arena, the National Committee for Quality Assurance (NCQA) developed the Health Plan Employer Data Information Set (HEDIS) in 1993, and in 1995, the Foundation for Accountability (FACCT) was established, to address issues related to health plan performance measures (Roper and Cutler, 1998). Quality-related organizations and programs such as these served as the foundation for the increased focus on health care quality that earned increasing attention within the health care industry throughout the remainder of the 1990s.

A final trend that emerged toward the end of the 1990s that related to the managed care marketplace was the push toward direct contracting strategies such as the development of the Buyer's Health Care Action Group (BHCAG) purchasing coalition in 1997 (Christianson, Feldman, Weiner, and Drury, 1999), as discussed by Wholey and Burns in Chapter Five. BHCAG created a new type of health care market in Minnesota that involved some of the largest employers in the state, including 3M, Honeywell, and Pillsbury. This program emphasized increased consumer choice and the release of comparative information about providers and hospitals (Burrows and Moravec, 1997). Whereas independent small primary care physician groups responded most favorably to this initiative, the response from managed care organizations ranged from supportive to ambivalent. The response from consumers was favorable, as shown by an enrollment increase from 116,000 in 1997 to 150,000 in 1999 (Christianson, Feldman, Weiner, and Drury, 1999).

The U.S. Health Care Workforce

A backdrop for the changes and issues enumerated in the previous section is the sometimes perplexing and always changing portrait of the U.S. health care workforce. The latter several decades of the twentieth century witnessed federal and state largesse that helped produce enormous increases in most of the professions and occupations in health care, including that of health administrators. Then, from the mid-1980s to the twenty-first century, the workforce continued to grow and evolve in shape as much a result of the workforce requirements of managed care plans as by explicit public or private policy formulation and implementation. In the 1990s, there was a renewed interest in the health professions (for example, medicine, nursing, dentistry), and a virtual explosion in the mid-level professional areas (such as nurse practitioners and physician assistants).

The interaction of changes in organizational arrangements for the delivery of health care and in the evolution of the workforce had a special place in the shaping of the 1990s health care system. The growth of the physician component of the workforce probably had a salubrious effect on managed care, that is, the purported "surplus" of physicians led to the availability of a large enough number of less recalcitrant professionals willing to work within the organizational constraints of managed care plans. And, of course, the practice of medicine within managed care itself was reshaped by the drive toward cost constraints, efficiency, and standardization of clinical practice.

The Council on Graduate Medical Education (1995), an Executive Branch advisory group of health professionals, suggested several important features in the managed care–physician relationship. Although controversial, many believe that continued managed care growth has only magnified and exacerbated the problem of a provider surplus, particularly among physicians. However, it may be possible that the historical imbalance between too few primary care providers and too many specialists may be rectified through the organizational device of managed care arrangements. Market pressures from the plans have had an impact in favor of medical student and resident choice of primary care medicine and less so for other specialties.

Many educational institutions have experienced severe financial difficulty as managed care plans erode their patient bases. That is, managed care plans, which historically have had little if any involvement with education and training, are underbidding educational institutions such as university medical schools with their higher unit costs stemming from their training mission. The impact of this pressure will be difficult to predict, but one effect might be lower clinical income for teaching organizations, with increasing budgetary burdens on university medical centers. This will probably translate into reductions in medical and other clinical faculty salaries, exacerbation of personnel conflicts, and even constraints on the ability of teaching organizations to meet their historic missions. There may even be a reduction in the number of training sites for health professional students.

Another possible result of managed care could be a shift to the kind of clinical practice that health plans require. Those educational institutions that have not already adapted to these new demands may place themselves at risk for organizational failure. The substance of clinical practice has included an emphasis on prevention, treatment of the whole person and not simply one or the other organ systems, prudent exercise of diagnostic and treatment approaches in which efficiency and cost-effectiveness are key, emphasis on "evidence-based" medicine in which preferred treatment approaches will have predictably positive and clear cut outcomes, and reliance on provider teams with more integration of different skill sets.

This discussion underscores several themes evident in the health care environment of the 1990s in the United States. These themes, which include marketplace and political uncertainty, a continued sense of cost consciousness, a drive toward technological innovation, a continuing presence of organizational adaptation, and turbulence in the workforce, suggest a matrix of conflicting forces, with no single way to predict their denouement. Within this matrix, health services organization theorists have before themselves an infinite number of research and analytical opportunities. At the very least, these events, issues, and themes are the crucible within which the authors of the present volume have mixed and combined their respective approaches to explain both general and particular phenomena. The next section outlines their efforts.

Emergent Themes

Each chapter in this book was written independently of the rest. Still, the following eleven chapters coalesce around a set of common themes, which were forced onto the awareness of the authors by the overriding events of the 1990s. Put another way, the convergence of thinking in a field of inquiry, of which the study of health care organizations is but one example, is influenced by the problems and issues in a historically grounded period of time. Our period of time is the decade of the 1990s, and the pressure of events, forces, and changes is something we have documented in this chapter. A brief overview of each following chapter's main contribution reveals the book's dominant themes.

W. Richard Scott in Chapter Two outlines a fifty-year evolution of the health care field, including its constituent market forces, in the San Francisco Bay Area. He concludes that the past half century has witnessed a large erosion of physician hegemony across a spectrum of traditionally clinical realms, notably in quality of care, and attributes much of this change to a declining institutional presence that has been successfully challenged by public and private controls, all couched within a triumphant "managerial logic." Scott's argument has an element of irony embedded in it, given that he is an architect of what is known as "institutional theory," a widely accepted theoretical posture that emphasizes rational myths, isomorphism, and legitimacy.

This chapter lays out the leitmotif of much of the rest of the volume: the place of institutional forces in the hurly-burly, barely ordered chaos of change in the health care sector of the 1990s. Much of what other authors of this volume present falls into three rough categories. First, the Scott argument is refined and supported, noting that although market and institutional forces run in parallel, market forces are gradually dominating organizational fields. Second, some authors suggest that the verdict is still out on whether there is a "winner." Rather, the real question is what new forms market and institutional forces have taken with what result. Finally, there is the point of view that takes the opposite tack: that institutional forces, in new clothes, have in fact emerged victorious over the putative power and discipline of market forces that have been so celebrated in the last quarter century of the previous millennium.

Jeffrey A. Alexander and Thomas A. D'Aunno build on the groundwork laid by Scott. In Chapter Three they explore and explicate several different competing possibilities of how market (or technical) forces interact with traditional institutional forces, raising the question as to whether the two can coexist, and, if so, in what manner. Although Alexander and D'Aunno do not gainsay that market forces have increased in strength and coverage across the nation, they do suggest that institutional forces have hardly been eliminated from the health care sector and have found new homes and new ways to exert themselves. In fact, they assert that in many areas of health care delivery, there is still very little resemblance to industrial and corporate sectors, implying that institutional forces have thwarted the intervention of market and technical forces. These observations led Alexander and D'Aunno to develop a typology of four different possible institutional and market relationships: of both as competing forces; of institutional dominating the shape of markets; of both offering parallel, nonconflicting presence and pressure on organizations; and of both forming a synthesis. Which of these possibilities might prevail, argue the two authors, is a function of the relative combination of agency in decision making, strength of values and interests, and variable resources and power. Such a matrix of factors appears to provide a template to understand the welter of organizational forms and their relationships to their environments or organizational fields.

Chapter Four, by Kenneth R. White, is a specific look at what happens when market forces and a highly focused institutional environment conjoin for a particular group of health care organizations, here hospitals and hospital systems guided by the Roman Catholic Church. Through his examination of the empirical situation of these organizations, he poses a paradigm that predicts the way organizations may react. Although the focus is highly specific, it offers a more generalized view of how other health care organizations change, adapt, and even fail, as a result of competing and conflicting values and pressures of the 1990s and 2000s health care sector.

Of the four possible interactions of market and institutional forces outlined by Alexander and D'Aunno, White's argument is that the behavior of Roman Catholic hospitals supports the idea of market and institutional forces in conflict. The rationale behind this stems from both the often unyielding value perspectives of the Church and the frequent trade-off choices between economic efficiency demanded by markets and social equity demanded by institutional pressures (Okun, 1975).

The shift toward a searching look at what markets *are* occurs in Chapter Five, by Douglas R. Wholey and Lawton R. Burns. Moving from a standard definition of an economic market, the authors demonstrate the power and creativity that results if one expands the definition of a market to what it is in its essential nature: a focus of exchange relations that emphasize economic transactions. Wholey and Burns aptly demonstrate how this "expanded vision" of health care markets permits a deeper and more nuanced explanation for the astonishingly different ways health care markets have evolved in the United States. Once this possibility is admitted, a torrent of interesting prospects arise that considerably widen the explanation of how and why markets and health care organizations interact. Notions of "micromarkets," of human agency via strategy, in short, of the panoply of human interaction and intention, can be brought into conventional discussions of markets that tend to be highly deterministic.

Stephen M. Shortell and Thomas G. Rundall in Chapter Six narrow the focus onto a description of physician practices in organizational settings and the ensuing relationships that have emerged between medical work and organizational arrangements. Their approach combines both deterministic and voluntary (agency) perspectives through a conceptual model that melds network theory and strategic adaptation, permitting a fresh view of physician-organization relationships, often consisting of activities, some of which are described in Chapters One, Ten, and Eleven especially, that fared very poorly in the 1990s.

Chapter Seven, by Jane Banaszak-Holl, Heather Elms, and David Grazman takes network theory into the realm of nonacute care, community-based services. In the tradition of the work by Levine and White (1961) and Levine, White, and Paul (1963), the authors have advanced our thinking about the importance of exchange networks in comprehending this often-neglected set of organizational arrangements. Conversely, the authors demonstrate that, in fact, exchange theory as expressed through network analysis is a critical way to understand the behavior and strategic intent of a large realm of health services delivery. This focus emphasizes that neither traditional organization theory nor conventional market analysis captures the activities of community-based services well, which may be a bellwether for an enriched understanding for the behavior of even acute care health service organizations.

The next contribution, by John R. Kimberly and Etienne Minvielle, opens up a "rediscovered" avenue of examination of health care organizations. In Chapter Eight, the authors revitalize and reassess the classic distinction of machine bureaucracy versus professional bureaucracy through the medium of the movement toward quality assurance and quality improvement in the delivery of health care. Kimberly and Minvielle aptly demonstrate how the problem of what to do about hospital quality, today translated into the term "patient safety," has caused the two traditional, and enduring, bureaucratic systems to deal with each other in a way not required in the past. One of the great strengths of their argument is to remind observers that health care organizations are still essentially bureaucracies, with all the functional and dysfunctional features of bureaucracies, as clearly articulated by Weber (Gerth and Mills, 1958) and Crozier (1964), among others. This organizational feature seems to have been forgotten in the hubbub of environmental change, strategic activity, health policy intervention, and, certainly, health care organization theory itself. We are reminded that to understand what creates good quality from poor quality, we need to return to an appreciation of how dimensions of bureaucracy (such as design, authority, work flows) may be critically related to whether good or poor quality care is delivered.

James L. Zazzali in Chapter Nine engages readers in a unique view of organization trust, a view that suggests that much of contemporary organization theory, from resource dependence to transaction cost economics, rests on unstated assumptions and reliance on the notion of trust. In fact, trust may not only be the one common piece to the disparate patchwork of perspectives that characterizes organization theory in health care, but may ironically also be one of the most underappreciated and unexplored features of most theoretical perspectives.

The next two chapters bring to closure the explorations of this volume. Chapter Ten, by James W. Begun, Brenda Zimmerman, and Kevin J. Dooley, concludes that chaos theory, or its derivative, complex adaptive systems, is a more fruitful alternative to understanding the behavior of organizations in the 1990s, and, by extension, in the present decade. Suggesting that traditional organization theory missed the mark on many organizational issues in the 1990s, the authors argue that the time is ripe for a paradigm shift. Their proposition rests upon the insights of biological sciences and other "hard" disciplines in their attempts to find coherence or explanation in the dynamics of change and evolution in extremely dense, complicated, and highly interrelated phenomena.

In Chapter Eleven, by Roice D. Luke and Stephen L. Walston, the authors also take aim at the inadequacies of current organization theory, but their conclusion is that one must employ an amalgam of existing theories, borrowing without shame from where the theory works and integrating the pieces into a new admixture that more accurately and faithfully reflects empirical reality, very little of which, they stress, conforms to theoretical predictions. They also add, as did Shortell and Rundall in Chapter Six, that strategic intent, human agency, and willful purpose must be part of the mix of any conceptual rationale if one is not to be off the mark about organizational activity. Strategy, they imply, is the "wild card," the element that makes the potage of diversity of health care environments and their constituent organizations what it is.

Finally, in Chapter Twelve, Mick and Wyttenbach discuss several underlying issues that emerge in most of the chapters. The first of these issues is the interplay between institutional and market forces and the multiple ways that this interplay is manifested. The second issue is a renewed look at the importance of the internal structure of health care organizations. Observers have placed so much attention on the effect of environmental and market forces on health care organizations that some feel that there has been an unjustified negligence of the role of intraorganizational design and dynamics in understanding contemporary problems of organizational performance. The third issue is the argument that no single organization theory, and perhaps even organization theory as we know it, is adequate to explain the multiplicity of organizational phenomena that have occurred in the past decade. The chapter provides a summary statement that challenges readers to use the book as a starting point for the improvement and application of theory for health policy, particularly as policy relates to organizations.

Macrolevel Themes

To recapitulate in a denser fashion several key themes that have emerged in these chapters, we point to the first: the "rediscovery" of the social basis of economic activity in health care. Throughout the book, readers will see various suggestions that economic activity within markets, however flawed, occurs in an *institutional* or *social* framework. In sociology, the terms are used together, as in *social institution*. What does this mean? Classically, the definition of a social institution consists of the notion of an interrelated system of roles and norms that specify appropriate and expected behavior toward the fulfillment of some need such as the provision of food or material goods, or, in the case here, of health care and, eventually, of healing, curing, and health (Theodorson and Theodorson, 1969).

It could be a framework, like that of George Herbert Mead (1934), that theorizes how specific individuals' activities are moderated by communal control through a notion of the "generalized other." The common activities, patterned and predictable behavior, taken together constitute a social institution. It could also be a conceptual scheme aimed more directly at economic activity, such as that of John R. Commons (1950), which portrayed the economy as a set of social relationships or a system of stabilized and regularized control of economic exchange. Commons contrasted this against the idea of the economy—or its markets—as a mechanism or organism. Finally, one might find in Parsons and Smelser's monumental work, *Economy and Society* (1956), an effort to understand market imperfections as directly related to their "institutional nature." That is, where markets are less than optimal, it is probably because of social relationships that have bound together in ways that influence how exchanges will and will not transpire.

In any event, the complex relationship between institutional environments and economic markets is a major preoccupation of authors throughout this volume. One way that several have tried to explore this relationship is through the lens of exchange theory adapted in various ways, most notably in the language of network analysis. Exchange is essentially a person's activities in relation to one or more other people, or an organization's activities in relation to one or more other entities, all motivated by the returns that such relationships are expected to bring from others. Exchanges can, therefore, be economic or noneconomic, with the boundary between them often vague. As noneconomic motivation becomes more salient in exchange relationships, that which accrues consists of obligations, favors, and "insider" connection. What results is that the descriptive and explanatory power of analysts of health care organizations in their respective environmental fields is largely increased. Although the idea that economic markets consist of social relationships is not new, it has been obscured in discussions about health care, especially in the health care policy realm, probably due to the astonishing pressure to find better ways to pay for, deliver, and maintain health care at some vague level of reasonable quality. With the mediocre results of so much market-oriented policy experimentation of the 1990s, the need for a recasting of how we look at the interplay of health care organizations and their environments has resulted. This has led, in our view, to a "rediscovery" of the social embeddedness of health care organizations in a matrix of crosscurrents, some economic, some social, some political, some cultural.

Second, although mostly implied in the majority of chapters, but explicitly recognized in that of Kimberly and Minvielle, there is a stress on the need for another "rediscovery" of the internal operations of health care organizations. This entails, first, an appreciation of the agency of health care leaders and managers in developing and executing strategy and in controlling their relationships with other organizations and entities. It also involves a new appreciation for the staying power of bureaucratic features of organization design and operation. That is, the notion of a hospital, nursing home, or any sort of health care organization as a mere end to larger ends, such as the production of health or the exercise of efficiency in delivering health care, is a flawed and incomplete depiction. Although there may be some validity in thinking of health care organizations as instrumentalities for the execution of wider health policy, there may also be a return to the idea of a health care organization as influenced by its own internal constituents and by the interplay of internal forces arising from the attempt to rationalize human behavior through organizational rules, regimen, structure, and operations. As pressure grows for more accountability in health care organizations in, for example, the realm of quality and patient safety, the rediscovery of these internal bureaucratic forces, small group behavior, and the complex of internal "trades" and exchange takes on new importance.

Finally, a dimension emphasized throughout this volume is the importance of including management agency as an ingredient in organizational activity; put another way, strategic intent cannot be neglected in analyzing health care organizational behavior. This point, although possibly hackneyed, deserves explicit mention because of the strong emphasis in earlier decades on a highly deterministic environmental and market effect on organizations, sometimes to the total exclusion of human intent and purpose. A thread throughout many of the chapters is that highly deterministic organization theory that posits the overriding force of environment circumstances has been inadequate in improving our understanding of organizational activity. This, too, is not a new issue: the argument about human agency and environmental determinism appears to endure, but with each swing of the pendulum, we gain more insight into just how complex is the interplay of each level of organizational life, from the individual to the macro-level organizational field.

Goals of This Book

In the 1990 volume on health care organization theory (Mick, 1990, p. xv), the editor quoted Scott, and it is worth repeating his argument that "The field of organizations has undergone enormous change in the past few decades. It is currently, I believe, the most lively and vigorous area of study within sociology, and perhaps within all of the social sciences. This is a source of both excitement and confusion. Much is happening in the field, and developments are occurring faster than our ability to assimilate them into coherent patterns."

We continue to believe that this remains a felicitous description of the ferment in health care organization theory. Thus this book attempts to whet the appetite of observers of both health care organizations and organizations more generally, especially those dominated by highly trained professions. Although we have teased out several underlying themes that exist in the various chapters, we also wish to emphasize that there remains a diversity and complexity of ideas that cannot be easily categorized or summarized. To attempt to do so would be to violate the richness of thinking that is expressed and to smooth over in a false way the differences that exist. Poole and Van de Ven (1989) suggested that differences and disagreements are the stuff of progress in analyzing complex human phenomena as expressed in organizational life. Our hope is that this book adds to the journey of discovery and rediscovery of what makes health care organizations what they are.

The Old Order Changeth

The Evolving World of Health Care Organizations

W. Richard Scott

Observers of health care delivery systems in the United States have been amazed at the extent and rapidity of change taking place during the past two decades. After watching for many years the numbing spectacle of systems displaying "dynamics without change," in Alford's (1972) cogent phrase, observers following recent developments and attempting to understand their characteristics, causes, and consequences suddenly have much to ponder.

The systems involved are complex and varied, the forces at work manifold and intricately interrelated, the speed of change alarmingly swift. Patients are concerned and confused; physicians, nurses, and other providers are beleaguered and, often, angry; politicians are uncertain and conflicted; managers and health care administrators are stressed and, sometimes, vilified; and investors and financial analysts are seeking to learn whether and how there are profits to be made out of illness. The former world of the independent physician ministering to the medical needs of his patients under simple fee-for-service arrangements, in sometime cooperation with nonprofit, independent community hospitals, seems a distant dream. These arrangements, so stable for so long—(from the 1920s into the 1960s)—appeared largely impervious to change. One would be hard-pressed to find a comparably stable instance among other arenas of social activity during the first half of the twentieth century. It would be equally difficult to identify a large system that has changed so quickly. The rapidity and multidimensional nature of the transformation attest to the truth of Greenwood and Hinings' (1996) generalization that highly institutionalized sectors, by definition, resist change, but when change occurs, they can become transformed rapidly.

How did it happen that the least changeable, most highly institutionalized sector of this earlier time began so suddenly to unravel before our eyes? That is the difficult question this chapter attempts to address. The question is sufficiently large and complex that any answer must be incomplete and partial. My analysis draws on conceptual and empirical materials assembled by a team of researchers working over a five-year period, reported in more detail in the book *Institutional Change and Healthcare Organizations: From Professional Dominance to Managed Care* (Scott, Ruef, Mendel, and Caronna, 2000). In this work, my colleagues and I attempt both to shed some light on changes occurring during the last half century in health care delivery systems in one metropolitan area of this country and to develop an analytical framework that can help to guide other studies of profound institutional change. While our systematic empirical data set only extends to 1995, the major trends we documented have continued up to the present time.

Conceptualizing and Measuring Institutional Change

This section proposes a framework for ordering our thinking about the complex world of health care organizations. We focus especially on ways of describing and understanding change.

Conceptual Framework

Most studies of health care organizations focus on a single organization or on a few organizations of the same type. Such studies can address important questions but are not very useful when we are trying to understand broader forces that necessarily affect, and work through, many diverse organizations. Our choice was to examine the *organizational field*, "those organizations that, in the aggregate, constitute a recognized area of institutional life: key suppliers, resource and product consumers, regulatory agencies, and other organizations that produce similar services or products" (DiMaggio and Powell, 1983, p. 4). (I employ the terms "field" and "sector" interchangeably.) We focus on selected types of providers of health care services but also include as important organizational actors in our study the purchasers of health care services (such as employers and governmental programs), fiscal intermediaries (such as insurance companies, health plans), and oversight structures (such as professional associations, regulatory agencies). Our interest is in examining changes in the health care field over an extended period of time.

A longitudinal focus on the organization field allows us to contemplate (1) diverse kinds of organizations; (2) changes in relations (exchange, competitive, ownership, contractual) among these organizations; (3) changes in the boundaries of organizations; (4) changes in the boundaries of organizational forms or populations (organizations of the same type) and the emergence of new types of organizations; and (5) changes in the boundaries of the field itself.

We embrace an open systems conception that emphasizes that if we are to understand changes in organizations and organizational forms over time, it is necessary to attend to changes in their environments, both in the material resources on which they depend and in the institutional frameworks on which they draw (Scott, 1998). The *material-resource environment* is "that facet of the environment most directly relevant to viewing the organization as a production system depending on and transforming scarce resources" (Scott, Ruef, Mendel, and Caronna, 2000). It includes factors affecting supply and demand (for example, numbers of physicians, insurance coverage of patients); technologies, including both specialized medical equipment and information processing; and the structure of the industry as it affects the flow of resources among competitors and exchange partners.

Of particular interest are the *institutional environments* that influence the structure and behavior of organizations. Although many analysts conflate organizational and institutional structures, we insist on the advantages to be gained by analytically distinguishing between them. Institutions are defined as regulative, normative, and cultural-cognitive frameworks that, in combination, provide stability and meaning to social life (Scott, 2001). Individual organizations can develop their own distinctive norms and beliefs— "corporate cultures"—that, in turn, provide value frameworks that affect their behavior (Selznick, 1949; Schein, 1992). However, we focus primarily on those wider symbolic frameworks operating at the field-level—or even the societal level—that provide legal guidelines, cognitive models, and cultural logics affecting the full range of organizations operating in that societal arena.

To examine changes in institutional environments, we found it useful to distinguish among three components: institutional actors, institutional logics, and governance systems.

> *Institutional actors* include both individuals and collective actors, such as organizations or associations, as they function to both create and carry (embody) institutional logics, as defined below. Changes in the number and type of institutional actors—for example, an increase in the number of health economists or a decline in the number of community hospitals—reflect significant alterations in the nature of an organizational field. We are also, of course, interested in examining changes in relations among actors.
>
> *Institutional logics* are sets of "material practices and symbolic constructions which constitute [a field's] organizing principles and which are available to organizations and individuals to elaborate" (Friedland and Alford, 1991). Changes in the prevailing logics, including rules (for example, should alternative practitioners be allowed to treat patients?) and belief systems (for example, should the federal government pay for

health care?), represent significant changes in an organizational field.

Governance systems are "those arrangements which support the regularized control—whether by regimes created by mutual agreement, by legitimate hierarchical authority or by non-legitimate coercive means—of the actions of one set of actors by another" (Scott, Mendel, and Pollack, forthcoming). We can learn much about the underlying processes of organizational fields by attending closely to the changing nature of power and authority structures.

The institutional environment and material-resource environment are interdependent, each affecting the other. Together they represent the dual facets of social structure—the rules or schemas and the human and nonhuman resources—as described by Giddens (1984) and Sewell (1992). Rules and schema need to be backed by resources to have effects; resources need to be linked to rules and schemas to have meaning and utility.

In our view, a sociologically informative portrait of significant changes in the health care field can be drawn by recording changes over time in institutional actors, logics, and governance structures and their interrelations and as they relate to changes in material resources. But it is also important to recognize that no organizational field is completely insulated from changes in wider social, economic, and cultural conditions. Some of the sources of change in organizational fields are endogenous to the system isolated for study, but others are exogenous, arising from outside the field to influence and penetrate it and, perhaps, alter its boundaries.

Empirical Case

To arrive at a feasible research design, we elected to limit our collection of data on health care organizations to selected populations located in a single, large, metropolitan area—the San Francisco Bay Area—and to focus on the most recent half century—1945–1995.

Five populations (types) of organizations were selected for systematic study: hospitals, integrated health care systems, home health agencies (HHAs), health maintenance organizations (HMOs), and end stage renal disease centers (ESRDCs). The populations were selected to reflect both more traditional forms (hospitals) as well as newer forms (HHAs, ESRDCs, and HMOs) and more diffuse forms (hospitals and integrated health care systems) as well as more specialized forms (HHAs and ESRDCs). The Bay Area is a large, rapidly growing metropolitan area—the population increased from 2.2 million to 6.1 million during the period under study—and is widely recognized to be on the cutting edge of innovation in health care delivery systems. Although it is by no means a typical or modal metropolitan area, it provides insights into how the health care system of one complex metropolitan community has been transformed in the past half century.

While we restricted our study of organizational actors to a single, metropolitan area, our examination of institutional logics and governance structures took into account developments at broader levels: regional, state, and national. Geographical boundaries may be employed to delimit the range and numbers of actors (individual and collective) affected by a set of forces, but should not be used to exclude from study those actors and processes that are producing and conveying the new rules, norms, and cultural models. Scholars attempting to understand the dynamics of organizational fields must attend to both horizontal (exchange and competitive) and vertical (hierarchical) influences and to both local and distant forces. Early studies of interorganizational relations within communities often neglected to take into account the important connections between branch and headquarter units or between local units and regulatory agencies at state and national levels (Scott and Meyer, 1983). Fields encompass both (local) organizational actors and relevant (perhaps nonlocal) governance structures, competitors, and exchange partners (Scott, 1994).

Charting Change in Health Care Organizations

Although, as noted, we view the various aspects of the material-resource and institutional environments to be richly interrelated, we think it helpful to suggest an order of causal priority in which changes in material resources, governance structures, and institutional logics are seen to bring about (and to be embodied within) changes in the types and distributions of social actors. Hence, we begin by describing observed changes in the numbers and types of individual and collective actors in the health care field, treating them as "dependent variables" to be explained by changes in available resources, institutional logics, and governance bodies.

Changing Distributions of Institutional Actors

Focusing on actors provides, we believe, a good descriptive account of changes in the social demography of a field. Both individual and collective actors are of interest, but rather than attending to their individuating features, we emphasize their institutionalized components: the *roles* of individuals, the *forms* of organizations.

Individual consumers of health care services during the period of our study were becoming much more numerous, more urbanized, and educated. As noted, the Bay Area population nearly tripled while the proportion living in urban areas increased from 80 to nearly 100 percent. The percentage of high school graduates increased from under 40 to over 80 percent. Health care providers were becoming more specialized. Whereas in 1945, less than 30 percent of the physicians were specialized, by 1990, more than 80 percent had qualified for such certification (Scott, Ruef, Mendel, and Caronna, 2000). Health care administrators became increasingly professionalized throughout the period, the locus and nature of their training undergoing change. Earlier administrators received their training primarily in schools of public health, whereas later ones increasingly elected business school settings.

Organizational forms are defined by institutionalized models that specify what types of work are to be done by what types of personnel in what ways. The models also prescribe what kinds of social functions are to be insulated from one another or permitted to interact. During the period of our study, traditional forms such as hospitals were confronted by new and competing models of health care delivery. Home health agencies, a reinvention of an earlier form of visiting nurse associations, emphasized home-based services as an alternative to expensive inpatient approaches. End stage renal disease centers began as a specialized service within hospitals but increasingly were provided by independent, freestanding units, an instance of the multiple and diverse services provided by a diffuse form becoming "unbundled" and allocated to specialist organizations. Both of these forms depended greatly for their development on new, improved technologies as well as on eligibility for Medicare funds. ESRDCs also were buoyed by an unusual, disease-specific federal funding program (Rettig and Levinsky, 1991).

For their part, hospitals were set upon from all sides, confronting competition from the new, specialized forms, reduced funding from health plans and federal agencies, and increased costs associated with higher patient acuity and advanced treatment techniques. Survival tactics included increased interdependence and collaboration with exchange partners, cooperation with former competitors, and the negotiation of contractual or ownership ties with the newly emerging delivery systems. These tactics often resulted in the creation of multiunit integrated health care systems—systems that varied enormously in scope, "size, geographical spread, formal structure, type of ownership, degree of control, importance and permanence of connections, and, generally, in extent of 'systemness'" (Scott, Ruef, Mendel, and Caronna, 2000). Hospitals, increasingly, are no longer freestanding, independent organizations but components of larger systems. Within the Bay Area, the number of systems increased from seven to twenty-five and the proportion of hospitals involved in systems from 30 to 70 percent.

Without question, the most innovative and controversial organizational form to emerge during this period was the health maintenance organization. Adapting and extending an earlier, prepaid direct services model that had long been condemned by the American Medical Association as subordinating medical decision making to economic criteria, HMOs were embraced by Washington politicians and policymakers in the early 1970s as a solution to reining in escalating health care expenditures (Starr, 1982). HMOs represent a *hybrid* organization that blends two or more elements from (formerly) distinct forms of organizations (Haveman and Rao, forthcoming). In this novel form, medical care delivery is combined with the insurance and financial function such that the economic effects of clinical decisions directly affect providers. Physicians practicing in HMOs are, to a variable degree, placed "at risk" financially for the medical decisions they make.

Increases or decreases in the number of organizations embodying a given form provide one of the simplest and most powerful indicators of change occurring in an organizational field. Ecologists have argued that the prevalence of an organizational form is a valid indicator of that form's cultural-cognitive legitimacy—its "taken-for-grantedness" as the appropriate arrangement for carrying out a set of activities (Carroll and Hannan, 1989). We extend this argument to suggest that comparing the relative density of organizational populations operating in the same field at the same time provides a good indicator of how these forms are faring in the competitive struggle for patients, dollars, and legitimacy. How were the five organizational forms doing relative to one another in the San Francisco Bay Area?

Eighty-two hospitals existed in the Bay Area in 1945 and eighty-two were still operating in 1992. (Of course, these were not necessarily the same hospitals.) In spite of the tripling of area population during this period, hospitals showed no net increase in numbers; indeed, those still surviving were shrinking, as their capacity utilization dropped from about 75 percent to under 65 percent during this period. By contrast, the number of HMOs increased from only one provider in 1945 (the original branch of Kaiser Permanente) to twenty-three in 1995; HHAs increased by nearly sevenfold, from twenty-one in 1966 to one hundred and forty in 1995; ESRDCs increased by more than fourfold, from ten units in 1969 to forty-five in 1993; and the number of integrated health care systems more than doubled, from seven in 1945 to seventeen in 1995. From the systematic data provided by our sample, community hospitals—the diffuse, traditional form—have been losing out to the newer, more specialized provider forms (Scott, Ruef, Mendel, and Caronna, 2000).

Our data also reveal a shift in ownership arrangements among health care forms. Two distinctions are important: public versus private ownership and, if the latter, nonprofit versus for-profit status. Public ownership of health care facilities shows a marked decline. Government-owned hospitals declined from 40 percent in 1945 to 15 percent in 1992. There are virtually no publicly owned forms among the new, specialized organizations. Hospitals continued to retain their nonprofit status, but among the specialized organizations (HMOs, ESRDCs, HHAs), the ratio of for-profits exceeded that of nonprofits in every case (Scott, Ruef, Mendel, and Caronna, 2000).

Finally, if we compare the extensiveness of relations among provider organizations, we observe growing interdependence among all of them. As noted, today's hospitals are much more likely than earlier versions to be affiliated with integrated health care systems. Similarly, both horizontal and vertical integration among the various types of organizations had increased. All three specialized organizational types—were more likely to be affiliated with "chains" of similar forms. Vertical integration—between hospitals, HHAs, HMOs, and ESRDCs—also had substantially increased during the period since 1980, either in the forms of contractual or ownership ties (Scott, Ruef, Mendel, and Caronna, 2000).

In sum, in our longitudinal case study of changes in the health care delivery systems of the San Francisco Bay Area, we observed an organizational field moving rapidly toward higher levels of specialization, concentration, private ownership, and for-profit orientation in its provider forms.

Although organizations and their leaders can by their actions influence the speed and direction of change, we view them primarily as reflecting rather than instigating change. Changes are more likely to emerge outside of organizations—this is particularly true of the kinds of organizations we are considering—as a consequence of changes in material resources, institutional logics, or governance systems. To move from the "how" to the "why" of societal change, we need to examine changes in resources, beliefs, and power.

Changes in Material Resources

Significant changes occurred on both the demand and supply sides of health care. Demand for medical services increased as larger numbers of individuals were covered by insurance plans—public, commercial, and employer-sponsored. Over time, purchasers have become increasingly concentrated, because of both the growing role of public programs and changes on the private side, including the growth of purchasing coalitions among employers and greater consolidation of health plans (Robinson, 1995). Major developments on the supply side include the increased specialization of individual providers, such as physicians and other health personnel as noted above, and the increasing ratio of physicians to the population. The physician-population ratio in the United States in 1945 was 120 physicians per 100,000 persons; by 1990, the ratio had increased to over 206 per 100,000. In the relatively affluent Bay Area, the ratio was even higher—over 300 per 100,000 (Scott, Ruef, Mendel, and Caronna, 2000).

Concentration among buyers in purchasing power (via medical insurance, employer associations, public programs) together with increased competition (because of greater numbers) and fragmentation in interests (due to specialization) among physicians reduced the economic bargaining power of the latter. These trends, in combination, worked to weaken the market power and political influence of physicians during the latter decades of the twentieth century.

Developments in health care systems were also greatly influenced by the expanding medical science base and associated pharmaceutical and technological advances. Medical care services became more efficacious and expensive. The new technologies were both more powerful and more portable, encouraging the decentralization and specialization of service settings. Developments in information technologies made possible the current, complex contractual arrangements among physicians, health care organizations, and funding units, including public agencies and medical plans.

Increased demand coupled with improved technologies and greater numbers of specialized providers have produced ever-increasing health care expenditures. Throughout the second half of the twentieth century, national health care expenditures have risen continuously, from accounting for 4 percent of gross domestic product in 1940 to almost 14 percent in 1995 (Scott, Ruef, Mendel, and Caronna, 2000). Since the early 1970s, annual increases in health care prices have regularly exceeded the consumer price index. Not surprisingly, much health policy since 1970 has been aimed at reining in health care costs.

Material resources—their availability, distribution, and scarcity—have clear effects on organizational fields. However, these economic effects are always mediated through a set of changing social mechanisms and cultural lenses. The "demand" for a doctor's services is never a direct function of physician supply, insurance coverage, and disease patterns. The institutional landscape intervenes to guide preferences and choices and to construct and constrain available solutions.

Institutional Logics and Governance Systems

Having described some of the important changes occurring in the numbers and types of individual and collective actors and in material resources, we now turn to examine the remaining institutional components: logics and governance systems.

Institutional logics are the belief systems and basic assumptions that motivate and guide the behavior of field participants. Changes in belief systems—cognitive and normative structures—constitute fundamental changes in institutional environments (Alexander and D'Aunno, 1990). To be active and in play, logics require carriers: individuals and organizations that affirm, embody, and act in accordance with the principles. Different logics tend to be associated with different actors. If their numbers and power increase, the logics they carry increase in prevalence and influence, and are instantiated in reconstructed governance systems. Our observations suggest that in the U.S. health care system three primary logics—associated with three different governance regimes—were dominant at different times during the past century.

Era of Professional Dominance, 1920s–1964

From the early part of the twentieth century until the mid-1960s, physicians enjoyed an unprecedented degree of "cultural authority" in the realm of medical care (Freidson, 1970a; Starr, 1982). This era of professional dominance was characterized by the preponderance of independent practice, with physicians able to insist that their professional autonomy be recognized in the structuring of hospital staffs and financing arrangements. The overriding logic during this period was a focus on *quality of care*, as defined by the physician. This value was employed to justify the physician's resistance to managerial and financial controls and to fuel the "medical arms race." The primary governance structures employed were professional systems, both formal and informal, operating at national, state, and local levels. The American Medical Association (AMA) served as the unified and unchallenged voice of organized medicine (Garceau, 1941). Public agencies played a secondary and circumscribed role. They functioned primarily to subsidize the development of infrastructure (for example, federal funding for medical research and for hospital construction following World War II) or to reinforce professional controls (such as state-level licensure systems).

These institutional arrangements were firmly in place for a half century and seemed unalterable. But signs of tension and weakness began to become evident. From the 1950s forward, health care expenditures began to slowly but steadily increase as physicians were unconstrained by financial or organizational controls in their pursuit of quality care. And after 1960, the unity of physicians began to erode. The growth in medical specialization resulted not just in heightened expertise (and expense) but also in increased fragmentation of physicians' interests. Membership in specialty associations soared while membership in the AMA began its decline (Scott, Ruef, Mendel, and Caronna, 2000). Thus, endogenous forces—unconstrained resource consumption fueled by the single-minded pursuit of medical logics and a growing fragmentation in the political interests of physicians—opened the gates to change.

Era of Federal Involvement, 1965–1982

The year 1965 was without doubt the high-water mark of the "Great Society" programs spearheaded by President Lyndon Johnson and a Democratic Congress. Responding to society-wide movements endorsing greater equity in many realms, including in health care more equitable access to services, Congress in 1965 passed the Medicare and Medicaid laws, providing publicly funded health care services to the elderly and the indigent. For the first time, the U.S. government was in the business of paying for direct health care services to large numbers of citizens. Almost overnight, the federal government became the purchaser of almost a quarter of all medical services. The medical profession was still sufficiently strong and unified to ensure that the payment mechanisms accommodated concerns for physician autonomy (Starr, 1982), but not strong enough to block legislation denounced by AMA leaders as leading to "socialized medicine." *Equity of access*—a political rather than a medical value—had joined quality of care as a guiding institutional logic.

Suddenly new types of actors (that is, new to the health care field)—politicians, federal policymakers, and administrative officials—were engaged in the health care sector and occupied positions of power therein. They created new public governance structures at all levels. Funds needed to be dispensed and accounted for, and, because the new source of funds stimulated increased expenditures, new types of regulative and rate-setting agencies were soon created. The total number of federal health-related regulatory agencies overseeing Bay Area health care organizations increased from under ten in 1950 to over ninety by 1975 (Scott, Ruef, Mendel, and Caronna, 2000). Physicians were obliged to share governance functions with bureaucrats, a situation leading to increased fragmentation in governance systems and inconsistent demands on provider systems. John W. Meyer and I (Meyer and Scott, 1983) argue that organizations subject to multiple and conflicting demands from institutional agents of their environments are likely to suffer reduced legitimacy. Health care organizations found themselves in an increasingly complex and conflicted environment.

Era of Managerial Control and Market Mechanisms, (1983–present)

As with the wider societal forces fueling the Great Society movement of the 1960s, the market-managerial era is primarily the product of broad (even international) changes in political ideologies of appropriate governance structures. Earlier models of "public utility regulation," which had not succeeded in containing inflationary pressures in health care, had become discredited as tools too easily captured by organized providers. They began to be replaced in the health care and other sectors, as a general wave of deregulation swept away many of the privileges previously enjoyed by the physicians' guild (Robinson, 1999). Faith was instead placed in market-based controls, as health providers were encouraged to compete on the basis of price and service. The new logic applied to health care stressed the central importance of *efficiency* in medical care delivery.

A secondary logic, also originating outside the health care sector, stressing the value of consumer choice and responsibilities, began to appear in health care discourse. It helped to legitimate the application of conventional market mechanisms in a sector formerly declared exempt from such "commercial" considerations. Policy designers introduced incentives to encourage first consumers (using copayments) then providers (using risk-sharing approaches) to reduce both the demand for and supply of medical care services (Melhado, 1988). Of course, the creation of a new health care delivery form, the HMO, was one of the principal mechanisms designed to alter physician incentives. While promulgated in the early 1970s, this form did not begin its period of rapid growth until the early 1980s.

More generally, however, a wide range of new organizational forms—including multispecialty groups, independent practice associations (IPAs), preferred provider organizations (PPOs), and physician-hospital organizations (PHOs)—have emerged that, to a varying but increasing extent, subject physicians to a wide variety of managerial controls (Robinson, 1999). Even traditional forms, such as community hospitals, are rapidly being incorporated within and subordinated to wider, organizational governance systems. Managers, long marginalized in the health care sector, have moved to center stage (Leicht and Fennell, 2001).

The rhetoric of deregulation and market mechanisms implies that public controls over the delivery of health care are being dismantled. Such is not the case. Except for a slight decline in the mid-1970s, public governance systems have continued to grow in numbers. Federal health-related regulatory bodies with authority over Bay Area health care providers increased from approximately 90 in 1975 to over 130 in 1995 (Scott, Ruef, Mendel, and Caronna, 2000). Thus, public controls continue to be exercised; only the mode of control has changed.

In sum, in this third (and current) era, professional autonomy is more circumscribed while public, market, and managerial controls have been greatly expanded. After decades of being treated as an exception to the structural models adopted by virtually all other industrial (including service) sectors, the health care sector increasingly resembles mainstream sectors in its organizational forms and institutional logics.

The dynamics of change we have observed involve both endogenous and exogenous forces. Professionals were dominant for many decades, but, over time, they proved to be unable to organize in ways that could curb insupportable cost increases or even to retain their own internal solidarity and political unity. Their declining political strength rendered them incapable of resisting two political tidal waves—both originating from outside health care—the first coming from the left, the second, from the right. First, liberal reformers, under the banner of reducing inequality, broadened access to health care but were then forced to erect complex regulatory systems to deal with the resulting financial crisis of escalating costs. In the second wave, conservative reformers, wrapped in the bunting of free markets, attempted to increase efficiency by restructuring incentives and relying on more conventional organizational (managerial) controls. Each of the three logics—physician-defined quality, equity of access, and efficiency—gave rise to and was supported by a different governance structure—professional association, public bureaucracy, private corporation—and carried by different types of actors, both individual and collective.

A Concluding Prescriptive Note

Having provided a brief description and analysis of the past movements and forces shaping health care delivery systems, I end with a few thoughts on where improvements might be sought. Departing from the bulk of this chapter—in which objectivity was the aim—my final comments reflect my own preferences and values.

While there is little question that the U.S. health care system has been radically transformed during the course of the past half century, few would argue that the changes represent unqualified improvement. Three social groups have been dominant at different times during the past fifty years, and each has been associated with a distinctive logic for guiding and gauging the performance of the health care system. Physicians placed ultimate value on quality of medical care—care defined in clinical terms, provided by physician to patient on a one-to-one basis. Nothing—other patients' needs, financial concerns, competition with other providers—was to be allowed to compromise this relationship. Public administrators, viewing health care less in individual and more in population terms, insisted that access to adequate (not, necessarily, optimal) care was an important right for every citizen, regardless of means. What good was high quality of care if its provision was restricted to the privileged few? Later policy analysts and managerial and corporate officers pointed to the inefficiency and waste built into pre-bureaucratic delivery systems—lack of coordination, redundancy, organizational slack, and overqualified providers—and insisted that the unleashing of market forces could bring discipline into an antiquated, craft-based nonsystem.

Who is right? What constituencies should prevail in this ongoing dispute? Surely, the answer must be: all of them! Each category of actors supports interests and values that should be incorporated into the design of a well-functioning health care system. Public advocates are correct to insist on the importance of equity of access. No system is adequate that does not meet the basic health needs of all, regardless of their ability to pay. While Medicare and Medicaid continue to provide an essential safety net for the elderly and poor, they do nothing to address the national scandal of 44 million Americans lacking health insurance. The working poor are currently excluded from appropriate access.

The significant role played by public funding to health care systems is illustrated by the effects that recent changes in Medicare policy have had on home health agencies, one of our organizational populations. The Balanced Budget Act of 1997 revised eligibility and coverage rules for HHA patients. Expenditures that had increased an average of over 30 percent per year between 1988 and 1996 suddenly experienced severe cutbacks, with payments falling over 50 percent between 1997 and 1999. As a result of this budgetary adjustment, "a substantial number of agencies closed, utilization fell, and the marketplace changed greatly" (McCall, Komisar, Petersons, and Moose, 2001). In a system in which all forms are heavily reliant on public funding, "modest" changes in reimbursement formula and eligibility criteria can have major consequences for the provider systems.

Physicians are correct that health care providers must be accorded sufficient discretion to attend to the unique needs of individual patients. This means that a physician should be involved in the basic decisions regarding health care. However, the direct services of specialized physicians are rarely required and, indeed, a large proportion of care episodes do not require the presence of even a general practitioner. The expertise of physicians needs to be better employed in informing and overseeing the decisions of other specialized but less highly-trained types of providers, such as physician's assistants, nurse practitioners, and home health personnel.

For the expertise of physicians to be better utilized, and to fulfill the hope that their services can be more equitably distributed, we need better-designed medical systems. Managerial logics that insist on the value of more economical methods of care delivery must be accorded high priority. Organizational arrangements can be designed to ensure efficiency and cost containment, but they can also make significant contributions to quality assurance. Health care providers need to attend to and learn from the remarkable results associated with the development of lean, quality-oriented, knowledge-based organizations in many arenas that enable specialized workers of varying skill levels to cooperate in the performance of exquisitely complex tasks. These organizations—often multiple organizations are involved, the work being managed across organizational boundaries—enable workers in a wide variety of settings not just to maintain but to continuously improve quality, often while reducing costs. These are *learning* organizations (Brown and Duguid, 1991; Cole and Scott, 2000; Womak, Jones, and Roos, 1990). Although health care systems lag far behind the best of these innovative forms, Robinson (1999) describes developments in multi-specialty medical groups, practice management firms, and physician-hospital systems that begin to push in these promising directions.

The ascendancy of managerial logics need not usher in an era of depersonalized, McDonaldized health care delivery. There are many modes of management and many ways to organize. It is essential that the values espoused by physicians be incorporated into management models so that the "bottom line" is not restricted to efficiency but incorporates attention to quality and quality improvement. Physicians themselves increasingly obtain managerial training and occupy managerial positions. And it is imperative that our definitions of efficiency and quality include the needs of all individuals, not just those currently able to pay. Health has a public as well as a private side.

But there remains a final, largely silent interest group. Among the types of actors who have shaped the logics and crafted the governance regimes, consumers (patients) and their interests have not loomed large. As noted, the consumer movements of the 1970s helped to raise consciousness in this constituency. More recently, highhanded practices by some overly greedy health care systems have aroused anger and elicited calls for greater consumer protections and expanded rights. These actions may result in the passage of a modest "patients' bill of rights" but are unlikely to usher in significant reform. An increased market orientation on the part of providers can also contribute. Some health care systems are beginning to compete for consumer loyalty on the basis of convenience, service, and quality (Herzlinger, 1997), but health care should not be reconstructed as a conventional service in which "the customer knows best."

Thus, much remains to be done if patients are to become full-fledged participants in protecting their own interests and health and in crafting an appropriate mechanism for their involvement. I encourage such efforts, believing that health care is too important to be left to the physicians, the bureaucrats, the managers, or even all of these actors working in concert.

3

Alternative Perspectives on Institutional and Market Relationships in the U.S. Health Care Sector

Jeffrey A. Alexander and Thomas A. D'Aunno

Institutional theory provides a convincing explanation for organizational isomorphism in the health care sector. Powerful actors in the institutional environment confer legitimacy on organizations that conform to deeply held, taken-for-granted beliefs about ways of organizing. Legitimacy, in turn, signals worthiness for receiving societal resources necessary for survival. Such institutional forces stand in marked contrast to the forces of the market that reward organizations for efficiency and effectiveness. Traditional, institutional forces that have dominated health care for the past fifty years include professional dominance and autonomy, public regulation of health care organizations, voluntary and philanthropic support of service organizations, and, perhaps most important, strongly held societal beliefs in health care as a right rather than a commodity. The central question this chapter addresses is How do the emergent technical and market forces in health care, as represented by managed care, cost containment, and corporate ideology, interact with and react to these traditional, institutional structures and beliefs? Answers to this question are important because they may provide a foundation for overcoming the inadequacies of both institutional theory and market economics in explaining the behavior and structure of organizations in the current, unsettled, and sometimes confusing health care environment.

Some argue that the influence of traditional institutional forces such as regulation, professional norms, and community control is weaker and therefore subordinated to the technical demands of the market (Thorpe, 1997; Ruggie, 1994; Hansmann, 1987). However, evidence shows that such institutional forces have not disappeared; rather, these forces interact with market imperatives to constrain and shape the structures and practices of health care organizations, including those originating in the corporate sector. As Scott and his colleagues have observed, "To a surprising extent, old forms and practices coexist alongside the new. These structures and practices are buttressed by the power of professionals and community leaders and they do not easily adapt to new ideas and new ways. Changes are not instantaneous in social systems: These structures exhibit much, perhaps desirable, recalcitrance and inertia" (Scott, Ruef, Mendel, and Caronna, 2000).

What does this coexistence look like in practice? Do the structures operate in parallel, as suggested by Scott and colleagues, or are domains of activity hybridized or even segmented between the new market-based forms of service delivery and the traditional, institutionally based structures? Finally, what conditions define the relationship of technical and institutional forces in the health care sector and in health care organizations? To address these questions, we build on two contemporary perspectives in institutional theory. The first view holds that institutional environments are neither monolithic in structure nor unitary in their effects, but instead are inconsistent, fragmented, and ambiguous (Friedland and Alford, 1991). The second view holds that organizations not only conform to institutional pressures but may also influence, resist, or evade institutional dictates. We posit that both perspectives form the foundation for organizational adaptation to market and institutional forces in the health care sector.

This chapter first reviews previous work that establishes theoretical foundations of the relationship between markets and institutions. This important body of work provides a basis for advancing four scenarios illustrating the expression of institution-market relationships in the health care sector, including their impact on organizational structure and practices. These scenarios and their real-world applications to the health care sector are explored at length. The chapter concludes with a discussion of how "old" institutionalism concepts of agency, values, and power determine the likelihood that one scenario will be more dominant than another.

Background

One of the most widely discussed changes in health care is the so-called "corporatization of American medicine," the penetration of the corporation into the voluntary health care sector and the extension of the voluntary health care organization into for-profit activities (Starr, 1982). The term broadly applies to various developments, such as the rise of for-profit enterprise in the delivery of health care, increasing market competition and consolidation among health care providers, and the introduction of measures to ensure accountability and consumer satisfaction. Both proponents and opponents of these developments have hotly debated the benefits and costs of health care corporatization (Burns and Robinson, 1997; Light, 1991; Lumsdon and Hagland, 1994; Mechanic, 1994).

Absent from this debate, however, is careful, analytical scrutiny of exactly how corporatization is transforming both the organization and delivery of health care in the United States. Unfortunately, with few exceptions, the ideologically and value-based positions taken by camps both for and against corporatization have sacrificed a dispassionate, objective picture of how corporatization interacts with traditional philanthropic and voluntary support of medical services and professional dominance (for example, Dranove and Shanley, 1995). Despite predictions in the late 1980s and early 1990s that the health care sector would come to resemble other segments of industrial and corporate America, today we see striking exceptions to these predictions. Not all physicians have become employees of large health care firms. Most have remained visible and powerful agents in the delivery of health care (Burns and Wholey, 2000; Bureau of Labor Statistics, 2000). Many local community-based boards still govern health care organizations, and these boards are charged with representing the interests of the community rather than investors (Alexander, Weiner, and Bogue, 2001). Perhaps most interestingly, although health care organizations are undergoing significant changes, they have not completely abandoned many of the traditional (and somewhat unusual) templates that made them a subject of great interest to students of organizations and sociology. Templates are patterns for arranging organizational behavior that specify organizational structure and goals and reflect a distinct set of beliefs and values. Accounting and law firms, for example, traditionally used templates that emphasized individual autonomy and equality among peers, what Greenwood and Hinings (1996) termed a "professional partnership model."

To address these apparent contradictions, we draw on two current streams of discussion in the literature of organizational change and institutional theory (that of relationships between markets and institutions and that of the relationship between the new and old institutionalisms). Although both perspectives inform our arguments, neither by itself convincingly explains the current situation in the health care sector. The literature on change in institutional systems, for instance, largely ignores the mechanisms and processes by which these changes occur (Thornton, 1995). Recent works point to shifts in institutional logics over protracted periods of time but do not convincingly explain why such logics have shifted. Likewise, this literature does not allow us to assess whether organizational sectors have reached equilibrium or whether current conditions simply indicate an ongoing process of institutional change and transformation.

The New and Old Institutionalisms

A key problem with using institutional theory to explain change in organizations is that its language is embedded in cognitive orientations and emphasizes taken-for-granted scripts, rules, and classifications. This has resulted in a problem of infinite regression to higher levels of abstraction, whereby institutions determine cultural scripts and organizational form and behavior. Indeed, the fundamental question that neo-institutional theory has addressed is, "Why are organizations so similar?" This perspective effectively rules out the role of individuals and organizations in effecting change and, more particularly, the informal network interests and value differences that characterize the "old" institutional perspective. At the level of the individual organization as well as at the field level, however, fields can be viewed as "arenas of power relations" (Brint and Karabel, 1991) in which field-level constituents engage in institutional war (Hoffman, 1999). The outcome is a political negotiation in which politics, agency relationships, and vested interests guide the formation of institutions that, in turn, guide organizational behavior. This dynamic bridges the two versions of institutionalism and, as we argue, explains much of the structure and behavior of organizations operating in the health care sector.

Recent discussions among organization theorists about differences between the old institutionalism and the neo-institutional perspective inform much of our work. Within the paradigm of old institutionalism, issues of influence, coalitions, and competing values were central, along with power and informal structures within individual organizations. By contrast, the new institutionalism emphasizes legitimacy, the embeddedness of organizations in fields, and the centrality of commonly held classifications, routines, scripts, and schema (DiMaggio and Powell, 1983; Meyer and Rowan, 1977). The new institutionalism has recently been criticized for its failure to account adequately for organizational change and agency among individual organizations and actors. Many authors in this area now advocate reconciliation between the new and old institutionalisms, with more emphasis on analyzing the internal dynamics of organizational change and the variation within fields with regard to the pacing and form that such change exhibits (Hirsch and Lounsbury, 1997; Fligstein, 1997; Selznick, 1996). Thus, rather than viewing change in organizations as the product of either externally determined, taken-for-granted structures on the one hand or the unfettered actions and decisions of organizational leaders on the other, greater emphasis is now placed on how organizational actors interpret and act on broad contextual pressures.

How well does this paradigm apply to organizations in the health care sector? Given the high degree of specialization and structural complexity of many health care organizations, it is not surprising that such organizations are highly differentiated in their interests and value orientations. These differences are expressed in terms of alternative ways of viewing the organization's purpose, the ways in which the organization might appropriately be organized, and the ways in which action might be evaluated (Alexander and Morlock, 1999; Mintzberg, 1983). For example, the provision of community benefit by nonprofit health care organizations may be interpreted by some as uncompensated care and by others as active community interventions to improve community health (Alexander, Weiner, and Succi, 2000). Such differences can arise as a function of vested interests and cognitive orientations of providers, regulators, or the community itself. Therefore, the contextual forces represented by the new institutionalism may be interpreted, acted upon, and regarded differently both within and across organizations (Oliver, 1991; Goodrick and Salancik, 1996). The likely outcome is variation in the form and pace of change experienced by health care organizations in the face of a changing institutional context. From a somewhat different perspective, it is reasonable to argue that the degree to which an organization is embedded in a strong institutional context will be directly related to the degree of inertia expressed toward significant or radical change in its structures and practices (Alexander and Scott, 1984; Alexander and D'Aunno, 1990; D'Aunno, Succi, and Alexander, 2000).

Not only do organizations vary in their responses to the institutional environment, but they are also actively engaged in shaping that environment. In our previous work, we argued that institutional practices could originate not only from the larger social environment in which organizations are embedded but also from individual organizations themselves (Alexander and D'Aunno, 1990; Greenwood and Hinings, 1996; Leblebici, Salancik, Copay, and King, 1991; Suchman, 1995). The work of Rosemary Stevens most notably exemplifies this perspective within the health care sector (Stevens, 1989). Stevens observed that hospitals themselves have shaped the operational definitions of institutional terms such as "public versus private," "voluntary," and even "industry." In working to shape a commonly held language consistent with hospitals' own interests (but within the framework of prevailing institutional beliefs), these organizations participated in shaping institutional norms and practices, not merely adapting to them. This interplay between broader context and intraorganizational dynamics explains the variation in which corporatization expresses itself within the health care sector (Oliver, 1991; Goodrick and Salancik, 1996).

Current Perspectives on Institutions and Markets

In the past decade, consensus among organizational theorists emerged regarding the importance of the interplay between market and institutional forces in understanding organizational behavior (for example, Singh and Lumsden, 1990; Scott, Ruef, Mendel, and Caronna, 2000; Baum, 1996; Wade, Swaminathan, and Saxon, 1998; Tucker, Baum, and Singh, 1992). Although there is clear agreement that both institutional and market forces jointly affect organizational behavior, there is less agreement on how these forces relate to each other and what their combined effects are on organizations.

Perhaps the most commonly expressed view is that institutional environments provide the context in which market forces operate (Baum, 1996). In this view, market forces are subordinate to institutional ones, in that institutional environments may prescribe the criteria and conditions under which competition occurs. This view is illustrated in a study by Wade, Swaminathan, and Saxon (1998). They examined how state legislation prohibiting the production and sale of alcohol (an institutional factor) influenced flows of resources and consequently the founding and closure of breweries in neighboring prohibition-free states.

In contrast, other researchers have implicitly or explicitly argued that market and institutional forces are of roughly equal importance but exert relatively independent or complementary effects on organizations (for example, Hannan and Carroll, 1992; Hannan and Freeman, 1989). Greenwood and Hinings (1996) proposed a model of radical organizational change in which market and institutional forces work primarily independently (although not exclusively) to promote such change.

Yet another distinct view is that market forces, at least under certain conditions, can promote change in organizational practices or forms that were previously institutionalized across a field (for example, Kraatz and Zajac, 1996; Leblebici, Salancik, Copay, and King, 1991; Oliver, 1992). Implicit in this view is the possibility that institutions and institutional forces can be subordinate to, or compete with, market forces. This work suggests that market forces can exert effects that are strong enough to call institutions into question and to undermine their usefulness and legitimacy. Kraatz and Zajac (1996) found that liberal arts colleges were more likely to make radical changes in their curricula (adding non–liberal arts courses and majors, such as business administration) to the extent that they faced decreased demand for traditional offerings as well as increased competition from other similar colleges.

Others have suggested that relationships between market and institutional forces may vary depending on key characteristics of organizational fields in which these forces are embedded (D'Aunno, Succi, and Alexander, 2000; Dacin, 1997). Specifically, market forces may be more likely to promote change in institutionalized organizational forms and practices to the extent that organizational fields have a fragmented structure of decision making (Meyer, Scott, and Strang, 1987; Scott and Meyer, 1983). Such fields can produce diverse and even competing regulations, norms, and cognitive models for organizations because actors pursue their interests independently, and there is no central authority to coordinate their activities or settle disputes.

When influential actors throughout a field promote a variety of regulations, norms, and cognitive models, an important result is a relatively wide range of accepted organizational practices and templates (Scott and Meyer, 1983; Friedland and Alford, 1991; Powell, 1990; Greenwood and Hinings, 1996; Hoffman, 1999). In such fields, organizations that are motivated to make changes due to market pressures have the opportunity to do so, even if it means that they are abandoning a template that was institutionalized across a field (Oliver, 1991; 1992; Ocasio, 1995). More generally, heterogeneous institutional environments support or even promote variation in organizational forms and practices, even in the absence of market forces that may motivate organizational change. Basing our proposal on earlier work (for example Scott, 1983; Carroll, Delacroix, and Goodstein, 1988; Alexander and Scott, 1984; Alexander and D'Aunno, 1990; D'Aunno, Succi, and Alexander, 2000), we argue that the health care field is now characterized by strong, heterogeneous institutional forces and relatively strong market forces.

Finally, Scott and his colleagues (Scott, Ruef, Mendel, and Caronna, 2000; Ruef and Scott, 1998) recently developed a view of markets and institutions that holds that market forces themselves represent a particular type of institutional logic and governance structure (see Chapter Two). In this view, markets do not exist separately from the institutional elements that compose them. Rather, markets are institutions that consist of a set of beliefs, values, and governance structures, as do other institutions. The substantive meaning of markets as institutions differs from the substantive meaning of other institutions (for example, in the health care field, markets prescribe efficiency, whereas other institutional logics or regimes prescribe the importance of access to care or quality of care), but they otherwise are equivalent.

Four Possible Relationships Between Markets and Institutions

From this discussion, we conclude that substantial variation in organizational responses to market and institutional forces may exist within the health care field as a result of key actors' agency, values and interests, and power and resources exercised in the field, and by the reciprocal effects of macro-context and micro-action at the organization level. We propose four possible scenarios by which market and institutional forces interact to influence the structure and practices of health care organizations. The scenarios are (1) institutional and market forces provide competing choices, (2) institutions shape markets, (3) institutions and markets operate in separate domains, and (4) institutional and market forces synthesize to create new structures and practices. This chapter discusses these four possible relationships in detail, with a specific focus on their implications for health care organizations. Figure 3.1 illustrates the interrelationships between these four scenarios.

Scenario 1: Institutional and Market Forces Provide Competing Choices

In this possible scenario, institutional and market forces act in direct opposition to each other, resulting in conflicting demands on organizations that require them to make choices in their responses; responding to one set of demands precludes responding to another (Oliver, 1991; 1992). For example, a community hospital may face

Figure 3.1. Four Scenarios Regarding the Expression of Institution-Market Relationships.

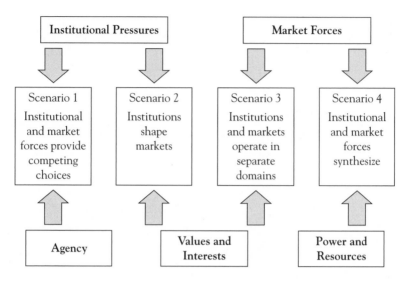

market competition that requires it to minimize costs and maximize revenues as much as possible. If the hospital responded fully to such market demands, it might, in turn, reduce the amount of care it provides to indigent populations, thus violating institutional norms that prescribe the provision of such care. In short, market demands for financial performance may conflict with institutional demands regarding access to care.

The potential for conflict between institutional and market demands on organizations concerns tradeoffs between organizational efficiency that markets reward and organizational ability to meet widely held societal expectations that define "effective" performance in a given field. Indeed, Meyer and Rowan (1977) emphasized this distinction in their now-classic statement of neo-institutional theory. In this view, efficient organizational performance is typically inconsistent with effective performance because conforming to institutional demands adds practices and structures to organizations that are costly to maintain. As a result, organizations that face both strong institutional and market forces also confront a series of difficult dilemmas that cannot be easily resolved.

Several recent instances of conflicts between market and institutional pressures affect the services, staffing, management practices, and structure of health care organizations. For example, rural hospitals often face pressure from local communities to keep maternity units open although they are infrequently used. The costs of maintaining these units preclude some hospitals from being as cost competitive as neighboring hospitals that do not offer maternity services. As another example, hospitals that reduce the number and skill-mix of their nursing staff to cut costs and improve efficiency may find that quality of care suffers. These examples show how health care organizations may find it difficult to respond adequately to conflicting pressures from markets that reward efficiency and institutional actors with values and rules that emphasize quality of, and access, to care.

Another prominent example of market-institutional conflict concerning hospital services occurred when many managed care firms across the nation tried to maximize efficiency in hospital obstetric care by limiting maternal and child length of stay in non-Cesarean ("normal") births to twenty-four hours. Such twenty-four-hour discharge plans ignored the fact that many newborns require eye exams and other checkups beyond twenty-four hours. Thus, parents under the twenty-four-hour plans often had to return to hospitals for some neonatal care; in cases when they failed to do so, infants experienced a higher rate of post-birth complications (Raube and Merrell, 1999). In response, many states passed legislation that required insurance firms to pay for at least forty-eight hours of hospital care for maternity patients. This case illustrates how pressures to maximize efficiency in a cost-sensitive market conflicted with institutional values about quality of care.

In the past several years, health care providers ranging from hospital systems to outpatient clinics have invested substantial resources to meet demands for improved quality of care, while, at the same time, trying to respond to demands for more efficient care. Although health care providers have employed a variety of approaches to improve care quality, they have often relied on total quality management (TQM) approaches (Westphal, Gulati, and Shortell, 1997). From the standpoint of efficiency, these efforts are costly. They require clinical and management staff to work extensively in teams on projects to improve care processes as well as administrative processes. As a result, at least in the short run, these efforts decrease the efficiency of health care providers at the very time when they must often try to reduce costs.

Similarly, the number of uninsured people continued to increase in the past several years and, as a consequence, it appears that health care providers face more pressure to provide care for which they may not be compensated. In urban settings, hospital emergency units face pressure to provide service for the homeless and for people with mental health and substance abuse problems who have no insurance or ability to pay for their care. Providing such care makes it more difficult to reduce costs in response to market pressures. In other words, organizations' efforts to conform to widely held values about access to and quality of care often conflict with market demands for efficiency.

Of course, increases in quality of care or access to care do not necessarily result in an increase in organizational costs and inefficiency. For example, improvements in the quality of many surgical procedures may reduce post-discharge complications for patients that, in turn, lead to lower costs for a hospital. Nonetheless, as these examples indicate, health care organizations often face complex tradeoffs in decisions about access, quality, and costs of care (Donabedian, 1980a; 1980b).

Scenario 2: Institutions Shape Markets

It is also plausible that institutional forces shape many key characteristics of markets that directly constrain or facilitate particular organizational practices and structures. This occurs primarily,

although not exclusively, through government policy and regulations. Because regulations often codify widely held beliefs and stem
from government initiatives, they can be viewed as institutional
forces (Carroll, Delacroix, and Goodstein, 1988; Edelman and Suchman, 1997). One important way that government regulation and
policy shape markets is by either increasing or decreasing the level
of competition that organizations face in local markets (Fligstein,
1996).

Government Policies

Government policy promotes competition through antitrust laws
that aim to prevent or break up monopolies among existing firms
(Dobbin and Dowd, 1997). For example, laws may reduce barriers
to entry so that firms that are new to a market can challenge established ones (Fligstein, 1990; Kelly and Amburgey, 1991; Dobbin
and Dowd, 1997). In contrast, policies can weaken competition by
regulating several aspects of markets, including the production of
goods and services, prices, and labor wages. Such anticompetition
policies often reduce organizations' uncertainty about resources and
provide them with a stable market environment (Fligstein, 1996).

Institutional forces can also shape markets in fundamental ways
through widely held beliefs, norms, and values about key elements
that are needed to construct and maintain markets, such as property rights, competition, and profitmaking. For example, in the
United Kingdom the use of markets to govern the provision of
health care services would violate widely held norms about individuals' rights to such care as well as the rights of care providers
to make a profit from their work. Rather than promote market competition, these norms provide the foundation for the National
Health Services (NHS), which, for the most part, does not operate
on market principles. Norms about property rights are critical
because they not only specify who owns organizational assets (public versus private ownership), but also shape the extent to which
these owners can, and will, use these assets to engage in competi-

tive behavior (Campbell and Lindberg, 1990). In the United Kingdom, for example, norms specify public ownership of health care
organizations and assets, and these rights inhibit competition.

Importantly, scenario 2 assumes that institutional pressures (regulation, norms, values, and cognitive models of organizing) in an
organizational field are strong enough to influence market characteristics. This assumption seems to fit the health care field, as many
analysts have observed that this field experiences long-standing and
powerful institutional pressures (for example, Alexander and Scott,
1984; Scott, Ruef, Mendel, and Caronna, 2000; Stevens, 1989;
Starr, 1982).

The 1983 Medicare Prospective Payment legislation effectively,
although perhaps not intentionally, stimulated competition among
hospitals to attract patients. Under this change in Medicare payment policy, hospitals often received reduced cash payments for services, which cut their budgets and contributed to cashflow problems
(Bazzoli, 1995). Hospitals tried to compensate by increasing their
service volume, but this in turn created more competition for
patients. Although market pressures might have been relatively low
for hospitals before 1983, they increased with Medicare reform,
marking an important change in institutional regulation.

This example also illustrates that institutional influences on
markets are likely to vary depending on the decision-making structure in an organizational field (Scott, 1983; Meyer, Scott, and
Strang, 1987). Because decisions about Medicare are made by a central, national-level authority (Congress), changes in Medicare regulatory (payment) policy can broadly affect local markets and
organizations within them. That is, to the extent that decisions
about regulation are centralized in an organizational field, we expect
their influences on markets to be more uniform and perhaps more
powerful. In general, decision making in the health care field is not
particularly centralized; instead, the health care sector has a relatively fragmented decision-making structure, giving rise to multiple, uncoordinated sources of authority and influence. In turn, the

extent to which institutional elements affect market behavior will often vary according to local-level factors.

State-Level Factors

Another compelling case in which institutional forces have shaped market behavior in the health care field illustrates these state-level factors. Certificate of Need (CON) legislation that many states enacted in the 1970s exemplifies government regulation that attempted either to prevent or to limit some types of market competition. CON laws made it difficult to purchase capital equipment or begin new construction because they required hospitals to demonstrate medical need for a particular service, facility, or technology. Hospitals and physicians competing to attract patients often purchase the latest medical technology, build new facilities, and begin new service programs; in doing so, however, their costs increase and expensive equipment often is underused (Feldstein, 1988). In response to such nonprice competition, many states passed CON laws in the 1970s. These laws limit technology competition and restrict offerings of new products and services.

To stimulate competition, many states either eliminated CON laws altogether or relaxed their stringency in the late 1980s and 1990s. The 1980s also witnessed procompetition legislation that focused on rural hospitals in several states. This legislation intended to promote competition by reducing barriers to entry into new markets for rural hospitals. Several states encouraged hospitals to diversify into nontraditional services (such as nursing homes) either in their current market areas or in other rural areas that lacked such services. This legislation assumed that diversification would enable rural hospitals to convert to provide more financially viable (less expensive to produce) services (D'Aunno, Succi, and Alexander, 2000).

Medicare Legislation and Court Decisions

At the federal level, Medicare legislation provides a third prominent example of how institutions can shape markets. In 1980, the

Omnibus Budget Reconciliation Act provided additional funds for home health care services with the goal of reducing inpatient care costs for the elderly (Scott, Ruef, Mendel, and Caronna, 2000; Ruef and Scott, 1998). In effect, this legislation created a new species of organizations (independent home health care agencies) that competed not only with each other for patients but with hospitals and nursing homes as well. This case shows how legislation that mandates funds to pay for services can create new organizations and markets for patient care. Also important to note is that after several years of growth in this market, the Balanced Budget Act of 1997 controlled escalating home health care costs by reducing funds for these services, thereby causing an increase in competition among the remaining service providers.

In our final example of how institutional elements influence markets, a set of court decisions in the early 1980s allowed physicians and other health care professionals to advertise their services. We now take such marketing for granted; advertisements for physicians, hospitals, and pharmaceutical medications are common in all media. In many ways, however, changes in regulation that allowed advertising contributed significantly to the development of nascent health care markets by informing individual consumers and health care professionals of alternative care providers and therapies. By contrast, many European countries do not allow direct advertising, such as from pharmaceutical firms directly to consumers (Rice, 2000).

Scenario 3: Institutions and Markets Operate in Separate Domains

A third scenario posits that institutions and markets operate in parallel fashion to affect organizational structures and processes. Under this scenario, market and institutional logics do not conflict because they operate in different domains (in terms of affecting either different and unrelated organizational behaviors and structures or different types of organizations altogether) (Amburgey, Dacin, and Kelly, 1994; Lumsdon and Hagland, 1994). The health care sector fosters parallelism because of the fragmented and ununified system of institutional actors and the existence of alternative organizational templates that such fragmentation creates.

Importantly, such parallelism is reinforced by the inherent difficulty in bridging and integrating separate domains that are demarcated by strongly held values, interests, or belief systems. For example, a for-profit eye clinic may define its values exclusively in terms of shareholder wealth, and its activities may be dictated by the drive for profit. In contrast, a religiously affiliated hospital may hold care for the underserved and health care as a fundamental human right as its dominant values. Because of these value-based differences, operational and strategic ties between these two types of organizations are rare. And because alternative organizational templates in the United States' health care sector have become more available in recent years, organizations need not conform to a single set of institutional norms or beliefs but can instead orient themselves to those most consistent with their own values and interests.

"Loose Coupling"

Institutional and technical segmentation can also express themselves *within* health care organizations. The idea that technical and institutional forces operate in different domains has its origins in Meyer and Rowan's (1977) notion of "loose coupling." In their view, institutionalized elements of an organization are separated from its technical processes, and these elements focus on conforming to broadly held societal beliefs rather than on improving internal efficiencies or effectiveness in the market (Alexander and Scott, 1984; Meyer and Rowan, 1977).

The classic example of loose coupling in the health care industry was the dual lines of control in health care organizations represented by administration on the one hand and by physician staff on the other. These dual lines of control operated in parallel but rarely intersected in a way that disrupted relative spheres of influence over issues related to operational control, resource allocation, and professional prerogatives (Scott, 1982; Alexander, Morrisey, and Shortell, 1986). These parallel structures often resulted in an absence of oversight by hospital management over the core production workers of the organization, the physician staff. Instead, administrative units were focused outward toward external stakeholders, with the goal of conforming to regulatory requirements and securing government funding for the hospital and its activities (Alexander and Scott, 1984).

Due to the fragmented and uncoordinated structure of the institutional environment in health care, each institutionalized element was often isomorphic with a specific actor, or set of actors, in the environment. These actors include regulatory agencies, accreditors, funders, or professional groups. To the extent that these external actors are uncoordinated and autonomous, health care organizations must mirror the somewhat fragmented and complex environment on which they depend in their own structures (Alexander and D'Aunno, 1990; Scott and Meyer, 1983).

However, powerful market forces now compel health care organizations to respond to pressures for efficiency and effectiveness. Although the medical profession has traditionally controlled these domains, health care organizations are increasingly designing structures and processes to provide control and administrative oversight to enhance both the market and technical capabilities of their organizations (Robinson, 1998a; 1999; Light, 1991). Despite these dual imperatives to conform to institutional pressures and respond to market forces, separate spheres of operation and organization are still evident, although different in form and content from those that have historically dominated health care organizations. For example, product line management is increasingly practiced in large health care organizations to make specific services more responsive to their particular markets and to promote efficiencies by pushing administrative accountability down to the production level of the organization.

However, such efforts rarely extend to dictating how medicine should be practiced within those structures. In fact, physicians rather than lay managers lead most clinical service lines, and attempts to bridge professional and managerial domains are rarely successful. For example, efforts to impose evidence-based medicine on clinicians have been notoriously difficult, primarily because they represent perceived external controls over a domain of activity traditionally protected by strong institutionalized norms and professional prerogatives (Waters and others, 2001; Shortell and others, 2001). Similarly, the recent, dramatic demise of Physician Practice Management Companies (PPMCs) points to the inherent problems of imposing the managerial logic of for-profit business enterprise on professional medical practices (Feorene, 1999; Robinson, 1999; Wholey, Christianson, and Sanchez, 1993).

Other studies (Alexander and others, 2001a; 2001b) further support the notion that separate spheres of activity are subject to either market or institutional pressures. Economic and strategic alignment between physicians and delivery organizations, for example, is promoted primarily through instrumental means, such as support services to physicians' clinical practices, not by attempts to integrate through administrative control or by participation of physicians or physician groups in organizational governance. These studies illustrate that both institutional and market forces exercise strong but separate pressures on health care organizations and that attempts to bridge domains have proven exceedingly difficult. Indeed, despite the market logic and resources devoted to developing integrated health care systems in the United States, few if any truly integrated systems have emerged. Rather, loose coupling among structures and processes within health care organizations continues to be the norm (Alexander and Scott, 1984; Alexander and D'Aunno, 1990).

A second major possibility in this third scenario is that different organizations (rather than different elements of organizations) will be more or less influenced by technical versus institutional forces.

This argument is predicated on the observation that health care organizations and health care markets are not uniform but instead differ widely in the extent to which they are susceptible to these different forces (Ingram and Simons, 1995; Sleeper, Wholey, Hamer, Schwartz, and Inoferio, 1998; Greening, 1994). Certain types of organizations can be influenced by both market competition and institutional forces. Others are more subject to institutional pressures than they are to market forces, and still others are dominated primarily by market pressures.

The local nature of health care markets and the diversity of providers operating within those markets give rise to these varying responses to institutional and market forces. For example, the severe managed care pressures in California have driven many health care organizations to adopt structures and practices that promote greater efficiency and effectiveness in the market (regardless of traditional institutional beliefs and norms). These changes include virtual networks designed to control the distribution channels for patients and health plan enrollees and the formation of large physician group practices (Robinson and Casalino, 1996). Similar types of organizations have not responded in the same way in other regions of the country where market pressures are less severe, where institutional forces are stronger, or where other organizational templates exist.

Conditions Fostering Parallelism

Parallelism is also promoted by competing values and ideologies within health care organizations that keep organizational responses to institutional and market pressures separate (Alexander and Scott, 1984; Meyer and Rowan, 1977). Historically, health care organizations have been viewed as exceedingly complex and increasingly specialized (Scott and Lammers, 1985; Stevens, 1989). We argue that this complexity is a strong catalyst for parallelism in many health care organizations, and that the values, interests, and agendas of specialized occupations and units within health care organizations facilitate the formation of parallel, institutional, and technically based structures. This is particularly true when no political interest or specialization dominates the organization, and when multiple specialties are necessary for the organization to survive and thrive. Although market and institutional logics may compete, neither has sufficient power to subsume or dominate the other. The result is a parallel set of structures in which each set of actors advances its own agenda within its own domain but lacks the power to force itself into a dominant position within the organization.

To the extent that adherence to institutional structures and practices results in legitimacy, and consequently improved flow of resources to organizations, and to the extent that market competition also influences resource acquisition and financial stability, parallelism will express itself in health care organizations. This is so because an organization must attend to the requirements of highly differentiated elements of its environment, including those emanating from the market and important institutional actors. Some organizations that depend equally on both express this differentiation through segmenting responses in different domains or areas of activity within their organizations. Others have specialized such that they are predominantly dependent on one or the other. This specialization allows them to adopt more uniform structures and practices to comply with a set of consistent demands from their environment.

There are numerous examples of parallelism in the activities of health care organizations. Most health care delivery organizations now engage in extensive marketing efforts to attract paying patients. These practices, adopted directly from the corporate sector, are designed to enhance organizational visibility among potential consumers. However, marketing does not extend to providing extensive product choice for consumers. This domain is left largely to the discretion of physicians and other professional clinicians. Also common to the corporate sector, but rare in the health care sector, is the notion of differentiating products or services based on ability to pay. Thus, marketing has increased as a response to market pressures but its domain is bounded and largely excludes activities that are antithetical to the notion of health care as a right, a long-held institutional belief in our country's health care system.

Scenario 4: Institutional and Market Forces Synthesize

Although institutional and market forces are often at odds, they do not necessarily engage in "institutional war" from which a clear, dominant winner emerges. Conflicting logics (such as market and professional) may result in a stalemate in which both camps are weakened and at least partially delegitimized (Scott, Ruef, Mendel, and Caronna, 2000). Such weakness allows new structures and practices to emerge, specifically those that reflect a synthesis or accommodation of both institutional and market logics. This scenario plays out when organizations dominated by traditional institutional beliefs and structures attempt to accommodate hard-to-ignore market and technical pressures for greater efficiency and effectiveness. Conversely, these integrative processes are also shaped by emerging market and technical forces adapting to a broader system of long-held institutional practices, beliefs, and structures (as discussed in scenario 2). We distinguish this scenario from the classic description of loose coupling whereby institutionalized elements of organizations are decoupled from each other as well as from the technical components of organizations. By contrast, our synthesis scenario suggests that, under certain conditions, institutional and market elements are so closely coupled they create new structures and practices that differ from both, at least in their pure forms.

Health Care Governance

Changes in health care governance provide our first example of this synthesis. Governance has been among the most highly institutionalized elements of health care organizations, reflecting the "agreeable fiction" of broad community control but somewhat loose system of accountability over hospital management and hospital operations (Starkweather, 1988). Boards tend to be large, community-based, and philanthropically oriented. These characteristics are all hall-marks of traditional institutional beliefs that health care is a vol-untary enterprise and fulfills social obligations to local communities. Data on hospital boards indicate that the structures characterizing this particular institutional form have remained largely unchanged over the past thirty years. For example, the size of hospital boards has remained disproportionately large relative to any measure of op-erations, largely as a function of its focus on community representa-tion and linkage (Alexander, Weiner, and Bogue, 2001). Similarly, board members remain largely unpaid and are drawn almost exclu-sively from the local community in which the hospital operates.

However, within this institutionally dictated framework, many changes reflect an organization's accommodation to institutional and market forces. These accomodations have focused on the nature of the relationship between the board and the hospital CEO. In response to increased market pressures and the need to be more strategically adaptable, CEOs are assuming a more central role on hospital boards and, in turn, boards are holding them more account-able for their actions. This change has been expressed in an increase in CEOs' voting positions on boards, the use of formal employment contracts with performance incentives, and the increase in the use of formal evaluations of the CEO by boards. Thus, health care gov-ernance has maintained much of the traditional framework dictated by institutionalized pressures but has, within that structure, adopted many of the practices demanded by market forces. This hybridiza-tion of the "philanthropic" and "corporate" models of governance is growing in popularity among hospitals and is now more common than either model in its pure form (Weiner and Alexander, 1993; Alexander and Weiner, 1998).

Physician-Organization Arrangements

A second example of the synthesis scenario is the so-called physi-cian-organization arrangements (POAs). These structures ostensi-bly were created to integrate and align the strategic and economic goals of providers and physicians to deal better with market pressures facing both (for example, managed care contracting). POAs include management service organizations (MSOs), physician-hospital organizations (PHOs), integrated delivery systems (IDSs) and foundation models. Each represents a structure and financing mechanism designed to preserve the traditional relationship and practices of physician groups and provider organizations while at the same time responding to the exigencies of market forces. Physicians, physician groups, and delivery organizations are all partners in POAs and contribute their own resources to these arrangements. The resulting organizations are distinct from either the physician organization or the delivery organization in terms of governance, membership standards, and performance expectations. The synthesis of institutional and market imperatives has allowed these new organizations to emerge and operate as quasi-independent entities while avoiding conflict and disruption of traditional practices and standards in the home organizations.

Managed Care

A third and final example of market-institutional synthesis relates to the development of managed care organizations. These organizations, which receive considerable government support, are actively moving away from the staff models that characterized HMOs early in the development of managed care. Staff model HMOs attempted to subordinate physicians to an administrative structure, along with the attendant controls, supervision, and externally imposed performance standards. These structures were initiated in the name of cost containment and "rationalizing" care. However, staff model HMOs proved difficult to manage and operate efficiently, owing largely to the conflicting cultures and traditions between organizations and physicians. Today we are witnessing a more synthesized approach to managed care that places more reliance on loosely structured networks of physicians who are oriented primarily to their own practices, or to small groups that engage with managed care firms on a contractual basis for part of their practice income. These so-called independent practice associations preserve much of the autonomy and discretion that physicians demand while at the same time offering managed care firms cost savings through discounted fee schedules. This new synthesis of market and traditional professional controls accommodates pressures to increase efficiency and cost savings as well as pressures to retain practices such as maintaining the locus of control for providing clinical services with the individual physician or physician group.

Which Scenarios Will Predominate?

We argue that each of the four theoretical descriptions of the relationship between market and institutional forces is plausible in the health care sector. We further maintain that the extent to which any one explanation is relevant to an organization, its local market, or its sociopolitical environment will depend on "old institutionalism" factors such as agency, interest, values, resource competition, and power. Such factors are relevant not only because of the general reciprocal relationship between macro and micro forces that shape institutional beliefs, norms, and values (see Scott, 1995, p. 142), but also because the health care sector is fundamentally a locally or regionally oriented activity. For example, the relationship between market and institutional forces in the San Francisco Bay Area may differ markedly from their relationship in Northern Ohio or the Boston area, because these areas differ in the relative power of insurers, providers, and consumers as well as in the political and economic contexts in which these groups operate.

The remainder of this chapter discusses the conditions under which each possible relationship between markets and institutions is likely to predominate. We provide examples to illustrate how these conditions or factors might affect market-institutional relationships. Specifically, we argue that three sets of factors will heavily influence how institutions and markets relate to each other in the health care field: the agency of actors, the actors' values and interests, and the distribution of resources and power among the actors.

Variation in the Agency of Actors

The agency of actors, that is, the extent to which they make conscious choices based on their interests, is likely to influence which of the four scenarios predominates in the health care field. An important assumption is that actors vary in the extent to which they express their potential agency (Fligstein, 1997; Hirsch and Lounsbury, 1997). On the one hand, actors in an organizational field may exhibit little agency: this condition is described by several neo-institutional theorists who argue that individuals and organizations often operate on the basis of traditional scripts and routines that are so taken-for-granted that they go unquestioned (for example, Zucker, 1977). In contrast, actors may be much more aware of the institutional rules under which they operate and, for a variety of reasons, may actively question institutional arrangements and seek to change arrangements that do not support their interests and values (for example, Leblebici, Salancik, Copay, and King, 1991; Newman, 2000; Hoffman, 1999).

For example, in the health care field in the past decade, one could argue that individual and organizational actors who expressed their agency primarily did so to promote market-based approaches that would weaken the role of institutional constraints on market behavior (Scott, Ruef, Mendel, and Caronna, 2000; Schmidt, 1999). In particular, the major payers of health care, including employers and public (Medicare and Medicaid) and private insurers, used their agency to develop "managed competition" and similar approaches that would use market competition to decrease costs and increase the quality of care. In contrast, institutional constraints on market forces were much less likely to be weakened or to change in local areas where actors accepted the status quo in institutional arrangements. Thus, the extent to which individuals, groups, or organizations are passive or active may matter a great deal in how markets relate to institutions (Oliver, 1991; 1992).

Values and Interests

Agency alone, however, cannot fully account for the conditions under which a particular scenario will predominate. The values and interests of actors who express their agency matter a great deal. The previous example illustrates that the payers of health care acted to weaken institutional arrangements to promote their interests in providing care in a more cost-effective manner. Employers and public and private insurers were not interested in institutional change per se or in weakening institutional rules per se. Instead, they wanted to develop market forces to promote their interests in cost-effectiveness.

Analyses of actors' agency must account for their particular values and interests (Selznick, 1949; 1996; Zald and Denton, 1963). Although agency signals the ability of actors to recognize that institutional elements are constraining their behavior, the particular interests and values of each actor tell us more about the direction of changes they will promote in both institutions and markets. In the health care field, actors whose primary interests lie in cost-effectiveness are more likely to promote market reforms at the expense of institutional constraints, whereas actors whose primary values focus on access to care are less likely to promote stronger markets at the expense of institutional rules.

Resources and Power

Actors may be aware of the ways that both institutions and markets shape their behavior, and may vary in their interests in supporting or opposing institutional or market influences on their behavior. However, the ability of actors to control resources and wield power in governance decisions may have the most impact on how institutions and markets relate to each other. This is because organizational fields are governed and influenced by actors who have authority and power to make critical decisions about institutional elements and their relationship to markets (Scott, 1983; Fligstein, 1996).

For example, antitrust laws and the courts that interpret and enforce them greatly shape local market competition in health care. Organizational actors that have the resources and power to influence such decisions are in a position to promote or inhibit the influence of institutional rules on market behavior. In general, actors' ability to express their agency and interests rests on their ability to marshal resources effectively (for example, advertising campaigns to influence public opinion about proposed legislation to regulate managed care competition).

The Case of Physician-Organization Relations

To illustrate how actors' agency, interests, and power can influence the relationship between institutional and market forces and, consequently, how organizations respond to these forces, we focus on the structures that define the relationship between physicians and organizations. Physician-organization relationships are a key domain in which agency, values and interests, and power and resources combine to shape organizational responses to institutional and market pressures. Physicians and the profession of medicine are largely responsible for the institutional beliefs, norms, and taken-for-granted practices that have shaped much of the health care system over the past fifty years (Freidson 1970a; 1986). Organizations, particularly large, corporate-structured health care systems, manifest much of the managerial logic and emerging market orientation fostered by competition, cost containment, and deregulation. Examining the variation in the interrelation of these two entities may shine a powerful light on the conditions giving rise to the different means by which institutional and market forces manifest themselves in health care organizations.

The purchase of physician practices by health care systems and the employment of physicians by these organizations are perhaps the strongest examples of market forces subsuming institutional practices and norms. Subjecting employed physicians to external control, regulating the conditions of employment, and replacing the loose peer or collegial form of organizations with administrative hierarchy can divest the physicians of much of the institutionalized prerogatives of autonomy, internal control, self-regulation and, in some cases, monopoly power. Scott (1982) referred to such structures as "heteronomous professional organizations." At the opposite extreme, many health care systems relate to physicians in a manner more closely approximating traditional, institutionally influenced practices in which physicians function as independent actors and organizations exercise little or no direct control over their practice behavior. Medical staff-hospital structures and independent practice associations are perhaps the most obvious examples.

Between these two extremes, however, lie a number of organizational permutations that to varying degrees represent the different relationships or scenarios between market and institutional forces. Some, such as PHOs, are syntheses of institutional and market elements while others, such as foundation models and IPAs, more closely represent examples of how traditional institutions shape the form and substance of markets. In many health care systems, a variety of organizational models have been adopted to reflect the reality that physicians associated with the same organization are not homogenous in their interests, power, or inclination toward action. Indeed, the mere existence of alternative organizational templates for structuring the relationship between physicians and delivery organizations supports our contention that institutional diversity has replaced the more monolithic notion of a single institutional system to which organizations must conform.

Which organizational template health care systems and physicians adopt will reflect the interplay of agency, values, and power and resources. For example, the absence of resources and the inability of individual physicians to engage proactively in collective action by forming large groups or marshalling political support (for example, against regulations proscribing the corporate practice of medicine) makes them vulnerable to aggressive actions and superior resources of health care systems. This will often lead to the purchase of physician practices and the adoption of more hierarchical relationships between physicians and organizations (Scott and Lammers, 1985), organizational forms that reflect institutional frameworks based on market logic and managerial control. The legitimacy of the outcomes of such institutional wars is by no means a foregone conclusion. However, because the playing field is occupied by alternative organizational templates (rather than just one), claims to legitimacy are much more easily made.

As our framework suggests, however, institutional shifts to more market-based logics are by no means a given. In states where physicians have been more successful in influencing regulation that supports traditional institutional practices and professional control, or where they are more active in wielding market power and resources, we might expect more loosely structured arrangements between physicians and organized delivery systems. Such arrangements are likely to emphasize flatter structures, greater autonomy, and discounted fees for service rather than capitated reimbursement. Certainly these arrangements are not well-suited for dictating to physicians specific clinical protocols or care-management procedures.

When the outcomes of the application of agency, values, power, and resources are less clear-cut on the part of physicians and delivery organizations, new structures that differ from both institutional and corporate archetypes may result. These are represented by PHOs, MSOs, or other hybrid or synthesized forms of physician-organizational arrangements. These structures operate separately from the health care system or hospital on the one hand and the physician group on the other. Although such separation is effected for both practical (operational) and legal reasons, it strongly symbolizes that neither the professional nor managerial logics will dominate, and that a new set of cognitive orientations and practices is expected. Physicians and managers who affiliate with these structures self-select according to their willingness to engage in network relations with each other and adopt practice patterns consistent with the goals and norms of the new entity (such as evidence-based medicine).

Of course, an impasse may also result in parallel institutional structures represented by the delivery system and the physician group. Here, the physicians are likely to develop organizations "in their own image," that is, with nonhierarchical governance and control structures characteristic of professional organization. The health care system, unencumbered by potential conflicting logics associated with maintaining a traditional medical staff, could structure itself based on organizational templates found in the corporate sector (Shortell, 1985). Functional relationships between the two are based strictly on contractual terms rather than on common interest, loyalty, or shared vision. Thus the agency, values, and power of various actors could greatly influence the choices that hospital leaders make as they respond to market and institutional pressures about their physician relations.

Conclusion

Opportunities to study the processes by which organizational, political, and professional agents attempt to lay claim to legitimacy by either reinventing or protecting the normative and cognitive foundations of institutional systems abound in today's health care environment. For example, the recent debates over a patients' bill of rights represent one battle in an institutional war whereby professional and market-based interests actively compete for legitimacy, invoking the established mantle of individuals' right to accessible health care to advance their own claims to institutional dominance. In the future, more battles are likely as the struggle for institutional dominance and legitimacy continues. This chapter emphasizes that the health care sector is neither monolithic nor static in its institutional makeup. Instead, there are several logics to which organizations might conform and there is a constant battle for institutional legitimacy being fought in the legislative and legal arenas, as well as in health care organizations themselves. Although market forces have clearly destabilized and, to some extent, deligitimized traditional institutional structures and practices, the result is not one of market dominance but of a rich variety of new relationships between market and institutional forces.

4

When Institutions Collide

*Hospitals Sponsored by
the Roman Catholic Church*

Kenneth R. White

For centuries, the Roman Catholic Church has been a major social actor in the provision of health services, particularly health care delivered in hospitals. Catholic-sponsored hospitals are a special case of organization in the health care sector, with two strong institutional environments defining their identity. Not only are these hospitals subjected to the institutional and technical environments that all contemporary hospitals face (Somers, 1969), but they also have the added institutional environment of the Roman Catholic Church. These institutional forces have interacted to form organizations that find it increasingly difficult to satisfy the opposing sources of demands on how the organization should perform.

Hospitals are important in the study of organizations. As complex organizations, hospitals provide fertile ground for study due to their wide variety of structures, missions, and ownership types. A great deal of research applying organizational theory has been conducted to explain the existence and structure of health care organizations (Mick, 1990), and as hospitals evolve and adapt to environmental forces, more knowledge is needed on the unique contribution of hospitals with varying ownership and control. Hospitals sponsored by the Roman Catholic Church are good examples of organizations that contend with environmental forces that may be unlike other hospital ownership types, as this chapter will describe.

The purpose of this chapter is to examine the collision of the demands on organizational activity that differing environments of the Roman Catholic Church and the contemporary hospital dictate. Powerful forces deriving from the Roman Catholic Church are pressuring Catholic hospitals to retain their distinctive mission of providing a church-sponsored work, while at the same time pressures from the hospital environment promote secular uniformity. This chapter analyzes assumptions of the institutional perspective of organizational study as they relate to organizations in multiple organizational fields, and various structural scenarios available to organizations. Finally, organizational implications are presented, as well as a discussion about research that describes the ways that Catholic hospitals have adapted to environmental pressures.

Background

The earliest Catholic hospitals were founded to provide charitable health care services for those who lived in their parishes (Farren, 1996). As society has become increasingly more secularized, the link between churches and their sponsored social institutions, such as hospitals, has weakened (Freeland, 1992). Catholic hospitals have shifted from being "ecclesiastical" institutions in the early part of the twentieth century to become the largest North American private, nonprofit sector effort delivering medical care, long-term care, and related health services to persons in need. Over time, the ecclesiastical presence has been eroded as the workforce in Catholic health care has shifted from one that is predominantly Catholic or has members of religious institutes to one that is more secular. Concomitantly, Catholic health care organizations have responded to market and regulatory pressures by changing their scope of services, organizational arrangements, and financing mechanisms (White, 2000). A challenge central to Catholic identity has been maintaining fidelity to religious values of providing comprehensive health care to vulnerable and underserved populations.

With declining numbers of Catholic religious orders and an increasingly secularized society contributing to changes in the Catholic health care tradition over time, as well as added market and regulatory pressures on all hospitals, it has been difficult to maintain a unique niche for Catholic hospitals. Yet as Catholic hospitals struggle to keep pace with economic, political, and legal pressures, while surviving as fiscally sound organizations, they continue to be faced with pressures from the Roman Catholic Church to maintain a distinctive Catholic identity (Catholic Health Association, 1998; Cochran, 2000; Hehir, 1995: Kauffman, 1990; Prince, 1994; Stepsis and Liptak, 1989; Sullivan, 1993).

Elements of Catholic Identity

Catholic health care has a few notable differences from health care controlled by other health care delivery systems (Cassidy, 1994; Sullivan, 1993; Vowell, 1992). The Code of Canon Law for the Roman Catholic Church grants the diocesan bishop the ability to determine the qualities necessary to identify an institution as Catholic, and thus as sharing in the mission of the Church. The moral responsibility of Catholic health care is outlined in the *Ethical and Religious Directives for Catholic Health Care Services*. The *Directives* describe procedures that are judged morally wrong by the United States Conference of Catholic Bishops. A section was added in 1994 (and modified in 2001) that deals with new partnerships between Catholic and non-Catholic organizations and providers. Specifically, ". . .[T]he purpose of the *Directives* is twofold: first, to reaffirm the ethical standards of behavior in health care that flow from the Church's teaching about the dignity of the human person; second, to provide authoritative guidance on certain moral issues that face Catholic health care today" (*Ethical and Religious Directives for Catholic Health Care Services*, 2001).

A revision of the *Directives* in 2001 was prompted by concern from the Vatican that Church rules were being misapplied in some partnerships in which the Catholic partner was not sufficiently distanced from the provision of services prohibited by the Church. The latest edition of the *Directives* reminds Catholic hospital partners that they "should avoid entering into partnerships that would involve them in cooperation with the wrongdoing of other providers" (Bellandi, 2001). Although the revisions appear to have stricter interpretation of partnership arrangements, some Catholic health care leaders believe that this makes potential nonprofit partners slower and much more cautious when it comes to partnering with Catholic hospitals (Bellandi, 2001).

Theologians and academicians have described Catholic identity as it is applied to the delivery of health care services (Cochran, 1999a; 2000; White, 2000). Common themes that emerge in describing Catholic identity are the ways the values of the Roman Catholic Church are combined, focused, and emphasized in the health care ministry (Wilson and Schindler, 1990); the responsibility to community, human dignity, and the call to justice (Marty, 1995); and the preferential service to the poor. Catholic identity may be realized in the provision of certain services that reach marginalized populations (for example, services for conditions that may be "stigmatized," such as HIV/AIDS, chemical dependency, psychiatric problems, and epilepsy) or services that promote the sanctity of life (such as perinatal services) and the dignity of death (for example, end-of-life services such as palliative care units, hospices, pain management). Conversely, being "Catholic" means *not* providing other services, such as surgical sterilization procedures (Weisman, Khoury, Cassirer, Sharpe, and Morlock, 1999), physician-assisted suicide, or certain counseling services that promote elective abortions.

Empirical analyses of Catholic hospitals compared to secular ownership types have shown that there are similarities on certain dimensions such as financial performance and other operational performance indicators (Prince, 1994; Prince and Ramanan, 1994; Tang, 1995; White, 1996; White and Ozcan, 1996; White and

Begun, 1998/99). However, in characterizing Catholic identity as the provision of certain mission-driven services that enhance fidelity to social justice and compassionate care, White and Begun (1998/99) have shown that there are certain differences between Catholic and non-Catholic hospitals. Furthermore, Catholic hospitals *are* able to differentiate themselves on the provision of certain services (White, Cochran, and Patel, 2002; Cochran and White, 2002).

The Institutional Perspective of Catholic Hospitals

Catholic hospitals may be viewed from an open systems perspective (Scott, 1995; 1998). In this way, one may depict Catholic hospitals as organizations responding and adapting to environmental forces, including, but not limited to, institutional pressures as predicted by the institutional theory perspective.

Institutional theory considers the organization as an adaptive organism responding to the characteristics and commitments of participants as well as to influences from the external environment (Selznick, 1948). This focus on the sociological aspects of organizations makes institutional theory useful for analyzing Catholic hospitals as "institutions" heavily imbued with values, rituals, myths, and ceremonies emanating from the tradition of the Roman Catholic Church and its sponsoring religious communities (orders of religious men or women). As explained by Scott and Meyer (1994), ". . .Hospital structures reflect standard forms created in the wider environment: The existence of such organizations depends in good part on the environmental institutionalization of such forms."

Institutional theory is particularly relevant for the study of Catholic hospitals, for several reasons: (1) because the *ownership* and *control* of Catholic health care are by the Roman Catholic Church, the institutional component of Catholic hospitals is strong; (2) hospitals face pressures for efficiency and effectiveness, and are required to exist in strong technical environments; and (3) sociological forces that shape organizations, such as values, traditions, and rituals, are considered. The institutional perspective considers the way an organization's culture explains its existence.

Technical and Institutional Environments

Relating the technical and institutional components in an environment helps define what, in fact, an organization and systems of organizations are (Scott, 1992). Meyer and Scott (1983) assert that it is important to distinguish organizations based on their degree of technical and institutional environments. Technical environments are those in which organizations produce a product of service that is exchanged in a market such that organizations are rewarded for effective and efficient performance. Institutional environments are characterized by the elaboration of rules and requirements to which individual organizations must conform in order to receive legitimacy and support. Institutional environments reward organizations that have correct structure and processes; technical environments reward organizations that achieve correct outcomes.

Several constructs of institutional theory are useful in the analysis of Catholic health care organizations. Isomorphism, or the tendency to become similar to other organizations that experience like environmental and institutional environments, is a central construct of the institutional perspective (DiMaggio and Powell, 1983). Other tenets of this theoretical perspective include deeply held beliefs and values of organizations, boundary-spanning activities, and the process of gaining legitimacy.

Isomorphism

Isomorphism is the notion that an organization will imitate other organizations in its environment where the same set of environmental pressures exists. Organizations not only compete for market position and specialized niches but also for political power and institutional legitimacy and for social as well as economic fitness. The evolution of hospitals evidences this point: while at one time hospitals were charitable organizations for the sick and injured, they have become more businesslike, with for-profit and nonprofit hospitals exhibiting similar attributes and espousing similar missions and goals (Griffith and White, 2002; Meyer and Rowan, 1977; Starr, 1982; Stevens, 1989). There has been a concomitant adoption of corporate management and governance structures (DeWitt, 1981).

DiMaggio and Powell (1983) described three mechanisms through which institutional isomorphic changes occur: (1) coercive isomorphism, which stems from political influence and regulatory pressures; (2) mimetic isomorphism, resulting from standard responses to uncertainty; and (3) normative isomorphism, associated with professionalization, or the formal educational process and the growth of networks across organizational boundaries. Organizations tend to model themselves after similar organizations in their field that they perceive to be more legitimate or successful. Abrahamson and Rosenkopf (1993) have used the term "institutional bandwagons" to describe the pressures of organizations to adopt an innovation, not because of their individual assessments of the innovation but because of the sheer number of organizations that have already adopted the innovation.

Beliefs and Values

Important in the study of Catholic hospitals is the construct of beliefs and values that sustain the legitimacy of institutions. Institutional theorists such as Meyer and Rowan (1977) have described these beliefs and values as "rationalized myths." They are *rational* in the sense that they are represented in elaborated systems of laws, professional standards, and licensure or accreditation requirements that are adopted as a way to accomplish an organization's objectives. They are *myths* in the sense that they are supported by widely held beliefs that cannot be tested. Institutional theorists purport that survival depends on conformity to rationalized myths (Alexander and D'Aunno, 1990; Meyer and Rowan, 1977; Mohr, 1992; Roggenkamp and White, 2001).

Throughout the history of Catholic hospitals, there have been redefinitions of its identity to keep pace with the changing contexts of society, religion, and health care sponsorship (Farren, 1996). An identity that began nearly two hundred years ago primarily as a social welfare ministry in response to urban need and Christian charity is now under pressure to define itself increasingly by its technical capacity. To maintain a connection to the Church, and to respond to technical pressures of modern hospitals, a special case of private, nonprofit health care providers has emerged.

Boundary-Spanning Activities

The way that Catholic hospitals organize for responding to the external environment and the various stakeholders is through boundary spanning. There are three forms of boundary-spanning activities. First, *boundary redefinition* occurs when a hospital joins one or more organizations that increase the organizational boundary. This is what happened when individual Catholic hospitals became members of multihospital systems in the latter part of the twentieth century, thereby increasing corporatization of hospitals (Alexander and D'Aunno, 1990). In addition, for Catholic hospitals, becoming members of multihospital systems may have started the trend to partner with hospitals in different locations as well as different religious community sponsors.

Second, *buffering* is a boundary-spanning activity that serves to protect an organization against disturbing environmental influences. Buffering activities are designed to protect the organization's technical core, or direct patient care in the case of health care. For example, buffering may involve augmenting or centralizing administrative structures to amplify the protective barriers surrounding patient care activities. Another method of buffering has been to develop offices of corporate compliance in response to pressures for more accountability in organizational ethics.

Third, *bridging* is a boundary-spanning activity that serves to connect organizations to other organizations. Bridging strategies involve creating linkages to other organizations through shared services and other product-exchange opportunities (Fennell and Alexander, 1987). As hospitals have merged or other partnership arrangements have been formed, more opportunities have existed for bridging in the last two decades of the twentieth century (White, 2000). For example, organizational structures may not involve changes in legal definitions but may involve partnership agreements for purchasing, negotiating with managed care companies, networking, and developing strategic health alliances (McCue, Clement, and Luke, 1999).

The three boundary-spanning mechanisms—boundary redefinition, buffering, and bridging—serve to extend the institution into its environment. This contributes to isomorphism, or becoming "like" other ownership types (Fennell and Alexander, 1987).

Legitimacy

Organization legitimacy is the essence of survival of hospitals sponsored by the Catholic Church. Although the legitimacy construct has been associated with institutional theory, Suchman (1995) pointed out that few have defined it. Moreover, there are contradictory uses of the term. In the strategic tradition, legitimacy is referred to as the way organizations use symbols to gain the support of society. The institutional school (for example, DiMaggio and Powell, 1983; Scott, 1992; Meyer and Scott, 1993; Powell and DiMaggio, 1991; Zucker, 1987) "adopts a more detached stance and emphasizes the ways in which sector-wide structuration dynamics generate cultural pressures that transcend any single organization's purposive control" (Suchman, 1995). In other words, legitimacy refers to the way the organizational culture explains an organization's existence

(Meyer and Scott, 1983; Suchman, 1995). This chapter is concerned with the aspect of legitimacy that derives from the distinct contribution of Catholic hospitals, which is necessary to justify a distinct ownership type.

Environments That Compete

The environments of the Roman Catholic Church and the contemporary hospital are often contradictory. Figure 4.1 describes the environmental forces that are impinging on Catholic hospital identity, as explained below.

Roman Catholic Church Environment

The Roman Catholic Church environment consists of elaborate theological structures, processes, and directives emanating from a highly centralized body, the Vatican. Cardinals, archbishops, or bishops interpret the policies of the Church for the local Catholic hospitals in their jurisdictions. In addition, the sponsoring religious

Figure 4.1. The Impact of Catholic Church and Hospital Environments on Catholic Hospital Identity.

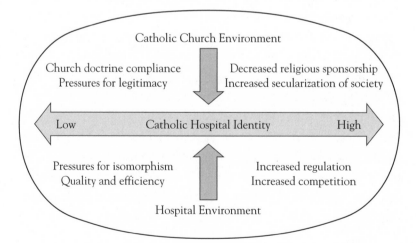

institutions, such as orders of nuns or brothers, impose their particular charism, or sacred mission, on the individual hospital. This layer of Church hierarchy provides a strong institutional environment that is unknown to secular hospitals.

Although the link to Catholic doctrine and the belief that health care is a right has remained central to Catholic identity, other environmental forces outside the control of the Catholic Church have affected Catholic hospital identity. The increasing secularization of society, the decreasing numbers of religious (nuns, priests, and others) who are leaders and providers of Catholic health care services, and the decreasing reliance on the Church to support its sponsored social works are forces that are reshaping the identity of Catholic hospitals.

However, because of the strong Catholic institutional environment, the pressure is strong to perpetuate a Catholic health care ministry. Therefore, debates about Catholic identity from the Church's perspective center on adherence to Church doctrine that encourages the provision of certain services in certain ways, while prohibiting others.

Secular Hospital Environment

The contemporary hospital has become a complicated amalgam of business structures and elaborate processes for delivering medical care, no longer dependent on philanthropy and church-donated labor (in the form of free services from priests, nuns, and others) for financial viability. The rise of technology, new inventions, and discoveries that aid in the diagnosis and treatment of diseases are central to the environment that has shaped the contemporary hospital. Furthermore, with the advent of federal and state programs to finance health care for the poor and elderly in the 1960s, philanthropy began to decrease. The often-opposing forces of increased regulation and market competition posed new environmental constraints on hospitals. Increased competition for lower-cost and higher-quality health care services was being demanded. Payers, employers, and policymakers wanted lower costs and higher quality, or at least more value for resources expended. The emergence of for-profit corporations into the market in the 1970s has added an additional burden with the increase in the provision of uncompensated, unpopular, or stigmatized care in nonprofit settings (LeBlanc, 1991).

What have emerged at the beginning of the twenty-first century are hospitals with a strong institutional environment *and* a strong technical environment. Like the strong institutional environment of the Roman Catholic Church, the hospital has elaborate administrative structures and bureaucracies. However, the hospital institutional environment has become more coupled to the technical environment due to the demands for increased quality, decreased cost, and compliance to the standards of regulatory bodies such as the Joint Commission on the Accreditation of Healthcare Organizations, the Center for Medicare and Medicaid Services, the National Committee on Quality Assurance, and others.

The Clash of Catholic Church and Secular Hospital Environments

The collision course of the competing Catholic Church and hospital technical environments is laid out in the definition of Catholic identity. As shown in Figure 4.1, Catholic hospital identity is defined by the various mission-driven constructs that are central to the sponsoring organization, within the context of Catholic doctrine. Ways that hospitals characterize their identity are to describe a commitment to social justice, effective and efficient stewardship of resources, the provision of compassionate care, and the treatment of all persons with dignity and respect.

While the institutional environment of the Church wants to maintain legitimacy by being able to describe a distinctive contribution to its health care ministry, the Church identity has become increasingly harder to define and maintain. Links to the Roman Catholic Church are fewer. The numbers of health care executives who are members of religious orders are decreasing; thus reliance on lay persons to carry out the sacramental nature of the ministry (Cochran 1999a) has placed additional threats to Catholic identity. The once-prominent religious icons and symbols are not as prevalent in Catholic hospitals as they had been in earlier hospitals.

The environmental pressures of the Roman Catholic Church and the modern hospital are summarized here. The strong institutional pressures of the Catholic Church are

1. To maintain legitimacy of Catholic sponsorship of hospitals and the adherence to Church doctrine

2. To infuse Catholic identity into hospitals that are increasingly being lead by laity

3. To promulgate the beliefs and values of the Roman Catholic Church through a sponsored social ministry that a more secular society may not appreciate

4. To retain sponsorship of Catholic health care organizations, as an extension of the healing ministry of Jesus Christ

The strong technical pressures of hospitals are

1. To compete in a market-based economy (isomorphic pressures)

2. To maintain legitimacy through regulatory body compliance and approval

3. To provide high-quality, low-cost health care services with acceptable outcomes

4. To improve health status of the communities being served and to satisfy the needs of all stakeholders (boundary spanning).

Together, the aforementioned institutional and technical pressures represent a collision course for competing, and often contradictory, environments for shaping the contemporary hospital. The way that Catholic hospitals may respond to this phenomenon is described in the next section.

Organizational Response to Environmental Collision

With strong institutional and technical environments in which to enact Catholic health care, organizations respond in their self-interest in different ways. This is akin to saying that Catholic hospitals have a strategy in order to survive (Luke, Begun, and Walston, 2000). Strategic adaptation to environmental pressures may be described as a continuum from low to high adaptation. The adaptation response may yield organizations that are very different from the traditional Catholic, acute care hospital.

If one considers the institutional pressure for Catholic identity and the technical pressure for efficiency and effectiveness as dichotomous dimensions, then a fourfold grid describes hypothetical organizational responses to environmental adaptation, as exhibited in Figure 4.2.

High technical, high institutional. In this scenario, the acute care hospital is likely to survive, although it will be increasingly harder to detect differences between Catholic and secular hospitals. If hospi-

Figure 4.2. Adaptive Framework.

		Catholic Institutional Pressure Adaptation	
		High	Low
Hospital Technical Pressure Adaptation	High	Acute care; rationalized myth	Acute care; ownership conversion
	Low	Change in business to Catholic-sponsored assisted living, long-term care, or other business	Closure, sale, or changed line of business

tals do maintain a distinctly Catholic mission, it will be because the deeply held beliefs and values and theological assumptions are integrated into the technical core.

High technical, low institutional. Here the acute care hospital does not adapt to the strong institutional environment of the Catholic Church, although technical adaptation is high. This organization has legitimacy as a hospital without the Catholic identity. In this case, an ownership conversion is likely to occur.

Low technical, high institutional. This organizational response is the Catholic hospital of yesteryear. With low technical pressures, it is not likely that an acute care hospital would survive because consumers and payers demand efficiency and quality. So a Catholic hospital would likely make the transition from an acute care hospital to a new organizational form. It may or may not be related to health care. In this scenario, Catholic identity is the prevailing strategic influence, thus meeting the needs of the community through a sponsored social ministry that could involve housing, assisted living, long-term care services, or other types of business.

Low technical, low institutional. This organizational response represents a shift from acute care and Catholic identity that could result in closure, sale, or changing the line of business. It would cease to exist as a Catholic organization because it would not be in compliance with the rational processes that define Catholic organizations (such as the *Religious Directives* and determinations by local bishops). It would cease to be a hospital because it would not conform to the high technical pressures required.

Catholic Hospitals Respond

The survival of Catholic hospitals qua *Catholic* hospitals depends on their ability to maintain legitimacy as a sponsored work of the Roman Catholic Church, while at the same time competing with secular hospitals in a market-based economy. Survival may involve a redefinition of what it means to be a Catholic hospital, a transition from sponsoring acute care services to providing other health care or social ministries beneficial to their communities and consistent with Church doctrine, or the abandonment of Catholic identity entirely. What actually is happening is a combination of the scenarios presented in the previous section, because the technical pressures are highly variable across the United States. For example, some states have stronger technical environments than others, such as California and Arizona as opposed to Arkansas or Mississippi. It is predicted that Catholic hospital identity would be stronger in states with lessened regulatory constraints on the technical aspects of health services delivery.

As exhibited in Figure 4.3, Catholic hospitals have adapted to Church and hospital environments in various ways. For heuristic presentation, the typology is simplified in Figure 4.3 (in reality the typology variables are continuous, not discrete as shown). The following sections describe ways that Catholic hospitals have adapted to the mixed nature of technical and institutional environments.

Serving Two Masters

Catholic hospitals that provide acute care services are adapting to high institutional and high technical environments by serving two

Figure 4.3. Adaptation of Catholic Hospitals.

Hospital Technical Pressure Adaptation	Catholic Institutional Pressure Adaptation: High	Catholic Institutional Pressure Adaptation: Low
High	Serving two masters (Church and hospital)	Changing identities (From Church to secular)
Low	Modifying missions (From acute care to other social ministry)	Acquiescing assets and identity (Closure or sale)

"masters" simultaneously. That is, pressure for efficiency, market share, and quality in the technical environment is one master. Another master is the pressure to provide the technical services in a manner that is consistent with and supportive of Church doctrine. This has created isomorphism *and* differentiation with secular hospitals on several dimensions.

Catholic hospitals have been shown to be similar to other hospital ownership types on certain dimensions. To date, organizational research has concentrated on ownership and performance, in terms of financial outcomes, efficiency, and returns to the community. Catholic hospitals have been shown to perform similarly to their secular counterparts as measured by return on assets, operating expense per discharge, and profit margin (Tang, 1995; White, 1996). Another dimension of isomorphism comes from normative sources. With the decline in the numbers of Catholic hospital–sponsored schools of nursing and other training programs and the concomitant decrease in religious men and women who transmitted Catholic values and normative processes, clinical providers are educated in secular colleges and universities. This has yielded nurses and other providers that may not have a uniquely Catholic perspective on providing health care.

Organizational differences exist in other areas involving service provision as it stems from mission-driven values that attempt to define Catholic identity. A commitment to social justice is carried out in the provision of health care to poor and marginalized populations. For instance, provision of charity care and certain socially stigmatized services (for example those for HIV/AIDS, mental health, and substance abuse) are ways to operationalize Catholic identity. Research has been conducted comparing provision of charity care and certain services by various ownership types of hospitals. Results suggest that Catholic hospitals *may* be differentiated from other private, nonprofit hospitals on these dimensions and would *likely* be differentiated from investor-owned hospitals (LeBlanc, 1991; LeBlanc and Hurley, 1995; White, 1996; White and Begun, 1998/99). However, they are second to large, public teaching hospitals in the provision of charity care and socially stigmatized services.

There are certain areas in which Catholic hospitals continue to differentiate themselves as distinctly Catholic. From the strong Catholic tradition of respect for life and the dignity of death, services that involve procreation and palliation are empirically different when comparing Catholic and secular hospitals. Catholic hospitals tend to provide more access to obstetric and pediatric services (White, 1996) while restricting services resulting in abortion and reproductive sterilization (Weisman, Khoury, Cassirer, Sharpe, and Morlock, 1999). At the other end of the life spectrum, Catholic hospitals are leaders in the provision of palliative care, pain management, and other end-of-life services (White, Cochran, and Patel, 2002).

For Catholic hospitals to continue serving the strong institutional masters of Church and hospital, two demands must be satisfied (Cochran, 1999b). First, they must continue to generate enough revenue over costs to fund charity care and form community outreach at levels that are higher than their secular counterparts. Second, the religious orders that originally established them must find ways to inculcate their charisms in the new lay leadership better than they have in the past (McCormick, 1994; 1995).

Changing Identities

The pressure to serve two masters (that is, Catholic Church and hospital) may be too great, resulting in a sacrifice of the Catholic identity. Pressures to continue providing hospital services override the requirements to remain Catholic. Such is the case with mergers, acquisitions, or other ownership conversions. The hospital remains viable, although the official Catholic identity is jettisoned. This has been seen in the declining numbers of Catholic hospitals from 640 in 1990 to 601 in 1999 (Place, 1999).

Modifying Missions

The pressure to imitate may reduce the level of organizational innovation and creativity (Jones, 1995). This, in turn, may lead to a hospital that may not be able to compete in a rapidly changing environment or one in which innovation is crucial. To maintain fidelity to a Catholic sacramental perspective (Cochran, 1999b), the organization may change from providing acute care services to providing transitional, continuing retirement care or ministry other than acute care hospital services. This has been witnessed in health systems becoming more involved in providing housing options for the poor, hospice care for the dying, residential services for the socially stigmatized (such as homes for those dying with AIDS), clinics in immigrant labor camps, addiction treatment centers, or outpatient mental health centers.

Acquiescing Assets and Identity

In some cases in which the institutional and technical pressures are too great, Catholic hospitals have been unable to survive as hospitals or as distinctly Catholic organizations. This has resulted in closures or acquiescence of Catholic hospital assets and identity. If sold, the new organization would face a different institutional environment determining whether the organization would continue to be a hospital.

Conclusion

According to institutional theory, Catholic health care will continue to redefine itself as the environment continues to change. In this way, traditions and rituals will take on new meanings. Promulgating rationalized myths will be even more important with the increasing secularization of society and the concomitant decrease in the use of religious icons and symbols, and the decline in the numbers of religious sponsors.

Institutional theory predicts that hospital ownership types, in their provision of services, will exhibit isomorphism (coercive, mimetic, and normative) to the extent that they share similar environments. However, organizations may face pressures for isomorphism from different organizational fields that are contradictory. Such is the case of Catholic hospitals. Powerful forces deriving from the Roman Catholic Church are pressuring Catholic hospitals to retain their distinctiveness, while, simultaneously, pressures for isomorphism are derived from environmental forces in the hospital industry (White, 1996, White, 2000). Institutional theorists have tended to assume that pressures for isomorphism affecting the organizational field are uniform across members of the field. In the case of hospitals with different ownership types, this is not true. Ownership type creates isomorphism pressures of its own, for uniformity within the ownership type. To maintain fidelity to the sacramental meaning of the Church, options other than acute hospital care should be investigated. A refined institutional theory should recognize the membership of organizations in multiple organizational fields, with pressures that may be conflicting.

5

. . . .

Understanding Health Care Markets
Actors, Products, and Relations

Douglas R. Wholey and Lawton R. Burns

H ow can we describe health care markets to help us understand why they operate so differently? In some communities, the health care provider market is dominated by hospital-based integrated delivery systems, whereas in other communities HMOs dominate. In between are a myriad of different types of markets, with each community seemingly having its own history and development path (Burns and Wholey, 2000; Wholey and Burns, 2000). In Minnesota, employers coalesce in the Buyers Health Care Action Group (BHCAG) to contract directly with providers, using HMOs as third-party administrators for claims processing and developing a separate clinical improvement group to provide a public good (Christianson, Feldman, Weiner, and Drury, 1999; Knutson, 1998; Robinow, 1997a; 1997b). It takes a single large purchaser, the California Public Employees Retirement System (CALPERS), to pursue similar direct purchasing in California (Kennedy and Jennings,

We thank the Center for Studying Health System Change for sponsoring this research. Prior versions of this research were presented at the Center for Studying Health System Change, the Lister Hill Center at the University of Alabama at Birmingham, and the Division of Health Services Research at the University of Minnesota. We appreciate the usefulness of the comments at these presentations and comments from Roger Feldman, Jon Christianson, Paul Ginsburg, Cara Lesser, and Joy Grossman.

1998). In many other communities, direct purchasing is not a feasible option.

An adequate description of markets that allows for comparative analysis requires clear conceptual definitions of markets and their related phenomena. This chapter outlines a relational and social network view of markets and its implications for the study of health care markets and organizations. We extend prior health services market-analysis research with concepts from organizational and economic sociology and from industrial economics to suggest some new avenues for understanding the reasons for differences across markets.

We view a market as a social structure in which producers enter into exchanges with consumers for a particular product or service. The three elements of the definition, *products*, *actors* (producers and consumers), and *exchange* suggest three ways of viewing markets. First, markets can be seen in terms of product or service characteristics. Economics provides a product-centric view of markets when it uses concepts such as elasticity of demand for a product or service or the cross-price elasticity between products. A sociological equivalent would be analyzing social relationships in terms of the functional purpose of the item being exchanged (Mauss, 1967). Second, markets can be seen in terms of the actions (decisions) of consumers and producers related to supply and demand of products of services. In health services research there is a burgeoning interest in understanding market functioning by understanding these decision processes (Hibbard, Slovic, and Jewett, 1997). Third, markets can be seen in terms of the exchanges, the characteristics of the relationship between a consumer and a producer in a market and of the social network structure of all the relationships among all producers and consumers. Market operation is a function of the characteristics of the product, the actors, the exchange relationship, and the interrelationships between markets. An example of the latter is the effect of labor market tightness on the operation of the health insurance market (Maude-Griffin, Feldman, and Wholey, 2001). The relational perspective, as a characteristic of both a particular market and the relationships among markets, has not been widely used in health services research to understand market functioning. This chapter shows how a relational perspective can be used to gain insights into health care market functioning.

The chapter is organized into five sections. The first two sections describe markets as phenomena and define the concepts being used. The remaining sections apply these concepts to three different levels of market phenomena. The third section, "Relationships and Markets," examines the way in which relationships affect market functioning via *relational characteristics*, that is, the nature of the relationships between any two actors. This section provides a microlevel analysis of relational strength and allocation of activities within a relationship. The fourth section, "Social Network Structure and Markets," adopts a macrolevel perspective to examine another way in which the pattern of relationships among actors in a market affects market processes. We develop the concept of micromarkets—segments of distinctive cliques of buyers and sellers—and argue that micromarkets influence market processes such as innovation diffusion, price competition, and information flow. The literature on network externalities is used to show how path-dependent historical processes and network externalities can shape the micromarkets. The fifth section, "Social Network Structure and Organizational Fields," extends the relational perspective to encompass the health care organizational field, the set of all health–care-related markets in a geographical area. This section describes how the structure of the organizational field and the interdependence of markets affect the functioning of each market within it. Table 5.1 shows the organization of our arguments.

Conceptualizing Markets

The word *market* has multiple meanings. Sometimes market is used to refer to all health care transactions within a geographical area, such as when we refer to the health care market in Minneapolis or

Table 5.1. Effect of Social Network Structure on Market Processes and Performance.

Market Social Network Structure →	Market Processes →	Market Performance
Relational Characteristics		
Longitudinality	Relational stickiness and stability	Patient outcomes
Integratedeness	Amount and diversity of information	Customized care
Comprehensiveness	Trust	Integrated care
	Cooperation and collaboration	Transaction and relational costs
Allocation of functions within relationships	Risk assumption	Elasticity of demand for product
	Development of expertise and capability to perform function	Scale and scope economies in performing funtions
		Uniformity in function performance across relationships
Social Network Structure of Markets		
Micromarkets	Information flows	Collusion
Associations	Innovation diffusion	Uniformity of products, quality, and prices versus cliques of somewhat similar but distinct markets
Purchaser coalitions	Competition, market segmentation, and bargaining power	
Quality and standards groups (such as ICSI)	Standardization or Coordination	Portability of insurance
	Standards enforcement (for example, NCQA/HEDIS)	Adoption of new ways of organizing (such as guidelines) and products
Network externalities and path dependence	Market dominance	Cross-elasticity of demand between "similar" products

Social Network Structure of Organizational Fields

Regular equivalence	Competition between equivalent actors	Diversity in choices of types of providers available to consumers (for example, IDSs, PHOs, HMOs)
Exchange, dependence, and power	Broker roles Competition over position in market social network structure rather than competition over products	Costs and benefits associated with broker roles Distribution of profits among participants in organizational field

Note: The presentation of the causal order is for didactic purposes. The Market Social Structure ⟶ Market Performance model was chosen because it is similar to the Structure ⟶ Conduct ⟶ Performance model in traditional industrial-organization (IO) economics. As the work in the new IO economics shows, the relationships are more complex, with significant endo-geneity.

in Los Angeles. Yet within a geographical area, there are multiple product markets. There are markets associated with health plans purchasing provider services, with employers purchasing health care coverage, and with self-insured employers purchasing administrative services only. Even for seemingly similar products there may be important institutional differences that affect market functioning. For example, health services can be provided by health plans that serve as intermediaries between employers and providers, while in the BHCAG model, health services are delivered by provider groups that directly contract with employers, with administrative services provided in a separate administrative services contract (Christianson, Feldman, Weiner, and Drury, 1999; Knutson, 1998; Robinow, 1997b). Because the multiplicity of meanings associated with the term *market* can impede cumulative research, it is imperative to define clearly the terms used to analyze markets.

We view markets as locations where buyers and sellers enter into exchanges of similar products. Similar products means that consumers view products as substitutable. From a product perspective, markets can be broadly described in terms of product differentiation and geographical location. While some markets may consist of only one distinct product, other markets may have a broad array of differentiated, substitutable products. The boundaries of markets are influenced by product differentiation, geography, and organizations. An example of product differentiation is a market where consumers can choose among indemnity health insurers, preferred provider organizations (PPOs), independent practice association (IPA)–type HMOs, and group or staff–type HMOs for health insurance coverage. Depending on patterns of substitutability among these products, these may be viewed as one or more distinct markets. An example of geographical differences is that of pharmaceuticals being more a national market than are primary care physician services. Finally, the market boundaries can be determined by institutions, such as when closed panel HMOs restrict the primary care physician choice or when states restrict occupational jurisdictions to particular professions. In sum, a market is the exchange of similar, substitutable products in a specific geographical area.

Markets are generally described using three components: products (similar goods), actors (buyers and sellers), and exchanges between buyer and seller. Products occupy a central place in economic views. Markets are defined in terms of product characteristics and the organizations that supply (or could potentially supply) close substitutes (Haas-Wilson and Gaynor, 1998; Morrisey, Sloan, and Valvona, 1988). Actors (buyers and sellers) making decisions also occupy a central place in health services research. Sellers, for example, make decisions about market entry and exit, pricing, and product differentiation (Wholey and Christianson, 1994; Wholey, Christianson, and Sanchez, 1992; Wholey, Christianson, and Sanchez, 1993). Consumers make decisions about which products to use, balancing quality and cost (Hibbard, Slovic, and Jewett, 1997). Exchange relations are the third component and have been less examined in health services research. The characteristics of exchange relations affect market performance. At one extreme are markets where the relationship has little value—producers and consumers easily switch between competing products and purchasers. At the other extreme are markets where relationships are highly valued. In a patient-provider relationship, for example, physicians and patients learn about each other and develop more efficient interactions and trust, which in turn may affect patient outcomes (Safran and others, 1998). Similarly, the accumulation of transactional data (such as claims) in a health plan–purchaser relationship over time allows reports and analyses specific to the relationship to be developed. The accumulated value from learning-by-doing makes some relationships sticky and costly to switch. The difficulty in switching gives these relationships economic value, which affects market functioning.

The next section formalizes our definition of markets and discusses some immediate corollaries of the definition. Although the conceptualization is more complex than typical market definitions, it allows a richer understanding of markets and suggests new avenues for research.

Markets and Social Structures

We define *markets* as social structures within which actors enter into exchanges for a product or service. *Social structures* are "(1) networks of interrelated status positions as well as (2) the cultural systems and roles with the positions in this network. Structure is thus evident when positions are connected to one another, such that our roles in one position are affected by, and conversely have an effect on, roles in other positions" (Turner, 1994, p. 51). A *status position* is the place an actor occupies in a social structure. Consumers and producers, for example, are status positions. The circularity in defining social structures and status positions is due to social structures and status positions being simultaneously defined—either both exist conceptually or neither exists. *Roles* refer to the behaviors expected of an actor in a status position. One part of the health care consumer role, for example, is choosing a physician or health plan. *Actors* are the individuals or organizations occupying a status position with its associated role. *Products* are the goods and services exchanged between actors in their roles of producer and consumer. *Exchange* is the process of exchanging a product or service between a consumer and producer, with *relationship* referring to characteristics of the exchange.

This definition explicitly differentiates between social structures and actors. Status positions and roles refer to social structures within which actors work. A key point of viewing markets as social structures is that corresponding to each position are roles, obligations, and expectations about decision-making behavior that actors in those roles fulfill. The social structural perspective specifies that behavior, action by particular actors, is constrained by roles and status positions. To understand behavior, therefore, role definitions and status position of actors must be described.

The sociological conceptualization of markets has some immediate implications for understanding market performance. Many analyses in health services research explicitly or implicitly assume a utility-maximizing actor. The view of markets as social structures suggests that this is an assumption about an actor's role and is not an inherent characteristic of the actor. It would be reasonable to ask, How well do actors fulfill this role? Research in behavioral decision theory shows that there are systematic anomalies from the normative decision-making model in individual behavior (Dawes, 1998). It is also well-known that individual decisions may be based on social identity (March, 1994) and organizational decisions may be based on actors simply following rules (such as mindlessly applying utilization review criteria). Separating role definitions from actors may allow us to determine when individuals can fulfill the expectations inherent in the role. This knowledge may allow us to design roles that better fit individual capabilities and behaviors and improve market functioning.

The relational view of markets also focuses attention on the involvement of actors in many status positions. Health plans, for example, occupy multiple status positions, roughly categorized along product, customer, and geographical dimensions. Many managed care organizations, for example, offer multiple products—such as HMOs, PPOs, self-insurance, and perhaps health plan management services—in the same market. They may also offer the same product in multiple geographical markets and tailor it to multiple customer segments, such as the Medicare or Medicaid enrollees (Grossman, 2000). Integrated delivery networks (IDNs) have diverse status sets, often operating in multiple product markets (including hospital care, ambulatory care, long-term care, insurance vehicles, "centers of excellence," carve-out products such as heart centers, and provider-sponsored organizations) as well as the same product markets (hospitals) in multiple geographical markets (Burns and Thorpe, 2000). The set of all these status positions for an actor is called an actor's *status set*.

The diversity of an actor's status set may produce *role strain*, which affects decision making and stress. Role strain results in conflict caused by the mix of possibly competing objectives among roles. One oft-cited example of role strain is the physician's multiple roles as patient's agent, self-interested economic agent, and society's agent (Eisenberg, 1986). Another example of role strain is the use of capitated payments in the physician-health plan relationship, which introduces an incentive structure that conflicts with the physician-patient relationship (Kao, Green, Davis, Koplan, and Cleary, 1998; Kao, Green, Zaslavsky, Koplan, and Cleary, 1998). Consumer trust in health plans (patient-plan relationship) may also influence a patient's trust in his or her provider, that is, the patient-physician relationship (Mechanic and Rosenthal, 1999; Sleeper, Wholey, Hamer, Schwartz, and Inoferio, 1998). Physician trust in hospitals may also influence receptivity to overtures from Wall Street or from venture-capital-financed physician practice management companies (PPMCs) that seek to lure physicians to establish free-standing specialty (or carve-out) hospitals (Burns and Wholey, 2000). Finally, the acceptance of capitated contracts by IDNs provides an incentive for physicians to minimize hospital days, while hospitals in the IDN have an incentive to use hospital days. Understanding status set diversity, the determinants of role strain, and its effect on decision making may suggest ways to improve market functioning.

Relationships and Markets

This section examines two aspects of relationships, lock-in and delegation. *Lock-in* refers to the situation when the relationship becomes valuable to both producer and consumer because of learning that is only useful to the particular relationship (relationship-specific assets). Lock-in affects the functioning of the market and may reduce the effectiveness of consumer choice as a basis of health system change. The second aspect concerns the delegation of tasks within a relationship. Health plans, for example, have the choice between delegating health care management functions such as utilization review to provider groups they contract with or performing the task themselves. The delegation decision has consequences for uniformity and cost of task performance within the health plan.

Lock-in: Relationship Strength, Switching Costs, and Consumer Choice

Relationships are characterized by their comprehensiveness, longitudinality, and integratedness. We illustrate these dimensions using primary care relationships. *Comprehensiveness* refers to a patient bringing all of his or her problems to the physician. *Longitudinality* is the duration of the ongoing personal relationship between the primary care provider (PCP) and patient (Starfield, 1992, p. 41). *Integratedness* is the integration of information necessary to treat a patient across time and across health care problems (Starfield, 1992, p. 79). As comprehensiveness, longitudinality, and integratedness increase, the patient and physician become tightly coupled, with significant amounts and diversity of information and emotional support flowing through the relationship. The result is an atmosphere of trust and its attendant benefits (such as cost and quality) (Safran and others, 1998). Over time, the relationship becomes stable and customized to the particular patient and provider. As a relationship becomes customized, the product becomes unique and nonsubstitutable, and the idea of choosing a new provider becomes anathema. These dimensions of relationships are not peculiar to the primary care relationship and are useful for characterizing many health care relationships.

During the course of many health care transactions, providers and suppliers gain transaction-specific information about their exchange partners (customers) that affects the ease of changing relationships. The health plan, for example, develops a historical file of claims from particular providers that can be used to analyze their changing performance. In some cases, purchasers and consumers will invest in specialized equipment, such as communication lines or specialized software that is usable only for the particular relationship. Plans and providers may invest in information systems specific to the provider-plan relationship that allows providers to know who is enrolled in a plan and what benefits the enrollee is entitled to. In addition to the economic investment, relationships become infused with value, emotionally laden, and institutionalized (Selznick, 1949). These investments result in stable relationships because of difficulties in transferring knowledge and other intangible assets specific to the relationship (high switching costs). While switching relationships is difficult, these strong relational characteristics can also result in transaction efficiency and trust. The development of trust is arguably the key ingredient for the effective functioning of strategic alliances and networks (Gulati, 1998). In fact, it is trust-based relationships that confer competitive advantage on alliances over both markets and hierarchies as modes of exchange (Podolny and Page, 1998; Powell, 1990). Within health care markets, stable and trust-based relationships are found to be critical for the success of physician-hospital alliances and their joint cost-containment efforts (ProPac, 1992; Shortell, 1991; Zuckerman and others, 1998), as well as critical in the primary care relationship.

Relationships vary in the extent to which the actors involved in the relationship become locked-in, and the degree that they are locked-in affects market processes (Klemperer, 1995). High switching costs result in a bilateral monopoly. What might have been a competitive market at the start of a transaction, such as an employer evaluating and selecting among many plans or a consumer choosing among primary care providers, turns into a small-numbers, oligopolistic market or a bilateral monopoly. The threat of high switching costs may dissuade purchasers from entering a relationship. The large investment required for information systems and the continued reliance on the system vendor, for example, may result in new technologies (such as computerized physician-order-entry systems for drugs) being slow to diffuse. Although this may be offset by producers and vendors engaged in aggressive price wars to entice consumers to switch relationships away from incumbents, high switching costs may give incumbents an incentive to diversify their product lines to maximize the likelihood that consumers will not need to switch to other producers. This may be one source of market diversification mergers and may be one reason that some physician groups diversify into new product lines, such as laboratory services or alternative medicine. It also may be a source of the "one stop" health plan that offers any and every insurance product and encourages employers to rely on the health plan for all their health insurance needs. As services and products become bundled, the nature of the consumer decision is transformed from one of buying individual products or services to one of purchasing bundles of products or services. Because of bundled products and services and higher switching costs, the impact of information and consumer choice on market functioning will be lessened. The health care market may be most competitive only when the initial decision to enter into an exchange relationship is made. Once the initial choice is made, markets take on a network structure reflecting long-term exchange relationships leading to a diminution of competitive forces.

Another implication of the lock-in process is that there is an inverse relationship between consumer choice, as emphasized in many current health policy recommendations, and relational strength. This tradeoff poses a policy dilemma: policies promoting consumer choice (for example, providing information) may result in less relational strength. For exchanges in which strong social ties are important, such as in the physician-patient relationship, the provision of information may be particularly harmful when it encourages switching behavior that minimizes the development of relational benefits. The situation may be exacerbated when an individual cannot easily evaluate the tradeoff between long-term gains from integratedness and longitudinality with short-term gains from switching. Information may also have an adverse effect when a relationship becomes strong. Illness, for example, may increase patient-physician relational strength and thereby decrease the usefulness of choice. Information that shows shortcomings in physician performance may pose a difficult dilemma for the locked-in patient and may result in patient skepticism, distrust, and cynicism. This may make patients more cautious in dealings with plan and provider, and diminish the effectiveness of treatment (Kao, Green, Davis, Koplan, and Cleary, 1998; Kao, Green, Zaslavsky, Koplan, and Cleary, 1998; Safran and others, 1998; Starfield, Cassady, Nanda, Forrest, and Berk, 1998).

Although relational strength appears to be an important factor in determining health care market functioning, we have limited empirical understanding of its determinants and consequences. We can observe that relationships vary in strength across health care markets, but we do not know what determines relational strength and we do not know how current policies designed to increase consumer choice affect relational strength. And although we have some knowledge of the effect of patient-physician relationships on patient outcomes and hospital-physician relationships on firm performance, we have much less knowledge on the effect of relational strength in many other types of relationships, such as the health plan–employer or health plan–provider relations, on market functioning.

Delegation: Task Allocation Within Relationships

The term *product* refers to the goods or services that are exchanged in a relationship. Physician services, for example, refer to the services provided by physicians to health plans. They may encompass a broad range of services such as utilization review, preauthorization, profiling, guideline development and implementation, managed care education, coverage decisions, formulary coverage, and outcomes research. Research shows that the allocation of these functions is not uniform but may reside with plans or providers under different conditions (Kerr and others, 1995). Health plans may delegate some functions to some provider groups, yet not delegate the same functions to other provider groups.

This variation in the delegation of functions suggests a few questions. First, what is the optimal delegation of functions between producer and consumer? When should a function be delegated to a subordinate organization? When should it not be delegated? Second, what determines the delegation of functions? Third, how does the delegation of functions affect organizational and market performance?

There are a variety of reasons for differences in allocating functions between actors in a relationship. Fiduciary responsibilities and potential legal liability may cause health plans to retain functions such as benefit design, benefit coverage, and formulary coverage. Similarly, the delegation of coverage decisions to provider groups may result in undesirable inconsistencies in coverage policies across enrollees in a health plan. Scale and scope economies are another important determinant of allocating functions. Research shows that a large panel of patients is required for reliable provider profiling (Hofer and others, 1999). This suggests that plans will be more likely to do profiling when they are larger in scale. But only a few, large medical groups may reach the scale necessary to perform the profiling function reliably. Scope economies through technological complementarity are another determinant of locating functions in the plan or provider. The organization that is performing claims processing, for example, may have specialized expertise in working with claims data that confers on it an advantage in performing provider profiling.

Transaction cost economics (TCE) provides a theoretical perspective on the allocation of functions in a relationship (Shelanski and Klein, 1995; Williamson, 1979; Williamson, 1981; Williamson, 1985). According to TCE, decision makers choose the least costly way to organize a transaction. In cases in which there is a large market for a transaction—for example, there are many sellers for products, services are well defined, it is easy to switch suppliers—markets and contracting are used. In cases in which organizations can write contracts specifying all possible outcomes of a purchasing decision, markets are the best way to organize transactions. Markets fail, however, under conditions of uncertainty, opportunism, and high asset specificity. TCE argues that organizations elect to make rather than buy when transactions are uncertain, when people behave opportunistically, and when transactions have high transaction asset specificity.

Although TCE is an attractive theoretical framework, it will need to be extended so that it will predict which actor in a relationship, the health plan or the provider group, for example, will incorporate a function. And TCE will need to be extended to cover how delegation affects overall market performance as reflected in prices, products, productivity, reliability, and uniformity in application of policies. These extensions are needed in health services research to understand the causes and consequences of allocating functions in relationships, such as between provider and consumer, between health plan and provider, and between health plan and employer.

Social Network Structure and Markets

The two aspects of relational effects, lock-in and delegation, reflect the "micro" perspective on relational effects. Social network structures reflect the "macro" perspective on relational effects. Social network structures are the aggregate of all relationships between status positions. We first discuss how social networks structure markets into micromarkets (distinctive groups of sellers and buyers) with more intense levels of interaction, price competition, and innovation diffusion. Then we consider how market structure reflects historical differences in development based on network externalities and path dependence.

Micromarkets, Product Innovation, and Price Competition

Micromarkets are distinct clusters of buyers and sellers that reflect durable, lengthy relationships. Table 5.2 uses a sociomatrix to illustrate micromarkets in plan-purchaser relationships. The sociomatrix shows all health plans selling health services in the rows and each purchaser in a column. The numeral 1 is entered in a cell to indicate whenever a plan sells health services to a purchaser. The top panel in Table 5.2 shows the sociomatrix as it might be coded in the field, with plans entered into rows and purchasers entered into columns following in some arbitrary order, such as alphabetical. It is difficult with a cursory examination to see an underlying market structure. The bottom panel in Table 5.2 uses social network analytic techniques, exchanging rows and columns with each other, to make cliques apparent. Each shaded area in Table 5.2 represents a micromarket. This technique is more fully explained in J. Scott (2000).

The conceptualization of a micromarket extends usual market conceptualizations. Much market analysis implicitly assumes that there is a fully connected market in which (1) all buyers can purchase from all sellers, (2) buyers can switch easily to other sellers, and (3) buyers and sellers are atomized. Micromarkets structure the larger market into blocks that (1) are segmented from each other, (2) consist of "sticky" relationships between buyers and sellers and, thus, less switching behavior, and (3) feature buyer-seller collectivities and alliances. These structures influence competitive processes, innovation diffusion, and market performance.

Micromarkets develop in a variety of ways. Organizations such as HMOs, for example, initially used closed panels of physicians who competed only with other physicians in the panel for the HMO's enrollees. The development of open-access HMO models with broad provider panels decreased the HMO's and health plan's financial and administrative leverage over providers. As a consequence, health plans may seek tight, preferred relationships with a subset of providers, in which they can exchange enrollee volume for greater influence and control. Health plans may also use more-formal partnership methods such as joint ventures or equity arrangements (Grossman, 2000). For their part, providers make a concerted effort

Table 5.2. Plan-Purchaser Sociomatrix.

Unorganized Plan-Purchaser Sociomatrix									
	Purchasers or Employer								
Plan	A	B	C	D	E	F	G	H	I	J
1	0	1	1	1	0	0	0	1	1	0
2	1	0	0	1	0	0	1	0	1	1
3	1	0	0	0	1	1	1	0	0	1
4	1	0	0	1	0	0	1	0	1	1
5	0	1	1	0	0	0	0	1	0	0
6	0	1	1	1	0	0	0	1	1	0
7	1	1	1	0	1	1	1	1	0	1
8	0	1	1	0	0	0	0	1	0	0

Organized Plan-Purchaser Sociomatrix									
	Purchasers or Employer								
Plan	H	B	C	F	E	I	D	J	G	A
1	1	1	1	0	0	1	1	0	0	0
6	1	1	1	0	0	1	1	0	0	0
5	1	1	1	0	0	0	0	0	0	0
8	1	1	1	0	0	0	0	0	0	0
7	1	1	1	1	1	0	0	1	1	1
3	0	0	0	1	1	0	0	1	1	1
4	0	0	0	0	0	1	1	1	1	1
2	0	0	0	0	0	1	1	1	1	1

to form preferred micromarkets (or networks) with health plans.
Thus, many systems want to become the "indispensable" sites for
patient care by developing greater geographical coverage (such as
multiple hospital locations in a market), PCP networks that attract
plan enrollees, and "must have" hospitals and physicians that
patients commonly prefer (Kohn, 2000). Status as a must-have hospital often reflects the institution's reputation or teaching status, or
presence of a children's hospital.

The development of relationships with significant switching costs means that markets come to consist of stable relationships. The segmentation of Indianapolis into four major hospital systems (Community Hospitals of Indianapolis, St. Vincent Hospital and Health System, St. Francis Hospital and Health Centers, and Clarian Health Partners) may reflect such a micromarket segmentation process of the market for health insurance, hospitals, and physician services (Center for Studying Health System Change, 2000b). One consequence of these micromarkets in Indianapolis may be the limited viability of managed care firms.

Producers or consumers may join together in associations with similar actors that structure their interaction. Some examples of associations include "joint operating agreements" (JOAs), under which hospitals seek to share (cooperate) with local competitors in some high-cost ventures to avoid duplication and rivalry, and rural health networks (Christianson, Moscovice, Johnson, Kralewski, and Grogan, 1990; Moscovice, Johnson, Finch, Grogan, and Kralewski, 1991; Moscovice and others, 1997). These associations affect market processes in two ways. First, some associations work collectively to develop innovative ways of structuring markets and work. Second, these associations and informal relationships pattern interaction and information flows among actors. Actors who are central in these networks may be more likely to be early adopters and opinion leaders (Coleman, Katz, and Menzel, 1966). In Minnesota, for example, a number of medical groups are members of the Institute for Clinical Systems Improvement, a collaborative effort to develop and implement quality improvements for clinical care.

Price-leadership models in economic theory suggest another common path of micromarket development: the segmentation of a market into core and peripheral sectors. Health plan markets often segment into two tiers: a small number of large plans concentrating enrollee market share, and a large number of small plans with relatively low enrollment (Grossman, 2000). Competition within each tier (in terms of products, customer segments, geographical markets) is likely to be more intense than competition between tiers.

Strategy researchers have developed a somewhat analogous term for these micromarkets called "strategic groups." These are organizations within an industry that are internally consistent and externally different from other organizations on one or more key dimensions of their strategy. Members of strategic groups are thus close competitors (Dranove, Peteraf, and Shanley, 1998). Researchers typically rely on observed differences in the markets and customers served to distinguish strategic groups, and thereby approximate clusters of buyers and sellers. Such groupings have been reported among both hospitals (Nath and Gruca, 1997) and nursing homes (Zinn, Aaronson, and Rosko, 1994). Some researchers suggest there are four strategic groupings of employers in local markets that are distinguished along two dimensions: whether the employers are in the service or manufacturing sector, and employers' relative size and leverage over HMOs (Center for Studying Health System Change, 2000b). The existence of these groups is theorized to be associated with variations in benefit packages, provision of information to and solicitation of feedback from employees, use of purchasing coalitions and brokers, aggressiveness in health plan bargaining, and efforts to change the local health care system. Thus, there may exist distinct micromarkets in the exchanges between employers and their labor force, employers and health plans, employers and purchasing coalitions, and employers and other corporate actors in the community concerned with local market reform.

This micromarket structure of markets affects innovation diffusion (Burns and Wholey, 1993; Burt, 1987; Coleman, Katz, and Menzel, 1966; Strang and Soule, 1998; Strang and Tuma, 1993) and causes variation in prices for ostensibly the same product (Baker, 1984). Micromarkets also shape the extent and intensity of competition within a geographical market because they structure the information flow to competing organizations. The purchasers within a micromarket are a mirror that reflects back to each plan what the other plans in the micromarket are doing. In Table 5.2, for example, purchaser A can play plans 2, 3, 4, and 7 off against each other as it bargains for lower prices. This bargaining process provides 2, 3, 4, and 7 information about each other's pricing behavior. It also can provide information about product development. Assume, for example, that plan 2 offers an open-ended product to purchaser A. A can then query plans 3, 4, and 7 about their interest in offering an open-ended product. The contracts established by plans 2, 3, 4, and 7 with purchaser A may establish precedents that can be used by purchasers J and G. Although these developments may diffuse across the market as a whole over time, their initial development and diffusion is likely to occur first within the micromarket. The types of innovation may also vary as a function of micromarkets. Routine, low-cost innovations tend to spread initially within networks of large, prestigious, centrally located organizations; radical, high-cost innovations tend to spread initially within networks linking smaller, more peripheral organizations.

Research shows that micromarkets affect organization performance (Uzzi, 1996; Yamagishi, Gillmore, and Cook, 1988), collusive behavior by organizations (Baker and Faulkner, 1993), organization reputation (Baker and Faulkner, 1993; Podolny, 1993), malfeasant behavior, and market performance (Baker, 1984). Micromarkets increase the possibility of collusive behavior, for example, by reducing the number of actors whose actions need to be coordinated. But malfeasance may be limited through the social monitoring that occurs during interaction in network structures. In terms of market performance, micromarkets increase the variance in prices observed for identical products, stock, and equities across a market as a whole (Baker, 1984). Paradoxically, prices become more heterogeneous, rather than more homogenous, as market size increases because micromarkets emerge. It is likely that where products are more dissimilar, such as in health care, the variation will be even larger.

In summary, micromarkets, associations, and patterns of relationships among actors affect variation in prices, product innovation, and process innovation in what is apparently a homogenous market. Social network analytic tools can be used to detect micromarkets—clusters of consumers and producers that have similar relationships or are groups of equivalent actors (Long, 1991; Wasserman and Faust, 1994). Micromarket structure can then be related to differences in products, prices, and innovativeness.

One important research question is the source of differences in patterns of micromarkets across communities. Following the organizational literature and the reported relationship between size and differentiation, we suggest that larger geographical markets and markets with lower population density may be associated with greater micromarket activity (or market fragmentation). Such markets may exhibit less competition overall and greater variation in prices and products across micromarkets. This view diverges from common economic arguments that the number of organizations in a market is associated with greater organizational rivalry and competition (Porter, 1980).

Network Externalities, Path-Dependent Processes, and Market Histories

Why do some multispecialty medical groups, such as Geisinger, Marshfield, or Mayo, become dominant health care providers, yet others do not? Why do some communities develop compatible technologies and agree on common standards? Why is the Wisconsin Health Information Network perhaps the only successful community health information network (Anonymous, 1997; Atkinson, 1995; Morrissey, 1995)? Why is it that provider groups in the Twin Cities can collaborate successfully to develop commonly used clinical guidelines? Research suggests that the structure of a market, and the relative power of actors in that market, often reflect "network externalities"; that is, the benefits that accrue to a user of a product is a function of the number of others using that product (Katz and Shapiro, 1985, p. 424).

There are two types of network externalities, "many-to-one" and "many-to-many." The oft-observed volume-quality relationship in medical procedures is an example of the many-to-one form. Quality in later relationships is higher because of learning that occurred in earlier relationships. The consumer gains the quality benefit of the producer's cumulative experience with other similar customers, and the producer gains a competitive advantage and dominant position by being able to refine and improve the product through learning by doing. Similarly, controlling for scale effects, the cumulative experience of behavioral health carve-out plans is associated with lower clinical costs (Sturm, 1999). These learning effects may be due to a variety of factors, including improved care management procedures, better patient monitoring techniques, and increased acceptance of carve-out network providers by patients. In these many-to-one examples, the provider remains constant over time while serving many different consumers who make independent decisions to purchase the product.

Many-to-many network externalities involve situations in which coordination between users of a technology and technological standardization increase the value of the technology (Katz and Shapiro, 1985; Katz and Shapiro, 1994). There are two basic forms of many-to-many network externalities. In the first, a technology's value to an individual increases as the number of others who have adopted increases. Telephones and fax machines are common examples. In isolation, they are not very useful. Their usefulness increases as the number of people who can be contacted increases. A second general form occurs with investment decisions regarding technology that will be used over a period of time. The initial investment involves both evaluating the current state of the technology and the future development of technology, such as software and support. The typewriter keyboard is a commonly used example for this process (David, 1985). The argument for the commonness of the QWERTYIUOP typewriter keyboard (standard layout of keys) is that as some organizations adopted a QWERTYIUOP keyboard and trained workers, it became cheaper for other organizations to use the QWERTYIUOP keyboard because there were workers available who were proficient with the technology. This reduced training costs for organizations and increased job opportunities for workers. This many-to-many argument is one of the reasons underlying the emergence of technological standards (Gilbert, 1992). These many-to-many network externality processes are at the core of the development of such technological standards as the Microsoft operating system. The producer gains a competitive advantage by promoting these technological standards in their product platforms, which then become adopted industrywide.

Many-to-One Network Externalities in Health Care

Positive network externalities result in a positive feedback process that permits an organization to become a dominant actor in a local market. This positive feedback can take the form of both a learning curve effect and a path-dependent process (that is, acquisition of resources in an earlier time period fosters competitive advantage in later periods) (Arthur, 1989). In the former, as a health plan accumulates enrollees, it accumulates experience and data that can be used to make better actuarial decisions about enrollee utilization and costs and thereby negotiate better premiums with employers as well as drive better bargains with providers (Wholey, Feldman, and Christianson, 1995; Wholey, Feldman, Christianson, and Engberg, 1996; Wholey, Engberg, and Bryce, 1999), all of which give it an advantage in competing for new members. In the latter, a health plan may have been established before the 1970s by consumer movements (such as Group Health Cooperative) or by employers faced with provider shortages (such as Kaiser), and thereby enjoyed the opportunity to increase enrollment without significant competition.

When path-dependent processes occur, current market structures are the consequence of a historical event that gave initial advantage to a particular technology or provider. The outcome of path-dependent processes is market variability, even though the network externality process is common across markets. At a given point in time, markets may look very different due to small differences in historical events that tip markets in particular directions. It is extremely likely that starting conditions and events will vary across communities, often being a function of social networks associated with community power structures. The implication is that there will be significant variation across communities in the dominance of various types of health care organizations and in the relative performance of the different types of health care organizations in each community.

Path dependence serves to explain why some types of IDNs are successful while others are not. IDNs such as the Carle Clinic (Champaign-Urbana, Illinois), Geisinger (Danville, Pennsylvania), Scott and White (Temple, Texas), and the Marshfield Clinic (Marshfield, Wisconsin) dominate their regional markets for several historical reasons. First, they inaugurated their health plans during the 1970s and have accumulated nearly three decades of experience with managed care. As their plans have grown, they have become the largest insurer in their local areas and have economically penetrated the practices of their affiliated physicians to a significant degree. Second, they operate in rural areas where they have been buffered from urban market competition. Moreover, their rural locations and growing regional dominance have deterred the entry of for-profit and national HMO chains. Third, these clinics developed historically around a core multispecialty group of physicians. Physicians are thus accustomed to practicing collaboratively in groups. Moreover, physicians have dominated the decision making of these IDNs, which are physician-centric, physician-led, and physician-governed (Burns and Wholey, 2000; Burns and Thorpe, 2000).

These conditions are not easily replicable by other IDNs today for several obvious reasons. Most IDNs are urban-based and thus exposed to urban health plan competition. There are few large multispecialty groups in the United States, they are not often found in rural markets, and they are not easy to foster or cobble together from smaller groups (Burns and Wholey, 2000). Finally, several years (if not decades) may be required to develop a cohesive physician culture.

The historically specific market development paths caused by network externalities and path-dependent processes sometimes result in a feeling that markets have few commonalities and cannot be easily compared. Some communities are dominated by hospital-based systems, such as Indianapolis, whereas others are dominated by HMOs, such as Minneapolis. Because these organizations have different attributes, one being dominated by hospitals and the other by managed care firms, they seem to be difficult to compare. One way to compare organizations across markets is by comparing organizations that have similar roles. An HMO, an integrated delivery system, and a globally capitated multispecialty medical group, for example, are similar when they perform the same role within the health care market as any organization that provides health services for a prepaid premium. Comparing organizations in terms of role similarity is one resolution of the difficulty posed by path-dependent processes for comparative analysis of markets. The implication for studying markets is that researchers require information on social relations, not just attributes of organizations, in order to determine which actors are performing similar roles that can be compared across markets.

Many-to-Many Network Externalities in Health Care

Coordination of information interchange in health care, such as claims or medical records, is an example of many-to-many externalities. A key source of coordination occurs when a major purchaser adopts a standard that becomes the de facto standard used by others, such as multiple payers and providers (Katz and Shapiro, 1994). Medicare has played a central role in standards development in the United States because of its adoption of data interchange standards that the private sector subsequently adopted (for example, the UB92 form for facility claims and HCFA 1500 for professional service claims). The Health Insurance Portability and Accountability Act (HIPAA) of 1996 is the latest round in this process that will standardize many health services transactions.

Absent the spur of a major purchaser such as the Center for Medicare and Medicaid Services (CMMS, formerly the Health Care Financing Administration or HCFA), the development of a common information interchange system at the community level is exceedingly rare, even though the benefits appear substantial. One exception is the Wisconsin Health Interchange Network, through which plans and providers have agreed upon common interchange formats that support the provision of health care services and insurance (Anonymous, 1997; Atkinson, 1995; Butera, 1992; Morrissey, 1995; Pemble, 1994). Another exception is the formation of Web-based information linkages among health plans, physicians, hospitals, and clinical labs in certain Pacific Northwest communities. Such linkages have been developed by an Internet startup organization called PointShare at the invitation of the corporate actors in these communities. The rarity of common interchange systems developing at the community level is due to the technological complexity of sharing health information, the lack of trust among actors, the difficulty actors have in adapting existing systems to a common standard, and the presence of organizations competing to have their proprietary standard become the agreed-upon system (Katz and Shapiro, 1994).

The path-dependence and network externalities arguments suggest that communities will have seemingly different configurations that are a function of historical starting points. Although the markets look different, their similarity can be analyzed in two ways. First, the processes underlying market evolution, path dependence, and network externalities are similar. Understanding what influences the operation of these processes may provide the policy levers to guide market evolution. Second, although the particular types of organizations in markets may differ, they may occupy similar status positions and have similar roles across markets. This role similarity supports the comparative analysis of markets. The next section discusses how equivalent roles can be determined within an organizational field.

Social Network Structure and Organizational Fields

The two previous sections limited the relational view to specific markets: actors exchanging "the same good." But each market is embedded in an organizational field, that is, "Those organizations that, in the aggregate, constitute a recognized area of institutional life: key suppliers, resource and product consumers, regulatory agencies, and other organizations that produce similar services and products" (DiMaggio and Powell, 1983). The health care organizational field in a geographical area consists of all actors involved in the financing and delivery of health care services. This includes health plans, hospitals, physicians, academic medical centers, alternative medicine providers, claims processors, and all those involved in health services (Scott, Ruef, Mendel, and Caronna, 2000). Each of these markets is interdependent on the others. This section explores how the interdependent structure of this organizational field affects the functioning of each market within the field.

Sociologists describe organizational fields using the concepts *institutional logics, actors,* and *governance structures* (Scott, 1995; Scott, 1998; Scott, Ruef, Mendel, and Caronna, 2000). Institutional logics are the material practices and symbolic constructions that "specify what goals are to be pursued within a field or domain as well as indicate what means of pursuing them are appropriate" (Scott, Ruef, Mendel, and Caronna, 2000). Actors are persons and organizations that are defined by the institutional logics and operate according to the principles embodied in the institutional logic. Governance structures refer to the mechanisms that legitimately enforce and modify the institutional logic (Scott, Ruef, Mendel, and Caronna, 2000).

We extend the definition of organizational fields, which does not include products (the objects being exchanged), by including markets, which does include products. This extension integrates models of economic processes in markets with sociological models of cultural and institutional structures and processes. The extension incorporates concepts related to products (such as elasticity and substitutability) and market functioning in theorizing about action in organizational fields.

The health care *organizational field* consists of all the interdependent health-care–related markets, institutional logics, actors, and governance structures that constitute a recognized area of institutional life. *Market interdependence* refers to the interdependency between the different health care markets in a health care organizational field. Examples of interdependent markets include (1) the labor-employer market and the employer-plan health services market, which are interdependent because employers are active as buyers in both markets, (2) the plan-hospital market and the plan-physician group market, in which plans are buyers in both markets, and (3) the plan-physician group market and physician group–individual physician labor market, in which the physician group is a seller in one market and a buyer in the other.

The social network structure of an organizational field can be described graphically by connecting all the actors who have a relationship. Figure 5.1 shows a simplified graph of the social network market structure that contrasts the conventional organization of health care markets with the BHCAG direct-purchasing model in Minneapolis. Each textual box represents an actor; lines connecting dyads represent relationships.

The social network structure for each market can be analyzed in two ways: in terms of interaction patterns and in terms of structural

Figure 5.1. The Hierarchical Structure of Markets.

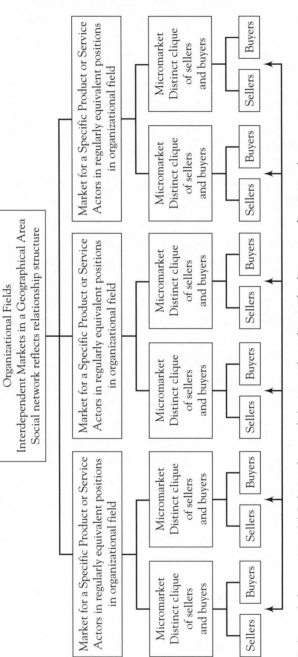

Relational characteristics (1) Relational strength (integratedness, longitudinality, comprehensiveness);
(2) Transaction organization

similarity (Knoke, 1990, pp. 11–16). On one hand, the interaction approach emphasizes the consequences of interaction and the ability to control interactions because of a central role in the social network. Actors who have relationships with each other are grouped together in a clique. It is argued that social influence, dissemination, information, and innovation diffusion occur within these cliques because of the strong relational cohesion. The structural approach, on the other hand, groups actors by the similarity in their relations with others. As Figure 5.2 shows, in the BHCAG market, the interaction approach would group primary care physicians 1, 2, and 3 with medical group or IPA 1 and group primary care physicians 4, 5, and 6 with medical group or IPA 2. The structural approach would group all primary care physicians (1 through 6) together because they have a common type of relationship with medical groups and IPAs and would group the medical group and IPAs together because they have common relationships with primary care physicians and with consumers. The interaction approach is useful for analyzing the use of power within markets, while the structural approach is useful for identifying actors who are competing because they are in similar markets.

These concepts are applicable to understanding market organization in organizational fields. For example, in Cleveland and Indianapolis, providers do not appear to be under as much financial pressure as are providers in other cities. One argument for the better performance of providers in these organizational fields is market interdependence associated with a tight labor market—the tight labor market results in employers seeking more open health plans, which means less pressure on providers. Although this explanation is attractive, it does not take into account that labor markets are also tight in many other communities, such as Seattle, Minneapolis, and most cities in California, where providers have not similarly benefited. So, the tight labor market explanation may be insufficient. An alternative explanation is that tight labor markets benefit providers more where providers are more centralized, where there

Figure 5.2. Market Interdependence and Broker Roles.

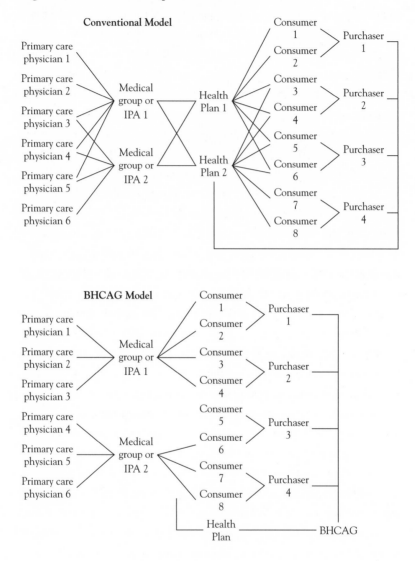

are more micromarkets, and where markets are less dense. The Cleveland area continues to consolidate into the Cleveland Clinic Health System and the University Hospitals Health System, and may have experienced decreased density in hospital markets since, 1998 (Center for Studying Health System Change, 2000a). In Indianapolis, the hospital market is segmented into four systems, which would also decrease density (Center for Studying Health System Change, 2000b). In both cases, perhaps lower density and more micromarkets allow providers to take advantage of the tight labor market because employers are more locked into existing relationships.

Market Interdependence and Market Power

Market analysts often refer to power in their explanation of market processes (for example, "hospital systems still dominate" [Center for Studying Health System Change, 2000b, p. 1]; "Health plans have focused on instituting premium increases and administrative efficiencies to enhance their financial performance and on responding to the increased market power of provider systems" [Center for Studying Health System Change, 2000a, p. 4]). The combination of the social network approach and exchange theory (Cook and Whitmeyer, 1992) can be used to understand power in markets. Examples are readily apparent. Contrast, for example, an HMO facing a monopolistic provider market with an HMO facing a competitive provider market, or an HMO in a community where there are only HMOs with an HMO in a community where PPOs occupy equivalent positions. The structure of these social networks influences HMO performance and profitability because they influence power (Yamagishi, Gillmore, and Cook, 1988).

Performance and profitability are likely to be a function of the power an organization derives from its position in a network and the patterns of its interdependence with others (Emerson, 1962; Thompson, 1967). For example, a health plan has power over a provider when the enrollees of the plan account for a large share of the provider's volume. Conversely, a provider organization gains power to the degree that it controls access to providers in a geographical area that a plan desires to serve. The relative level of power between a plan and a provider is the ratio of the two dependencies (provider on plan, plan on provider)—that is, which party needs the other more. Some Wall Street analysts have dubbed this the "kick butt ratio" (Marsh and Feinstein, 1997). Actors with greater power are able to use that power to obtain lower prices or higher quality products (Feldman and Wholey, 1999).

Because network position influences profitability, the structure of the social network becomes a valued commodity that organizations contest. Among interdependent markets, changes in one market often spur changes in related markets. Growing monopoly or monopsony power in one market spurs efforts to achieve similar, countervailing power by organizations in upstream and downstream markets. Burns and Wholey suggest that such a scenario may describe hospital system-building and physician network-development efforts to counteract the growing bargaining power of consolidating HMOs (Burns and Wholey, 2000). Such efforts are aimed at reducing a "domino effect": employers form purchasing coalitions to negotiate HMO rate reductions, which leads HMOs to consolidate in order to leverage premium increases (upstream) and reduce provider reimbursement (downstream) (Grossman, 2000; Kohn, 2000).

The BHCAG market experiment in Minneapolis illustrates how market interdependence can be restructured to change the incentives facing actors. Figure 5.2 contrasts the conventional organization of health care markets with the BHCAG direct-purchasing model. Social network research shows that brokering positions, such as that occupied by health plans in the conventional market, are valuable because they provide a base of power that actors can use to make money (Burt, 1992a; 1992b; Yamagishi, Gillmore, and Cook, 1988). The market restructuring by BHCAG moves health plans from this lucrative position into a less lucrative position as a third party administrator. These differences are solely structural changes in relationships. Accompanying these structural changes are changes in the logics of action within the market, such as new ways of reimbursing physicians and structuring consumer choice. For example, primary care physicians can gain access to consumers through only one medical group. Moreover, removal of brokering roles affects the economic returns to the occupants of such roles. Consequently, diagramming the social-network-structure markets and identifying broker roles should be a core activity of health services market description so that comparative market analysis can be performed.

One question of obvious interest is whether the BHCAG experiment can be replicated in other geographical markets. An analysis of network structure and interdependence in the Twin Cities suggests it may not. One factor facilitating BHCAG's emergence is the social network structure of corporate headquarters in the Twin Cities—the historical working relationships among CEOs and their collaborative efforts with the provider community (stemming back to the Twin Cities Health Care Development Project in the early, 1970s) (Anderson, Herold, Buler, Kohrman, and Morrison, 1985). Another unique characteristic is the large number of multispecialty groups in the area, which reflects the social network structure of professional organization, and their experience with managed care. Physician intermediary organizations—whether they be groups or IPA networks—may be essential for both direct contracting (as in the Twin Cities) and full-risk capitation and delegation of medical management (as in Southern California). The presence of intermediaries enables the development of risk-adjusted provider profiles, care management processes, and utilization management incentives.

Roles and Regular Equivalence

Health care markets vary in which specific types of organizations— IDNs, HMOs, or PPOs—dominate. But these different types of organizations may occupy equivalent roles. Identifying equivalent actors because of their roles provides a basis for comparing the relative performance of diverse actors and organizations across communities. If an input-output matrix for a community were developed that included IDNs, PPOs, and HMOs in the rows and columns as well as factor, or input, and product, or output, markets, it is likely that these input-output matrices would differ across communities, with IDNs being dominant in some communities and HMOs dominant in others. It is also likely, though, that the IDNs, PPOs, and HMOs would be seen to be equivalent. If they may possess similar linkages to physicians and seek to serve the similar customers (especially if the IDN has its own health plan), then they occupy similar roles (enrolling members, contracting with physicians) and are substitutable. For example, some markets (such as Indianapolis) have a small number of large IDNs that contract with a large number of small health plans, each of which accounts for only a small percentage of the IDN's patients. In other markets (such as Philadelphia), the situation is reversed. Although the particular types of actors that occupy equivalent positions differ, the overall market structure may be similar across communities.

Social network theorists have developed the concept of structural equivalence to group actors into similar roles (Lorrain and White, 1971). Organizations and actors are structurally equivalent when they have similar relationships to other specific actors in the network. Regular equivalence is more useful for determining roles in markets because it requires only a similar pattern of relations to other actors (Long, 1991; Wasserman and Faust, 1994). Although a mother and father are structurally equivalent because of their similar relationship to their particular children, they are not structurally equivalent to other mothers and fathers because the children differ. But mothers and fathers would be regularly equivalent because they share a similar pattern of relationships to their children. It is this similar patterning of relationships that is useful for understanding roles in markets. Whereas an IDN, an HMO, and an IPA are different types of managed care organizations, they are similar because they occupy a broker role between consumers and physicians. In Figure 5.2, a regular equivalence approach groups all primary care physicians, in contrast to the interaction approach which groups medical groups or IPAs with the physicians associated with them.

Analyses of regular equivalence can determine whether new types of organizations constitute breakthrough organizational innovations that reorganize health care (Robinson, 1998b) or just an equivalent, alternative approach (Burns and Thorpe, 2000). There have been recent efforts to restructure markets and remove HMOs as an intermediary using provider-sponsored organizations (PSOs) and new forms of health insurance such as Definity, a plan in which employees have reimbursement accounts funded with untaxed contributions that are used to pay for health care. These involve new ways to pay providers (global risk payments), new relationships between hospitals and physicians (as they split these global fees), new methods of supporting consumer choice of health plans, and new skill sets (for example, the medical management and actuarial functions once performed by HMOs) (Wholey and Burns, 2000). It may be that PSOs, PPMCs, and IPAs are simply equivalent vehicles that merely rehash already existing organizational structures rather than reorganize health care delivery in breakthrough, innovative ways. Given the plethora of new organizational forms in health care financing and delivery, researchers should seek to identify the degree to which "new" organizational types are really innovative ways of restructuring health care or just new ways of bottling old wine. Are they new ways of organizing health care management functions (such as medical management) in the market or merely contests among differing organizational forms for the control of these management functions (Kohn, 2000)?

Market Interdependence

Organizational fields consist of multiple markets. The interdependence among these markets affects the operation of specific, individual markets in two ways. First, supply-and-demand conditions in one market influence the types of products demanded in other markets (Maude-Griffin, Feldman, and Wholey, 2001). Employers faced with tight labor markets and employee complaints (enrollee—employer exchange), for example, have induced health plans to develop more consumer-friendly products. These include POS, PPO, and IPA models (employer–health plan exchange) and more consumer-friendly physician services such as free choice, open-access panels (health plan–physician exchange), as less restrictive health plans are seen as more desirable. At the same time, health plans may be scaling back some of their traditional utilization management activities (health plan–physician exchange) to develop instead more direct interactions with members, such as health education classes, and condition-specific case management within existing disease-management programs (health plan–enrollee exchange). Enrollee and employer pressure may also prompt health plan efforts to reduce friction and instability in their provider networks, for example, by downstreaming risk to providers.

Explicit modeling of market interdependence is a key to understanding health care market processes, as has been demonstrated in analyses of the effect of the labor market on HMO premium cycles through unemployment (Maude-Griffin, Feldman, and Wholey, 2001). Burt has pioneered more complicated analyses of market interdependence(such as the social network structure of markets in organizational fields) with his analysis of input-output matrices (Burt, 1988; Burt and Carlton, 1989). These techniques could be extended to the analysis of health care markets to predict which types of markets will strongly influence the delivery of health care services in an organizational field.

Conclusion

Markets are social structures in which individual and organizational actors enter into exchanges for a product. There are three core components to understanding markets: products, actor decision making, and exchanges. The views are complementary. This chapter has explored the potential gains in comparative market analysis from viewing markets as relationships. Our core argument is that the relational characteristics of exchanges, relationships within markets (micromarkets), and relationships between markets (interdependence within organizational fields) affect organizational performance, malfeasance, trust, product innovation, and market performance.

Relations vary in their comprehensiveness, longitudinality, and integratedness. Some relationships are comprehensive, longitudinal, and continuous while others are temporary, transitory, and simple. Stronger relationships have higher switching costs, which gives the relationship greater economic value but which encourages price wars and product differentiation. Strong relationships are associated with the structuring of markets into relatively stable social network structures (micromarkets) that pattern price competition and product innovation. The pattern of relationships can both encourage and discourage malfeasant behavior. Although social relations support collusive behavior, they also support the monitoring of the activities of the actors who share a relationship. The pattern of relationships is market specific because network externalities and path-dependent processes lead to the historically specific development of each market. Markets are also interdependent, whereby the functioning of related markets and the location of a market in the social network of all markets influence the functioning of that market. Network positions thus have economic value: actors that occupy broker positions, such as plans between providers and purchasers, have the possibility of extracting profits from their position.

The analysis of relational and social network structures and their effects is particularly suited to in-depth community analyses. These analyses include both micro and macro components. The micro component measures relational characteristics. When employers purchase health services from a plan, the comprehensiveness, longitudinality, and integratedness of the relationship should be assessed. In terms of comprehensiveness, the types of services, such as claims paying, provider profiling, employee profiling, and risk adjustment, can be assessed, as can the pattern of delegation of functions. Longitudinality, the length of the relationship and magnitude of switching costs, can be measured. In terms of integratedness, the responsibility for coordinating the exchange can be assessed. Does it reside with the plan, the purchaser, or some committee? Who takes the risk, and who gleans the benefits? Once the relational characteristics of markets are measured, researchers can be begin to examine how market organization affects market performance.

Focusing on relationships rather than on actors also provides a rich description of the social processes that create products and markets. Plans, for example, are involved in many decisions, including benefit design and care management processes. Although these could be viewed as attributes of the plan, they are more appropriately viewed as a consequence of relationships. Benefit design and prices are based in the plan-purchaser relationship. Care management processes are based in the plan-provider and plan-patient relationships. Understanding each decision requires understanding the actors in the relationship, their power, and their interests. How much are coverage and benefit decisions influenced by plan or purchaser organizations? Does the plan develop a product that it then sells to purchasers? Do purchasers specify the product and request prices from plans? How do these relations and exchanges vary across particular relationships and across communities? How much does each actor in a particular relationship influence the exchange and how does this influence vary across communities?

The macro component to social network analysis measures network structure. The degree to which micromarkets affect the level of competition and diffusion of products and innovations needs to be studied. At the organizational field level, social network techniques can be used to identify equivalent actors. Different types of organizations, such as IDNs, PPOs, or HMOs, can be compared across markets because they occupy equivalent roles in the health care organizational field. Analysis of input-output tables allows the identification of regularly equivalent markets, such as markets with similar factor and product markets. This will allow researchers to more easily identify different types of organizations that occupy equivalent roles. The assessment of centrality and brokering is likely to provide important insights into where health care profits flow.

As well as posing a variety of important research topics, this chapter poses two important policy issues. First, there is a tradeoff between consumer choice, as emphasized in many current health policy recommendations, and relational strength. On one hand, greater choice is associated with lower relational strength. Illness, on the other hand, may increase patient-physician relational strength and thereby decrease the usefulness of choice. Information may thus have an adverse effect when a relationship becomes strong, for example by disclosing shortcomings in physician performance. This may decrease treatment effectiveness. This tradeoff between choice and relational strength needs to be explicitly considered in policy decisions.

Second, the social structure of markets affects competition because the location of positions confers economic advantage. Developing a strong relationship with a patient, for example, is to a provider's advantage. It increases the switching costs for the patient and increases the provider's power in the relationship. The provider is not highly dependent on any given patient, whereas patients are typically dependent on one or a few providers. Similarly, broker roles, such as that of HMOs, may confer power advantages in some situations. In Indianapolis and Cleveland these broker roles appear to have provided hospital-based health plans with significant economic advantages. The consequence of positions having economic value is that competition occurs not over tradeoffs between quality and prices, as described in the ideal typical market, but over occupancy of positions that confer economic advantage.

6

$\cdots\cdots\cdots\cdots\cdots\cdots\cdots\cdots\cdots\cdots\cdots\cdots\cdots\cdots\cdots$

Physician-Organization Relationships
Social Networks and Strategic Intent

Stephen M. Shortell and Thomas G. Rundall

There is an increasing need for physicians and physician organizations to change in response to new demands for the promotion of cost-effective care and the implementation of new care management processes, particularly to meet the chronic illness needs of a growing number of people. In this chapter, we develop a social network or strategic adaptation perspective as a complement to economic explanations for examining the behavior of physicians and the organizations with which they are affiliated. This combined perspective is consistent with evolving applications of complexity science to the study of health care organizations.

Background

There is an extensive literature on the development and evolution of the medical profession over the past century (for example, Freidson, 1970a; 1970b; Light, 1993; Starr, 1982; Stevens, 1971). There is also an extensive literature on the organization of health care delivery and numerous empirical studies of the performance of

This chapter has benefited from the comments of Carol Caronna, Rob Burns, Jill Marsteller, Steve Mick, Dick Scott, and Doug Wholey, for which we are most appreciative. We also thank Jackie Henderson for her assistance in manuscript preparation.

health care organizations—primarily hospitals and health systems (Bazzoli, Chan, Shortell, and D'Aunno, 2000; Cutler, 2000; Rundall, Starkweather, and Norrish, 1998; Shortell, Gillies, Anderson, Erickson and Mitchell, 2000; Snail and Robinson, 1998). In the past decade or so, growing attention has been given to the interface between these two large areas of inquiry; specifically, to the changing roles of physicians and the medical profession at large within the context of changing organizational forms for health care delivery and increased demands for performance and accountability (Alexander, Morrisey, and Shortell, 1986; Alexander, Burns, and others, 1996; Alexander, Vaughn, and others, 1996; Burns and Thorpe, 1993; Davies and Rundall, 2000; Mechanic, 1996; Morrisey, Alexander, Burns, and Johnson, 1999; Pauly, 1980; Shortell, 1991; Shortell, Waters, Clarke, and Budetti, 1998; Zuckerman, and others, 1998). A central theme in this stream of research has been the issue of control over professional work and the associated issue of trust among the parties involved. No longer freestanding professionals, physicians have seen their ability to control their work (including its clinical dimensions) steadily eroded by societal forces involving employers, payers, health plans, consumer groups, and regulatory bodies demanding both cost containment and improved quality and outcomes of care. Hospitals and health systems, which at one time were viewed as "doctors' workshops" and "protectors" of physician interests, are now subject to severe financial and public accountability pressures frequently resulting in action that is in direct conflict with physician interests. Health plans that formerly were passive intermediaries paying for physician services have become active managers of the premium dollar directly overseeing the "appropriateness" of services physicians provide.

Physicians have responded, however slowly, by becoming more organized. The percentage of physicians belonging to groups has increased steadily over the past four decades, and represented approximately one-third of all nonfederal physicians in 1997 (Havlicek, 1999). But about 80 percent of the approximately 20,000 group practices in the United States involve nine or fewer physicians, with only 246 practices being composed of fifty physicians or more (Havlicek, 1999). Approximately 45 percent of physicians are now employed at least on a part-time basis (Kletke, Emmons, and Gillis, 1996). Approximately 5 percent have joined unions to protect their economic interests (Cochrane, 1999; Hoff, 2000). Thus we have seen a marked shift from the autonomous model of organization traditionally characterizing the medical profession to more conjoint and heteronomous models in which physicians must share control or are subjected to the administrative controls of bureaucratic organizations (Scott, 1982).

This shift has important consequences for both the internal work of physicians within their various practice arrangements and their ability to exert external influence in the health care marketplace at large (see Burns and Wholey, 2000; Robinson, 1999). Among the internal issues are physicians' ability to retain control over clinical decision making and to adopt and implement new technologies (diagnostic and therapeutic) and clinical or organizational process innovations (for example, electronic medical records, care management systems, disease management programs). Among the external issues are the ability of physicians and physician organizations to develop relationships that enable them to secure the resources needed to retain clinical control over their work through the ability to exert market power with purchasers and health plans and by forming partnerships with other organizations that provide needed access to capital. These internal and external issues have taken on particular importance in recent years, given the increased demands to hold the profession and the health care system at large accountable for the provision of more cost-effective "value added" care (Emanuel and Emanuel, 1996; Institute of Medicine, 1999; 2001; Millenson, 1997; Shortell, Waters, Clarke, and Budetti, 1998). In brief, physicians and physician organizations need relational ties both to do their work and to create an external environment conducive to doing their work.

Given this changing landscape of physician practice, this chapter addresses two issues of growing significance: (1) the ability of physicians and physician organizations to form successful ties or partnerships with others; and (2) the ability of physician organizations to adopt, implement, and diffuse clinical process innovations such as new evidence-based clinical practices. To address these issues, we need to shift attention away from analysis of individuals and individual organizations that are the subjects of so much health services research to an analysis of *relationships*. Further, while recognizing the importance of economic motivations and influences on these relationships, we chose to underscore the importance of *social relationships*, consistent with Pfeffer's (1997) call for more work on social models of explanation. In particular, we suggest that a marriage of social network theory and strategic adaptation theory provides some fresh perspectives and a useful lens for addressing the questions posed. Specifically, we will argue that the position of physician organizations within networks, various characteristics of the networks themselves, and the strategic intent of the networks provide important understanding regarding the formation of successful partnerships and the adoption and implementation of clinical process innovations.

Network and Strategic Adaptation Theory

In this section, we highlight those tenets of social network theory and strategic adaptation theory most relevant to our argument. We then use these tenets to develop a set of sample hypotheses for investigation and conclude by suggesting how such research might be undertaken.

Network Theory

Network theory emphasizes the importance of social relationships among actors. It notes that all behavior, including economic behavior, is embedded in social relationships.

Network theory has been used at both the micro and macro levels of analysis. At the micro level, it has been used to explain work-related behaviors and perceptions (Ibarra, 1993), turnover (Krackhardt and Porter, 1986), job-seeking behavior (Granovetter, 1973), and promotion (Burt, 1992a). At the macro level, it has helped to explain the diffusion of innovations throughout an organizational field (Burns and Wholey, 1993; Galaskiewicz and Wasserman, 1989), the adoption of poison pill antitakeover defenses (Davis, 1991), philanthropic contributions (Galaskiewicz and Wasserman, 1989), and organizational survival (Baum and Oliver, 1991; D'Aveni, 1990). Although largely unexplored to date, network theory also holds potential for understanding the restructuration of entire organizational fields (for example, Scott, Ruef, Mendel and Caronna, 2000) and markets (Wholey and Burns, 2000). Further, it plays a potentially key role in the study of complex adaptive systems (CAS) based on understanding the dynamic, nonlinear pattern of relationships among agents (Waldrop, 1992; McDaniel and Driebe, 2001).

For present purposes, six dimensions of network theory are of particular interest. These are (1) embeddedness, (2) centrality, (3) strength of ties, (4) direct versus indirect ties, (5) structural equivalence, and (6) structural holes. Figure 6.1 provides a concrete illustration of these core concepts, as described in the following paragraphs.

Embeddedness or *density* refers to the number of different ways in which two or more organizations are linked to each other, particularly in regard to their social relationships. As Uzzi (1999) notes: "social embeddedness is . . . the degree to which commercial transactions take place through social relations and networks of relations that use exchange protocols associated with social, non-commercial attachments to govern business dealings" (p. 482). At an individual organizational level, embeddedness refers to the number of ties that the organization has to other organizations within the network. At the network level, it refers to the extent to which dyadic relationships within the network are connected to each other. It is

Figure 6.1. Simplified Community Health Care Network.

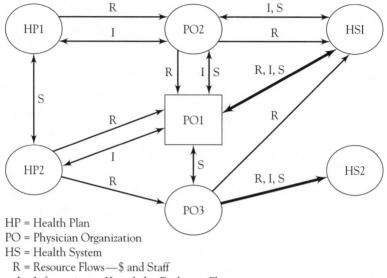

HP = Health Plan
PO = Physician Organization
HS = Health System
  R = Resource Flows—$ and Staff
  I = Information or Knowledge Exchange Flows
  S = Social Support and Encouragement

Note: First count all double-headed arrows between organizations. Each double-headed area counts as two relationships. There are seven double-headed reciprocal relationships resulting in fourteen connections in the figure. In addition, there are three additional nonduplicative unidirectional relationships—between HP2 and PO3, between PO3 and HS1, and between PO3 and HS2. This results in seventeen total connections.

important to note that embeddedness is defined without reference to the strength of the relationship between the entities. As discussed below, ties may be of varying degrees of strength. In Figure 6.1, at the individual organizational level, PO1 is more heavily embedded than PO3. Counting *any* sort of relationship as *one* tie (resource, information, or social support), the overall embeddedness of the network is seventeen ties or connections out of a possible forty-two ties [$N(N-1) = 7 \times 6 = 42$] or 40 percent. This can be assessed by counting the number of arrows coming in and going out of each PO. Embeddedness has been associated both with innovation output

(Shan, Walker, and Kogut, 1994) and with offering greater potential to transfer knowledge associated with greater resource sharing and joint problem solving (Gulati, 1995a; Uzzi, 1997).

Centrality refers to a given organization's position within the network. Generally, the greater the amount of resources or influence exerted by a given organization, the greater that organization's centrality. In network analysis, this is often measured by resource flows, information flows, and social ties. As shown in Figure 6.1, PO1 exhibits the highest degree of centrality in terms of the number of other organizations that provide PO1 with resources, information, and social ties, and vice versa. Centrality may also be thought of in terms of being in the middle of relationships or having ready access to others who are connected (Nohria and Berkley, 1992). Using these criteria, inspection of Figure 6.1 reveals that PO1 would still be viewed as the most central in the network. Centrality has been found to be related to a number of behavioral outcomes for organizations, including whether or not a particular innovation is sustained over time (Podolny, Stuart, and Hannan, 1996).

Strength of ties refers to the degree or magnitude of resource flows, information flows, and closeness of social ties among organizations in the network. Strength is often achieved through frequency of interaction. As such, ties are dynamic in that weak ties can be converted to strong ties and vice versa as a function of changes in the frequency of interaction over time. As shown in Figure 6.1, PO1 has a strong reciprocal (indicated by the bold arrow) relationship with HS1 while PO3 also has a strong but unidirectional tie with HS2. Further, whereas PO1's relationship with HS1 is exclusive (among the HS types), PO3's relationship with HS2 is nonexclusive, given that it also has a resource flow relationship with HS1. For example, PO1 might be a salaried group practice owned by HS1 whereas PO3 may be strongly identified with HS2 and admit most of its patients to HS2 hospitals, but it may also admit some patients to HS1. At the individual level, Granovetter (1973) found that weak ties were more important for individuals finding jobs than strong ties. This was explained by the fact that strong ties usually operate within the same social networks and thus provide redundant information. Weak ties, in contrast, link individuals into a more diverse set of contacts and therefore provide less redundant information and more useful job leads.

Ties may also be considered as *direct* or *indirect*. A direct tie between two or more organizations is not mediated by a third party. Indirect ties involve relationships between two or more organizations that are mediated by other organizations. In Figure 6.1, for example, neither of the health plans has a direct relationship with either of the health systems but, rather, have indirect ties; HP1 with HS1 through PO2 and HP2 with HS1 through PO1 and HP2 with HS2 through PO3. HP1, however, has direct resource and information flow ties with PO2 while HP2 has such ties with PO1 and a direct resource flow tie with PO3. As shown, PO2 and PO1 have various direct ties with HS1 and PO3 with both HS1 and HS2. Also, there are direct social relationship ties between the two health plans. Other things being equal, direct ties are expected to be stronger than indirect ties. The addition of a given organization's direct and indirect ties, of course, generates its degree of embeddedness within a given network. Ahuja (2000) has shown that both direct and indirect ties have a positive impact on an organization's rate of innovation.

Structural equivalence refers to situations in which two organizations (say, A and B) have a tie or contact with a third organization (say, C) or provide a third organization with the same indirect contacts, but A and B have no direct relationship with each other. For example, in Figure 6.1, both HS1 and HS2 have a resource flow relationship with PO3 but no direct relationship with each other. They are also "structurally equivalent" (Burt, 1992a) because PO3 gets nothing unique from either one; HS1 and HS2 may compete with each other for PO3's patient admissions.

Finally, the situation described above in which A and B have a tie to C but not to each other, and in which they provide C with different indirect contacts constitutes a *structural hole* between A and B. In the case of Figure 6.1, this exists for HS1 and HS2. Burt (1992a) suggests that this presents a potential opportunity for an intermediary to emerge to mediate transactions between the two parties to its own advantage. Alternatively, the intermediary may play an important entrepreneurial role in developing new transactions that might not occur to each party separately. We suggest that this could include bringing the two organizations (A and B) closer together to produce cooperative activity that might be of benefit to both parties and to the network at large. For example, a local foundation might provide a "community health improvement" grant to the two systems to coordinate better primary care and health promotion activities that might involve PO3. The ability to fill structural holes in a given network may also play an important role in transferring knowledge and learning. Ahuja (2000) has shown, for example, that structural holes have a negative impact on organizational rates of innovation.

Strategic Adaptation Theory

Social network theory has been criticized for inadequate attention to the *content* of the ties between two or more actors or organizations. As Fligstein and Brantley note in regard to relationships between corporate board members, "We should abandon our concentration on . . . directors as a source of network data, in general, and financial linkages across boards of directors, in particular, unless their possible relevance can be specified theoretically" (1992, p. 304). We would argue that network theory concepts, as presently discussed and defined, reflect largely *structural* properties of networks and neglect *content* properties inherent in the social relationships themselves. We argue that this content is provided in part by institutional forces in the environment (Meyer and Rowan, 1977; Scott, Ruef, Mendel, and Caronna, 2000) as well as within the network itself as these forces are "sensed" into meaning (Weick, 1969; 1995) by key actors in the network. These external and internal forces are reflected in an organization's strategic adaptation: the behavioral actions taken by organizations to shape their environment and performance. These actions incorporate the notions of (1) strategic intent (see Shortell and Zajac, 1990); and (2) the actual number, type, and scope of activities undertaken by network members (Alter and Hage, 1993). By *strategic intent* we mean the purpose for which the network exists and the motives, goals, objectives, and expectations of the individual actors, units, or organizations constituting the network. We suggest three primary categories of motives for such relationships: (1) instrumental, (2) institutional, and (3) altruistic. *Instrumental ties* involve an exchange of resources between two or more parties to achieve each party's specific goals and objectives, particularly in regard to economic gain and survival. For example, a physician organization may agree to affiliate with a specific hospital or health system in exchange for clinical and managerial support services, including information technology support (Alexander and others, 2001a). *Institutional ties* involve relationships in which the purpose is to achieve greater conformity with existing norms and expectations for greater legitimacy and credibility (Suchman, 1995). These norms and expectations may come internally from the network itself or externally from the environment outside the network (Cooper, 2001). For example, a given physician organization may adopt a specific clinical information system because it is used by everyone else in the network and it is "taken for granted" that everyone will conform. From an external perspective, a physician organization may apply for certification by the National Committee for Quality Assurance because this provides the physician organization with credibility and legitimacy. This, of course, may be further reinforced if it is also the norm or expectation of the network at large that such certification occurs. *Altruistic ties* involve relationships and behaviors that are in the name of a higher belief or value beyond the organization's own economic survival or need to appear in conformity with external expectations. The behavior or relationship is undertaken because it is the "right thing to do."

For example, two physician organizations may share resources to continue a comprehensive disease management program for congestive heart failure patients even when it costs the organizations money and there is no internal or external pressure to do so. The strategic intent categories instrumental, institutional, and altruistic are somewhat analogous to others' descriptions of strategic alliances as being service alliances, opportunistic alliances, and stakeholder alliances (Zuckerman and Kaluzny, 1991).

In addition to understanding the strategic intent of the network and of its participants, it is important to know something about the actual activities in which it is engaged (Alter and Hage, 1993). For example, to what extent do network members exchange services, staff, technology, and information? How narrow or broad are these exchanges? How frequently do they occur? How capital intensive are they? In brief, the impact of the structural characteristics of networks (such as embeddedness, strength of ties, centrality, structural equivalence, structural holes, and so on) may depend on both the strategic intent and the scope of activities undertaken by the network. This is supported by Ahuja's (2000) recent research suggesting that the optimal structure of networks depends on the objectives of network members.

Building on the just-discussed definitions and framework, we turn to developing the rationale for some preliminary hypotheses regarding successful physician partnerships; adoption, implementation, and diffusion of clinical process innovations; and overall network effectiveness.

Forming Successful Partnerships

We define a successful partnership as one that achieves the intended objectives for the involved parties both at a given point in time and over time. Historically, health care has been a loosely coupled (Scott, Ruef, Mendel, and Caronna, 2000; Weick, 1976) field comprising six thousand or so individual hospitals; seven hundred thousand physicians, many of whom are in solo or small partnership practices; thousands of suppliers; hundreds of health plans; and myriad other entities. These entities are tied together through a complex, pluralistic, largely decentralized decision-making process in regard to insurance coverage, payment, and service delivery. In the past decade, there has been considerable consolidation among hospitals, health plans, and suppliers and growing recognition on the part of physicians of the benefits of joining together in groups and various practice associations. There has also been movement to establish relationships across sectors as perhaps best exemplified by organized or integrated delivery systems that comprise significant hospital, physician, long-term care, and, sometimes, health plan components. As in other fields, work is increasingly accomplished through partnerships of various forms (for example, strategic alliances, joint ventures, coalitions, or consortia) both within given sectors, such as hospitals, physician organizations, or insurance plans, and between sectors. Although economic theory and economic rationales can help us understand some of the reasons for these relationships and their performance, we suggest that network and strategic adaptation theory helps us to obtain a fuller understanding of partnership processes and outcomes. In particular, we suggest how strategic intent interacts with various characteristics of networks to influence partnership success.

Hypotheses About Partnership Success

As previously noted, *strategic intent* has to do with the purpose of the alliance or partnership. We distinguished between instrumental, institutional, and altruistic motives. These relationships may exist for either pooling of resources or actual exchange of resources for trading purposes (Nielsen, 1986; Shortell and Zajac, 1990; Zajac, D'Aunno, and Burns, 2000). In *instrumental partnerships*, resources are pooled or exchanged to achieve each party's specific strategies and objectives, the most fundamental of which being survival. Thus physicians may agree to sell their services to the hospital or hospital-led network or system in exchange for clinical and managerial support services and assistance with information technology improvements.

In the case of *institutional partnerships*, resources are pooled or exchanged to meet certain expectations of the network or from the larger environment or both, to maintain credibility and legitimacy. For example, physicians may agree to staff the hospital emergency room or outpatient clinic in return for the hospital's support of a primary care residency program. This enables each to achieve certain legitimacy and credibility objectives—in this case, care for the poor and uninsured on the one hand and support of medical education on the other hand.

In the case of *altruistic partnerships*, resources are pooled or exchanged to achieve a shared social mission. For example, physician organizations may join a community health coalition and agree to commit a certain number of days of "free" care per week.

Scope of activities, as previously noted, refers to the number and types of resources pooled or exchanged. For example, a given relationship between physicians and hospitals might be based on exchange of staff only or direct monetary exchange (limited scope). Or the relationship could involve many different activity forms, including the exchange of money, staff time, technology, and information across multiple levels of care activities such as acute care, primary care, rehabilitative care, and so on. The latter situation, of course, would represent a broad scope of activity for the partnership.

Finally, *embeddedness*, as noted earlier, involves the number of different ways that two or more organizations are linked to each other. For example, a given physician organization may have multiple linkages to a health system through belonging to a physician hospital organization (PHO), accepting patients from a system-owned health plan, and serving on a systemwide advisory council.

Using these concepts of network and strategic adaptation theory, we suggest that the success of a partnership involving physician organizations is contingent on the *strength of ties* that exist given the strategic intent and scope of activities of the partnership. Further, we suggest that this relationship is modified by the degree of embeddedness existing within the relationship.

The first premise is that the strength of ties will be more important for instrumental and altruistic partnerships than for institutional partnerships. Instrumental partnerships almost always involve an exchange of resources to advance specific objectives. Such an exchange requires *trust* on the part of the parties involved. Trust, in turn, requires strong ties in the form of close, ongoing, permanent relationships that permit the opportunity to exchange information and knowledge, make joint decisions, and build experience in working together (Langlais and Cutler, 2001). In like fashion, the joint pursuit of social mission objectives (that is, altruistic partnership) requires strong linkage among the parties involved to sustain the commitment, particularly when they face many competing demands and economic forces. Thus, contrary to the "strength of weak ties" argument in explaining microlevel job-search behavior (Granovetter, 1973), we suggest it is the "strength of strong ties" that explains successful instrumentally and altruistically motivated partnerships involving physician organizations.

In contrast, partnerships motivated primarily by conformance or legitimacy considerations, or both, (in other words, institutional partnerships) will find weak ties sufficient to achieve and maintain conformance or legitimacy needs. Frequent interaction is less necessary to maintain these objectives than in the case of primarily instrumentally or altruistically motivated partnerships. Instead, one is able to use occasional meetings and selective reassurances to maintain needed conformance and legitimacy. These arguments and premises lead to the following hypotheses:

H1A: *The ratio of strong to weak ties among physician organizations will be positively associated with success for instrumental and altruistic partnerships.*

H1B: *The ratio of strong to weak ties among physician organizations will be unrelated to success for institutional partnerships.*

Our second premise is that the scope of activities matters for all types of physician-organization partnerships. Specifically, a larger scope of activities of the partnership is likely to be associated with more successful partnerships. This is because increasing scope increases interdependence between the partners as they engage in more activities together. Kanter (1989), among others, has high-lighted the importance of interdependence to successful strategic alliances. But increasing scope also increases the opportunity for building trust, which, as argued above, is particularly important for instrumental and altruistic partnerships. Much as a diversified portfolio enables an investor to balance gains and losses, so a more diversified scope of activities among partners enables them to bal-ance their experiences of trust as well as distrust. A relationship based on one activity only or on very few dimensions (for example, direct financial exchange) can erode completely if one or the other parties reneges or is perceived to renege. But that same relationship based on multiple sets of exchanges or activities such as staff, endorsements, or technical assistance can endure even if one of the parties is forced to withdraw direct financial resources. They can still maintain trust by providing support in kind. A greater scope of activities also provides those partnerships, based primarily on insti-tutional motives, a greater number of opportunities to demonstrate conformance to expected norms and opportunities to be perceived as "legitimate." However, a greater scope of activities also places more demands on the partnership's management and governance capabilities (Weiner and Alexander, 1999; Mitchell and Shortell, 2000). Thus the following hypothesis is contingent on the overall management and governance capabilities of the partnership:

H2: *The greater the scope of activities involved in the physician-organization partnership, the greater the degree of partnership success, contingent on the management and governance capabilities of the partnership.*

Our third premise, derived from the first two, is that the scope of activities undertaken is particularly important for weak-tie partners. Without a number of activities to spread the tie or linkage across, weak-tie partners are more vulnerable to dissolution. Paradoxically, however, it would appear that weak-tie partners are *less likely* to have a broad scope of activities than are strong-tie partners. This follows from the second premise that greater trust is achieved by having relationships across a wide variety of activities, resulting in stronger ties. Also, one would expect network members that have strong ties with each other to be more likely to undertake new initiatives than those with weak ties. Thus, physician-organization partnerships with weak ties are particularly challenged to engage in a wide scope of activities, but we suggest that such behavior is critical to their success.

H3: *Weak-tie physician-organization partnerships with a broader scope of activities will be less likely to dissolve (that is, more likely to succeed) than those with a narrower scope of activities.*

Our fourth premise builds on Scott, Ruef, Mendel, and Caronna's (2000) notion that the current era of medicine is largely dominated by the logic of managerial control and market forces. However, the degree to which this exists (as might be measured, for example, by the extent of managed care penetration and local competition between and among physician organizations, hospitals and health systems, and health plans), varies across the country. We believe that this variance will be associated with both the *type* of physician-organization partnerships found in each market and the scope of activities undertaken. In turn, we suggest that the *alignment* of both partnership type and scope of activities with the "competitiveness" of the local market will be associated with partnership success.

Specifically, we expect that instrumental physician-organization partnerships will exist more frequently in markets dominated by the managerial logic of managed care competition than will institutional or altruistic partnerships. This is because instrumental partnerships are primarily focused on achieving economic viability, particularly important in markets emphasizing managed care competition. In regard to scope of activities, the organizational strategy literature suggests that diversification of organizational activities contributes to organizational survival by spreading risk (Montgomery and Porter, 1991; Scherer and Ross, 1990). The organization invests in, and gains returns from, a variety of markets and product lines. Such diversification of activity in physician-organization networks serves to protect the network from external economic threats. Also, in environments dominated by managed care competition pressures, organizations are motivated to exert control over a greater scope of activities related to their core processes so as to protect or buffer them from external demands. Diversification or increased scope of activities is likely to be particularly important for instrumental partnerships. Given these arguments, we hypothesize that

> H4A: *The greater the degree of managed care competitive pressures in a given market, the greater the percentage of physician-organization partnerships that will be of an instrumental as opposed to institutional or altruistic nature.*
>
> H4B: *The greater the degree of managed care competitive pressures (that is, managerial logic) the greater the scope of activities undertaken by the physician-organization partnership, particularly instrumental partnerships.*
>
> H4C: *The greater the degree of alignment or "fit" between the strategic intent and scope of activities of the physician-organization partnership and the extent of managed care competitive pressures in the local market, the greater the success of the partnership.*

Our fifth premise is that the previously discussed relationships involving strength of ties, strategic intent, and scope of activities will also be influenced by the degree of embeddedness of the network. Embeddedness increases the opportunity for learning and social interaction across the multiple linkages. In highly embedded networks composed of multiple direct and indirect linkages among partnership members, the ratio of strong to weak ties decreases as it becomes increasingly difficult to maintain strong ties throughout the partnership. In such partnerships, the importance of weak ties grows, as they are a source for introducing new ideas and transferring learning from one partner to another. For example, for a given partnership, embeddedness based on a relatively greater percentage of weak-tie linkages provides cost-effective opportunities for learning. Such opportunities may be particularly important for instrumental partnerships dependent on rapidly incorporating new knowledge into their strong-tie relationships. Thus our fifth hypothesis:

> H5: *In highly embedded networks, there will be a positive association between the ratio of weak to strong ties and partnership success. This relationship will be stronger for instrumental partnerships than for other partnerships.*

To summarize, the strength of ties that physician organizations form interacts with the purpose or strategic intent of the partnership to influence likely success. Strong ties will be positively associated with success for instrumental and altruistic partnerships but unrelated to success for institutional partnerships. But strong ties are difficult to maintain in highly embedded networks. For these networks, weak ties that facilitate access to new information and ideas will be positively associated with success. Scope of activities will be positively associated with success across all partnership categories contingent on network governance and management capabilities. Finally, the strategic composition of partnerships in a given area will be influenced by market forces with greater competition favoring more instrumental partnerships, and a partnership's success will also be a function of its ability to align its strategic intent and scope of activities with the demands of the local market. These relationships are shown in Table 6.1.

One aspect of successful physician partnerships is likely to be their ability to adopt and implement advances in evidence-based medicine; that is, clinical process innovation. Thus we turn our

Table 6.1. Summary of Partnership Success Hypothesized Relationships.

		Type of Partnership Based on Strategic Intent		
Network Characteristics		Altruistic	Institutional	Instrumental
H1A and B	Strength of ties	+	0	+
H2	Scope of activities	+	+	+
H3	Scope of activities × Weak ties	++	++	++
H5	Highly Embedded Networks × Weak ties	+	+	++
Environmental Characteristics				
H4A	Managed care competitive pressures	0	0	++
H4B	Managed care competitive pressures × Scope of activities	+	+	++

		Competitive Pressures	
		High	Low
H4C	Strategic Intent—more instrumental and high scope of activities	+	0
	Strategic Intent—more altruistic and low scope of activities	0	+

Note: 0 = neutral or no effect, + = positive relationship, ++ = very positive relationship.

attention to examining how social networks and strategic adaptation concepts might interact to influence adoption and implementation of clinical process innovations.

Adoption and Implementation of Clinical Process Innovations

There has been growing interest in improving the quality and outcomes of care as a result of research demonstrating wide variation in process and outcomes of care on multiple fronts (Chassin, Galvin, and the National Roundtable on Health Care Quality, 1998; Institute of Medicine, 1999; 2001; Schuster, McGlynn, and Brook, 1998). As scientific knowledge advances, a major challenge is getting physicians and other health professionals to use such knowledge in everyday practice to reduce unwarranted clinical variation and eliminate underuse, misuse, and overuse of procedures. There is growing realization that these efforts must address multiple levels of the organization, involve committed physician and administrative leadership, be based on reliable data fed back to physicians in a supportive environment, and be reinforced by the organization's culture, performance appraisal, and reward systems (Eisenberg, 1986; Ferlie and Shortell, 2001; Greco and Eisenberg, 1993). Much of this improvement activity has centered on the adoption, implementation, and diffusion of evidence-based practices developed by the Agency for Health Research and Quality and various professional associations and specialty societies. Evidence-based practice involves the use of multiple care management practices such as clinical guidelines, protocols, clinical pathways, case management, disease management, and demand management systems. These have been complemented by or incorporated as part of efforts to apply continuous quality improvement philosophies, models, and techniques to clinical practice (Batalden and Mohr, 1997; Berwick, Godfrey, and Roessner, 1990; Blumenthal and Edwards, 1995; Blumenthal and Epstein, 1996; Blumenthal and Kilo, 1998;

Marszalek-Gaucher and Coffey, 1993). Collectively, we will refer to all of these efforts as *clinical process innovations* (CPI).

Despite the efforts just described, the field has largely failed to come to grips with the complexity and embeddedness of physician-organization relationships that makes threshold improvements in quality and outcomes of care difficult to sustain. We suggest that network and strategic adaptation theory can provide insight into these issues and lead to more informed change initiatives.

Hypotheses About Clinical Process Innovation Implementation

For purposes of this discussion, we will treat the adoption and implementation of CPI by individual organizations within a network separately from the diffusion across organizations in a network. We realize, of course, that one can also examine the diffusion process within individual organizations.

As before, we suggest that strategic intent matters and argue that physician organizations adopt and implement CPI for the three basic reasons that also motivate partnership formation: instrumental, institutional, and altruistic. *Instrumental adoption* involves the decision to adopt and implement a particular innovation because it will put the organization in a more efficient and competitive position for survival and success. *Institutional adoption* occurs when organizations adopt and implement CPI to respond to pressures from others or to satisfy at least the minimal requirements of outside bodies, consistent with the normative, coercive, and mimetic pressures suggested by DiMaggio and Powell (1983). *Altruistic adoption* and implementation involves organizations that adopt CPI because it is "the right thing to do for our patients," regardless of whether or not it will save costs, position the organization better for success, or meet the demands of the institutional environment. Altruistic organizations tend to be strongly mission driven.

The position of an actor within a network (that is, its centrality) is associated with adoption of innovations (Coleman, Katz and Menzel, 1966; Rogers, 1995). The general explanation focuses on the central actors' greater prestige, power, authority, influence, and resources. More central actors are viewed as early adopters, trend-setters, and innovators. Others look to them for what to do. We believe that this is also likely to be true for the adoption of CPI by physician organizations, but this will also be influenced by the content of the ties among the actors in terms of their *reason* or strategic intent for adopting.

In the case of both instrumental efficiency and altruistic motives, more central organizations will be more likely to adopt and implement CPI, but for different reasons. In the instrumental case, the central organization has a strong motive to maintain its position of dominance, influence, and leadership by acting to maintain or enhance superior performance and competitive position. It will view CPI as an important means of achieving these ends and it is likely to have the resources to commit to its implementation. In the altruistic case, the central organization tends to epitomize the values of the network and its visibility as the central player sends strong signals to others in the network regarding these values. To maintain its position of "moral leadership" within the network, the central organization will be motivated to adopt CPI early because it is "the right thing to do for our patients."

However, in the institutional case, we suggest that less central organizations will be early adopters and implementers. This is because the network wishes to buffer or protect its more central organizations from innovations that are not viewed as either key to efficiency or contributing to mission and values (Thompson, 1967). Nonetheless, because of the salience of the innovation in the larger institutional sphere requirements on the part of others for action, the network will "try it out" in a minor way, in some of its more peripheral organizations. This signals some degree of compliance and acceptance, but without committing substantial resources or making significant changes in its more central organizations. The central organization may play a support role to the peripheral organization, but it will largely adopt a "wait and see" attitude. We particularly expect this to be the case with tightly connected networks in which the network can exert more influence than might be true in more loosely connected networks (compare with Leblebici, Salancik, Copay, and King, 1991). Given the preceding, we suggest the following two hypotheses:

H6A: *Under conditions of instrumental or altruistic motivational ties, centrality will be positively associated with adoption and implementation of CPI.*

H6B: *Under conditions of institutionally motivated ties, centrality will be negatively associated with adoption and implementation of CPI.*

The positioning of organizations within a network may take place following multiple criteria such as availability of resources and staff, possession of general or specialized knowledge or expertise, or the ability to provide social support and encouragement. Most studies of network centrality assume that the focal organization is central on *all* dimensions. But this need not be the case. It is possible, for example, that organizations that are central in regard to resources may not be central in regard to specialized knowledge or social support. This raises the interesting question of whether networks with a focal organization that is central on a greater number of or, indeed, all, dimensions are more or less able to implement and diffuse innovations across the network than networks in which centrality itself is more diffuse. For example, some organizations are the central player for resources, but others are central for knowledge and still others for social support. In other words, in adopting and implementing an innovation, do network members primarily turn to a single member for help or to different members depending on the needs involved? To reduce the transaction costs (see Williamson, 1981) involved, we suggest that they will turn primarily to a single centrally positioned organization in the network provided that organization is seen as "central" on a number of different dimensions. This leads to our seventh hypothesis:

H7: *The adoption, implementation, and diffusion of CPI in a network will occur more quickly the greater the extent to which the central organization is seen as "central" on multiple dimensions involving resources, knowledge transfer capability, and social support.*

In the context of successful partnerships, we argued that a broader scope of activities that ties organizations together within a network provides greater opportunity to build trust and gain experience in working together. In the case of CPI, we emphasize the value of trust for learning and the ability to transfer new ideas (Huber, 1991; Levin, 2001). For example, physician organizations that are involved in multiple activities or exchange relationships, such as sharing staff, facilities, information systems, contracting, and patient referrals, have a more extensive base for sharing new ideas. They may, possibly, have even greater motivation to do so than those whose ties are limited to a single activity. We believe that a broader scope of activities will be associated with greater adoption and implementation of CPI regardless of the motive or strategic intent (that is, instrumental, institutional, or altruistic). Thus we hypothesize that

H8: *The broader the scope of activities shared by physician organizations within a network, the greater the likelihood of adoption and implementation of CPI.*

Generally speaking, for a given organization, the stronger its ties to other organizations in the network, the more likely it is to adopt and implement innovations. This is particularly true if the focal organization is strongly tied to the central organization in the network, which has motives for adopting the innovation or has already done so. This is because the process of adopting and implementing something new in an organization usually involves substantial change requiring significant knowledge, experience, support, and resources associated with more central organizations. Weak ties do not provide a sufficiently strong "transmission belt" for adoption and implementation. This argument is consistent with Banaszak-Holl, Elms, and Grazman's suggestion in Chapter Seven that integration across cliques (that is, strong ties), rather than across all network members, will be positively associated with learning. We believe that this relationship will be particularly strong for instrumental and altruistic intentions but perhaps less so for institutional purposes. Institutional motives involve more symbolic adoption and implementation for which strong ties or exchanges may be less necessary and potentially redundant and inefficient. Weak ties characterized by more superficial knowledge and learning exchanges will suffice. Given the above, we suggest the following hypothesis:

H9: *The stronger a given physician organization's ties to its network, particularly in regard to the central organization, the greater the likelihood of the physician organization adopting and implementing CPI. This relationship will be stronger for instrumental and altruistic motives than for institutional motives.*

Central organizations can clearly play a key role in the adoption and implementation of innovations. This role, however, is influenced by the relative strength of the central organization's ties to other organizations in the network and the ability of the central organization or some other entity to meet what may be competing needs and interests of network members. Specifically, consistent with Burt (1992a), physician organizations having no relationship with each other may each have a tie with a third organization (for example, an organized delivery system) and depend on it for support and resources to adopt and implement CPI. Which of the two organizations is most likely to adopt and implement CPI will depend on the relative strength of its tie to the central organization and the availability of alternative sources of support. Due to the potential competition for resources, this can result in suboptimization and disharmony for the network as a whole. Thus, an opportunity exists to "fill the structural hole" by providing support, knowledge, and resources to bring the two organizations together in a way that strengthens the innovative capacity of both organizations and thereby enhances the capabilities of the network as a whole. At the organized-delivery-system level, examples include the development of centers or institutes for clinical effectiveness such as those that exist at Intermountain HealthCare in Salt Lake City, Henry Ford Health System in Detroit, and the Lovelace Clinic in Albuquerque. Examples also exist within given market areas that cut across delivery systems, such as the Institute for Clinical Integration in Minneapolis-St. Paul, which brings together clinical leaders from competing physician organizations and health systems to develop and implement care management practices for a number of chronic and acute illnesses. At the national level, the Boston-based Institute for Health Improvement serves as an "intermediate bridging" organization by sponsoring disease-specific and problem-specific continuous quality improvement collaboratives that bring together a diverse array of health care organizations from across the country. The foregoing suggests the following hypothesis:

H10: *The greater the number of structural holes among physician organizations within a network, the stronger the association between the presence of an entity that can fill the structural hole and the adoption and implementation of CPI.*

The arguments and hypotheses thus far have focused primarily on the adoption and implementation of CPI at the individual or focal organization level. But network theory can also help explain differential adoption, implementation, and diffusion of CPI throughout the network. This involves considering the relationship between strategic intent and the strength of ties. The key assumption is that learning about new ideas is as likely to be facilitated by having many weak contacts, even though they may be of a superficial nature, than by having strong ties that are likely to provide redundant information or a more narrow perspective and knowledge base. Thus, in general, networks characterized by a higher ratio of weak to strong ties among physician organizations will be further along in adopting CPI innovations than those with a lower ratio of weak to strong ties. But we believe this will only hold for networks in which the strategic intent of diffusing CPI is primarily instrumental or institutional, *not* altruistic. For altruistic purposes, strong ties are needed to provide the motivation for adoption and spread of CPI throughout the network. These arguments suggest the following hypotheses:

> H11A: *Under conditions of instrumental or institutional motivational ties, a higher ratio of weak to strong ties at the network level will be positively associated with greater adoption of CPI at the network level.*
>
> H11B: *Under conditions of altruistic motivational ties, a higher ratio of weak to strong ties at the network level will be negatively associated with greater adoption of CPI at the network level.*

However, although a greater ratio of weak ties to strong ties at the network level will be associated with adoption, we suggest that a lesser ratio of weak ties to strong ties will be associated with actual *implementation* and *diffusion* of CPI throughout the network. This is consistent with our earlier hypothesis, H9, regarding the probability of a given organization implementing CPI. The rationale is that frequent interaction of a substantial nature is needed to implement CPI. Thus

> H12: *A lower ratio of weak to strong ties will be positively associated with the* implementation *and* diffusion *of CPI across the network.*

Finally, we suggest that the "managerial logics" of the external environment will also influence the strategic intent for adopting CPI. The greater the presence of managed care and competitive pressures, the less likely that physician organizations will adopt CPI for legitimizing purposes or simply because it is the "right thing to do" (altruistic purposes) and the more likely they will be focused on the need to reduce costs. Legitimacy is still important but relatively less so given the dominant pressure for financial viability. Given this, we hypothesize that

> H13: *The greater the presence of managerial logics and competitive pressures in the institutional environment, the greater the ratio of clinical process innovations adopted for instrumental purposes relative to institutional and altruistic purposes.*

To summarize, centrality will be positively associated with adoption and implementation of CPI for instrumental and altruistic ties, but negatively associated for institutional ties. Further, the greater the extent to which centrality exists on multiple dimensions (such as resources, knowledge, and support), the greater the degree of adoption, implementation, and diffusion across the network. Broad scope of activities will be positively associated with adoption, implementation, and diffusion among all categories of strategic intent, as will strong ties at the individual physician-organization level, particularly for instrumental and altruistic ties. At the *network level* we distinguish between *adoption* and *implementation* and *diffusion*. We suggest that a greater ratio of weak to strong ties will facilitate adoption of CPI but that a smaller ratio of weak to strong ties will facilitate actual implementation and diffusion. We also suggest that networks with a large number of structural holes will require entities to fill these holes in order for adoption, implementation, and diffusion of CPI to occur. Finally, we believe that adoption of CPI for primarily instrumental purposes will be associated with markets with high managed care penetration and competition. These hypothesized relationships are shown in Table 6.2.

Table 6.2. Summary of Clinical Process Innovation Implementation Hypothesized Relationships.

		Type of Partnership Based on Strategic Intent		
Network Characteristics		Altruistic	Institutional	Instrumental
H6A and B	Centrality	+	–	+
H7	Multiple dimension centrality	+	0	+
H8	Shared scope of activities	+	+	+
H9	Strength of ties to central organization	++	+	++
H10	Structural holes and presence of a mediating entity	+	+	+
H11A and B	Weak or strong tie ratio (for adoption)	–	+	+
H12	Weak or strong tie ratio (for implementation)	–	–	–
H13	"Managerial Logics" and competitive pressures	0	0	+

Note: 0 = neutral or no effect, – = negative relationship, + = positive relationship, ++ = very positive relationship.

Measurement, Research Design, and Analysis Implications

The main purpose of this chapter has been to suggest how social network and strategic adaptation theory can inform understanding of the behavior of physician organizations and the networks with which they are associated. Based on network and strategic adaptation arguments, we have suggested a number of hypotheses for testing in regard to partnership success and adoption, implementation, and diffusion of clinical process innovations. These raise a number of data collection, measurement, study design, and analysis issues, a few of which are briefly highlighted in the following text.

To examine many of the hypotheses advanced in this chapter, there is need to compile a national data set on physician organizations (both for groups and for independent practice associations) similar to that which exists for hospitals and health systems. This would include collection of information on practice size, type of practice, ownership, governance, staffing, finance and resources, compensation approaches, relationships with hospitals and health systems, contractual relationships with health plans, and related items. Currently, the American Hospital Association (AHA) annual survey database can be used to assess some models of relationships between physician organizations and hospitals (American Hospital Association, 2001). For example, this survey collects information on the number of physicians who have a relationship with the hospital through one or more of the following arrangements: (1) independent practice association (IPA), (2) group practice without walls, (3) management service organization, (4) open physician-hospital organization, (5) closed physician-hospital organization, (6) equity model, or (7) salaried group model. These arrangements could be used as proxies for the strength of the tie between the physician organization and the system, with the IPA being the weakest tie and the salaried group model being the strongest tie. Also, the first four arrangements primarily involve a pooling of resources for the purpose of managed care contracting, whereas the latter three involve the exchange of resources to achieve a potentially broad range of objectives. The AHA survey also contains information on whether the hospital or health system owns a health plan and whether the plan has an HMO or PPO product, or both. Here, an HMO product would be viewed as a strong tie and the PPO as a weaker tie. Thus, using the AHA database, one can begin to map some of the relationships between and among the physician organization, the hospital, and the health plan. However, the AHA database does not contain information on physician organization size or service offerings that would produce some insight into the centrality of the physician organization within the network. Neither does it contain information on referral relationships or other relationships between and among physician organizations that would permit construction of measures of network embeddedness, structural equivalence, cohesion, structural holes, and direct and indirect ties.

It is important to acknowledge that even the collection of more comprehensive data on physician organizations will not provide sufficiently sensitive measures of many of the concepts relevant to the network- and strategic-adaptation-theory-derived hypotheses developed in this chapter. Thus, there is a need to supplement such data with original primary data collection on the relevant variables of interest in well-defined samples of physician organizations, hospitals, health plans, and related health care organizations of interest in given markets or geographical areas. For example, recent work has drawn on organizational identification theory (Dukerich, Golden, and Shortell, 2002; Dutton, Dukerich, and Harquail, 1994) to examine the degree of commitment and identification that physicians have with health systems and the consequences of the relative strength of such ties for the implementation of evidence-based care management practices (Shortell and others, 2001; Waters and others, 2001). Examining the impact of social network ties among organizations participating in quality improvement collaboratives is another promising area for research (Marsteller and Shortell, 2001).

To examine those hypotheses related to strategic intent, it is necessary to combine use of available secondary data and primary quantitative data with qualitative research methods. Qualitative methods are better suited for teasing out the underlying motivations for particular actions, whether they be of an instrumental, institutional, or altruistic nature (Devers, Sofaer, and Rundall, 1999). It is important to obtain these perspectives from all partnership organizations in the network and not only from the focal organization that may be of primary interest. There is need to understand better what network characteristics really matter to organizational leaders and what motivates their behavior.

Finally, it is of interest to note that most network research has been of a cross-sectional nature with relationships captured at a single point in time. Relatively little is known about the evolution of networks over time. The ability to build longitudinal data sets coupled with periodic in-depth fieldwork could shed considerable light on such issues as the relative stability of networks, as well as changes in other network characteristics such as size, embeddedness, centrality, strength of ties, structural equivalence, and the extent to which new organizational arrangements arise to fill structural holes.

Summary and Conclusion

The main theme of this chapter has been the importance of examining the *relationships* of physician organizations within networks of health care, financing, and delivery systems. In the future, physician organizations will have to develop successful partnerships, and they will need to adopt, implement, and diffuse various clinical process innovations as part of restructuring clinical care. By combining concepts and arguments developed from social network theory (such as embeddedness, centrality, and strength of ties) with explicit consideration of strategic intent and motives, we have proposed an integrative framework for addressing the issues raised. This is consistent with the evolution of complexity science applications to further the understanding of health care organizations (Begun, 1994; McDaniel and Driebe, 2001). Using this framework, we have developed a number of illustrative hypotheses regarding the possible behavior of physician organizations in regard to partnership success: adoption, implementation, and diffusion of CPI. Testing even some of these hypotheses will require using a creative combination of secondary and primary data collection and quantitative and qualitative research methods. But we believe devoting greater attention to the social influences operating inside and outside physician organizations can complement more explicit economic analysis of such behaviors and thereby lead to potentially more informed policy and practice.

7

Sustaining Long-Term Change and Effectiveness in Community Health Networks

Jane Banaszak-Holl, Heather Elms, and David Grazman

Organizational networks remain central in providing health care to community populations. Organizational networks—community-based health systems or community health networks (CHNs)—have been characterized as diverse groups of organizations linked together to serve the complex health needs of specialized populations collectively and are unique in their combination of private and public members and in their collection of diverse stakeholders (Mitchell and Shortell, 2000). Historical developments in medical care, chronic care, public health, and social services have dictated that the services necessary to care for any one person be provided across multiple organizational settings, and that those services be paid for through multiple streams of insurance, public funding, and private coverage.

Many observers of community-based delivery systems have concluded that a lack of adequate system-level planning and coordination has resulted in unnecessary fragmentation and duplication of services across settings, and, for some individuals, gaps in service or inaccessibility to existing services (Bolland and Wilson, 1994; Oliver and Montgomery, 1996; Provan and Milward, 1995). Having embraced this view, policymakers have sought to improve overall system efficiency and effectiveness through greater planning, structure, and centralization of community networks, often implicitly taking a markets-and-hierarchies approach to community health networks. This approach assumes that community health networks will sustain superior performance if they embrace the qualities of well-functioning markets and hierarchies, thus applying to community health networks prescriptions developed in the context of markets and hierarchies (Flynn, Williams, and Pickard, 1996).

Organizational theory, however, suggests that networks are a distinctive organizational form—and thus that the characteristics of efficient and effective *networks* differ from the characteristics of efficient and effective *markets* or hierarchies. We use this literature to suggest an alternative to market-and-hierarchy approaches to sustaining community health networks, emphasizing learning as an incentive for participation when participants have neither a market nor hierarchy to foster cooperation and maintain control. We suggest that policymakers recognize community health networks as the distinct organizational forms they are.

Network forms are unique in the extent to which they facilitate learning among individual participating organizations. The effects of this learning on the performance of networks and their constituent organizations, however, remains unclear. Hence, policymakers should develop appropriately distinct methods for emphasizing the importance of learning in sustaining network participation and cooperation. They should also work with network organizations to evaluate the impact of network membership on both network performance and the performance of member organizations.

Neither Network nor Hierarchy

Powell (1990) highlights the distinctive features of networks and contrasts them with those of market and hierarchical governance structures. Hierarchies use explicit and implicit controls on individuals' behavior to ensure that individuals act effectively as agents for their principals, and markets use competitive dynamics to ensure the effectiveness of agents (Williamson, 1975; Jensen and Meckling, 1976). Networks, in contrast, use the requirements of social interaction, including reciprocal and collaborative patterns of communication and exchange, and normative, rather than legal, sanctions to ensure performance on behalf of both agents and principals (Powell, 1990). These distinctions are obviously not exclusive, as networks will use the legal sanctions available through formal contractual arrangements, and both markets and hierarchies will use normative sanctions through informal organizational relationships and social communication in markets.

However, it is the predominant role of reciprocity, collaboration, and normative sanctions that makes networks unique forms of exchange and transaction. Rather than arms-length (market) or authority-based (hierarchical) relationships, networks are complex, multidimensional, resilient relationships dominated by horizontal exchange and characterized by preferential and mutually beneficial actions (Powell, 1990). Network relationships assume that each party is dependent on resources controlled by the others and that there are mutual gains to be achieved through either the pooling or the exchange of resources.

Parties are expected to forego the pursuit of self-interests that would detract from the gains of exchange or pooling, although in some cases free ridership and even deception may occur on behalf of some organizational members. The ability of organizational members to maintain their network membership when engaging in deceptive or free rider practices will depend on the extent to which the network has developed structures for maintaining control and monitoring membership. The degree to which CHNs are characterized by such behavior, or by such control and monitoring mechanisms, remains unclear. The possibility of free ridership and deception only emphasizes further the need to explore what benefits individual network members gain from participation.

Researchers differentiate pooling networks, those that develop among organizations that provide the same goods or services, from exchange networks, those that develop among organizations that provide complementary goods or services and within which organizations are mutually dependent for resources (Zajac, D'Aunno, and Burns, 2000). For the most part, community health networks are predominately exchange networks, as community health networks work to integrate health care across different organizational settings. As members of exchange networks, community health network members may actually have a more difficult time cooperating than they might as members of pooling networks, as exchange network members' work cultures and market needs differ from those of pooling networks, varying not only across professional settings but also across social, medical, and chronic care sectors. In addition, the incentives that network member organizations need to ensure continued participation vary more across exchange networks than across pooling networks and, hence, some of the difficulties associated with sustaining network participation discussed here will be less important in pooling networks. However, in both pooling and exchange networks, networks generally include both market and hierarchical incentives. For example, a CHN might include both a membership-based incentive for participation and a performance-based one.

The Development of Networks in Health Care

Network research suggests several factors that encourage network development. These factors describe the health care environment well. Although markets develop when transactions are straightforward and nonrepetitive, and require no specific investments, hierarchies tend to occur when transactions are complex, recur frequently, and require specific investments. Networks develop when exchange is social, that is, dependent on relationships, mutual interest, and reputation (Powell, 1990; Zajac, D'Aunno, and Burns, 2000).

Health care transactions are certainly not straightforward—the relationship between input and output is generally complex and ill defined. Transactions are repetitive and require specific investments—particularly in the form of relationships between patient and provider, and among providers. These relationships, however, are usually based on mutual interest and reputation. Thus health care is characterized more closely by the conditions leading to hierarchy than to market—but it is additionally characterized by several important factors encouraging networks. Professionals, and physicians in particular, prefer minimal organizational controls over many aspects of their work (Scott, 1982). In addition, government financing of health services, and more narrowly of medical services, has developed through a number of agencies, and, more important, these government agencies depend on nongovernmental governance structures to ensure appropriate delivery of services (Milward and Provan, 2000).

Networks are also more likely to occur within industries in which the desire for future relationships discourages opportunism and makes individuals both more likely to cooperate and more interested in punishing those who do not cooperate (Axelrod, 1984; Powell, 1990). These industries are frequently markets in which the quality and reliability of products and services, rather than price and quantity, are of overriding concern, as in many service industries (Starkey, Barnatt, and Tempest, 2000). Market incentives in service industries, although good at reducing costs, are risky mechanisms for ensuring quality, as information about quality is difficult for buyers to obtain. Hierarchies, though perhaps better than markets at ensuring quality, impose higher administrative, supervision, and personnel costs than markets (Starkey, Barnatt, and Tempest, 2000). The costs of hierarchy become insurmountable when organizations attempt to integrate across too many steps of the production chain relative to industry standards (Conrad, Mick, Watts-Madden, and Hoare, 1988; Mick and Conrad, 1988). Networks instead externalize hierarchies' in-house activities, thus reducing the costs of integration, but at the same time guarantee minimal quality by promising the benefits of repeat contracting (Starkey, Barnatt, and Tempest, 2000).

Participants in health care markets value long-term relationships to a relatively high degree, and they are increasingly concerned with the quality of services provided. Markets do not appear to provide either. But whereas vertical integration appears to be increasingly difficult to implement successfully in most industries, changing norms in health care favor continuity of care and demand greater integration of the multiple steps of health care production—across preventive, acute, or long-term care, and even social services. This integration is, however, presumably a costly endeavor even at low levels. The development of new integrated health services in particular, then, will benefit from a network structure. Networks are also most likely when know-how is important to production or provision—when jobs are dependent on intellectual capital or craft-based skills acquired through education, training, and experience (Powell, 1990). Know-how typically includes tacit knowledge that is difficult to codify and share. Network structures emphasize lateral forms of communication and mutual obligation, and hence are particularly well-suited for knowledge sharing within highly skilled labor forces (Powell, 1990). Professionals in industries other than health care, including architecture and engineering, exhibit network-like features as well (Von Hippel, 1987; Powell, 1990). Engineering, for example, is characterized by the informal trading of proprietary know-how among technical professionals in competing firms (Von Hippel, 1987). Organizations that employ predominately professionals are often highly porous; within such organizations "work roles are vague and responsibilities overlapping, and. . . . work ties both across teams and to members of other organizations are strong" (Powell, 1990, p. 309). In fact, networks are a common way in which large production firms, such as pharmaceutical companies, acquire know-how and research and development capabilities without directly hiring many professionals (Powell, Koput, and Smith-Doerr, 1996). Know-how is important in health care, because health care professionals typically work with a large number of other professionals, both within and outside their employer, and health care professionals will seek to share their knowledge and know-how in the interests of patients.

Networks are additionally likely in situations characterized by uncertainty, as they are particularly nimble at responding to fluctuations in demand and other unanticipated changes, situations in which hierarchies often remain inert (Kranton and Minehart, 2000). Networks reduce uncertainty through ready access to information, reliability, and collaboration. Markets do not provide such access. Networks thus resolve contingencies that perplex other organizational forms. They are more adaptive and suited to coping with change, given more sophisticated communication channels and thus greater ability to disseminate and interpret new information. The more that competitive advantage depends on firms' ability to innovate and quickly translate ideas into products or services, the more likely network forms of organization will arise and flourish; whereas if competitive advantage is based simply on price, networks will not develop or endure. Thus Powell, Koput, and Smith-Doerr (1996) and others have suggested that networks tend to develop in quickly changing, rapidly developing fields—in which innovations occur quickly—and when knowledge is so sophisticated and widely dispersed that no one firm has the capability for success.

The rapid rate of change, development, and innovation in health care is often noted (see, for example, the chapters of this book by Alexander and D'Aunno; Begun, Dooley, and Zimmerman; Shortell and Rundall; and Scott), and given the fragmentation of service provision (in which patients generally see multiple specialists), no one provider or organization has the ability to determine a successful outcome solely. Part of the complexity of health care environments, and of network industry environments more generally, comes from marked changes in government regulation and market competition. Starkey, Barnatt, and Tempest (2000) offer the U.K. television industry as an example of an industry witnessing marked changes in structure in response to regulatory and competitive change—and a concomitant move from hierarchy to network.

Health care researchers have suggested that as health care markets become more turbulent and more heavily regulated in the future, and individual health care needs become more complicated, community health networks will continue to increase in prevalence (Milward and Provan, 2000; Proenca, 2000). Given its propensity to engage change and uncertainty, the network structure may be the best organizational structure to address future population health care needs.

As suggested in the foregoing, industries other than, but similar to, health care have also been historically dominated by network structures. In addition to other professional industries (architecture, engineering), craft industries encourage network development because each product tends to be somewhat unique, and because craftsmen use nonroutine search procedures to solve exceptional cases—that often depend heavily on intuition and experimentation (Perrow, 1967; Powell, 1990). Relationships between buyers and suppliers tend to be stable and continuous as a result. For example, in the construction sector, many professionals and trade workers coordinate their contributions to build unique, highly complex products such as skyscrapers through relationships between general contractors and subcontractors. These relationships do not rely on standardized responses and tend to be both stable and continuous over the long term and infrequently established through competitive bidding (Eccles, 1981). The parallels to community health are striking: products (patient diagnoses and treatments) are unique, physicians rely on nonroutine search techniques to solve exceptional cases, and resulting diagnoses and treatments necessarily depend on intuition and experimentation. The relationships between primary care physicians and specialists are also strikingly parallel to those found in the construction sector—stable, continuous, and not on the basis of competitive bids.

At a more macro level, CHNs additionally resemble many regional economies and industrial districts that have been viewed as operating most successfully as network structures (Powell, 1990).

Given the geographical basis of community health networks, these examples may be particularly helpful as comparable structures. At the international level, countries such as Sweden and Japan have encouraged much greater integration of suppliers and buyers within their countries and the sharing of risks and resources as well as the pooling of information (Hagg and Johanson, 1983; Westney, 1988). By developing integrated national markets, these countries have been better able to compete in global markets. It is possible that locally dominant CHNs may make some local health care markets better places to receive service and may explain some of the local area variation in health care services.

The Efficiency and Effectiveness of Networks

Because networks develop under different circumstances than do markets and hierarchies, and have different structural characteristics, the efficiency and effectiveness of networks cannot be evaluated from a market or hierarchy viewpoint. Community health networks, for example, have been criticized for redundancies in service provision and the frequency of network contact occurring between organizations. Models of market efficiency dictate minimal contact and as little overlap as necessary to provide services. Baum, Calabrese, and Silverman (2000) have found, however, that similarity in the scope of activities among biotech network participants increased firm performance as measured by the number of patents filed and the firm's level of R&D spending. Group solidarity is often strengthened by similarity of partners and by repeated and frequent contact, which can strengthen trust among participants and lead to clan-like governance structures (Hechter, 1987; Ouchi, 1980). Cohesive groups, or those in which ties are "relatively strong, direct, intense, frequent and positive" (Wasserman and Faust, 1994), are characterized by frequent contact between network members and can enhance learning through extensive feedback and greater ease of understanding among network partners (Ingram and Roberts,

2000; Uzzi, 1996). Likewise, ongoing, complementary activities, including staff pooling or joint production, often lead to greater information sharing, the development of trust, and the emergence of common values (Buckley and Casson, 1988; Coleman, 1988; Krackhardt, 1992; Larson, 1992; Uzzi, 1997).

At the same time, researchers have also emphasized the benefits that can be found in weak ties (Rowley, Behrens, and Krackhardt, 2000). Weak ties by definition are non-redundant and not cohesive, and often connect rather distant parts of a network. Consequently, weak ties are generally associated with access to novel information (Burt, 1992a; Granovetter, 1973), in part because weak ties link network members to others unlike themselves (Banaszak-Holl, Allen, Mor, and Schott, 1998; Wholey and Huonker, 1993). Rowley, Behrens, and Krackhardt (2000) found that in dense networks, strong ties are negatively related to firm performance (though only at $p < .10$)—suggesting that redundancy may not always promote network effectiveness. Likewise, Mitchell, Baum, Banaszek-Holl, Berta, and Bowman (2000) have found that links to similar others can reduce organizational learning because these links provide information that, although it may be easier to understand, is already known to some extent by the other party and therefore does not lead to dramatic service or product changes that increase market value. Overall, little research has been done on which types of ties within community health networks provide the most benefit to individual members (for progress in this area see the chapter in this book by Shortell and Rundall) and on when or if redundancy in communication within a network is beneficial.

Conflicting theoretical arguments and empirical evidence about the link between network structure and performance imply that better information and refinement are needed in our models of community health networks. In addition to the previous arguments and evidence suggesting the value of both strong and weak ties, there remains disagreement about the value of integration. Further refinement and elaboration of the structure of CHNs, by identifying differences in the types of ties that link organizational members and the subgroups that interact, may resolve some of the existing conflicting evidence on the effectiveness and efficiency of community health networks (Roussos and Fawcett, 2000; Shortell, 2000; Wagner and others, 2000).

Researchers began evaluating health care networks by examining the extent of integration across all organizational members (Alter and Hage, 1993; Dill and Rochefort, 1989). The basis of integration can be any kind of ongoing contact, usually face-to-face, among network members that would not just promote a particular client's needs but encourage systematic shared resolution of client problems. For example, governing meetings that require participation of more than two organizational members is a common form of network integration.[1] Greater integration has been expected to increase network and firm performance. More recent evidence indicates that network effectiveness may be less associated with integration across the whole network than with integration between and among small, overlapping subsets of firms, sometimes linked by a coordinating organization (Provan, 1983; Provan and Milward, 1995; Provan and Sebastian, 1998; Gargiulo and Benassi, 2000). Provan and Milward (1994) have found that the availability of a few key central agencies can radically change the structure and efficacy of community health networks.

Provan (1983), for example, suggests that federations offer substantial benefits—in part because while interacting with the federation's central organization, individual organizations reduce their direct interaction with one another. Federations thus tend to reduce the number of direct ties between organizations substantially while increasing the number of indirect ties between organizations through the federation management. At the same time, federations may

1. We emphasize communication among at least three organizational members because a meeting of two members will not necessarily promote network communication nor will such decisions necessarily be taken as effective network governance.

also reduce the number of direct ties to nonfederation organizations. Federation affiliation thus allows participants to reduce complexity by reducing their need to manage multiple direct relationships and additionally allows affiliates to focus on their primary areas of expertise—rather than on managing a network.

Similarly, Provan and Milward (1995) analyzed networks of organizations involved in the delivery of mental health care and found that centralization was a key network characteristic affecting performance. That is, when influence over mental health decisions was highly concentrated in a single core agency, client outcomes were best. Relatedly, Provan and Sebastian (1998) found that integration within network cliques improved performance in the delivery of mental health services, but integration across the entire network did not. In their study, the most effective network structure of the three studied had the fewest cliques, but each clique had several key agencies that coordinated with other parts of the network. It was the presence of the few links across network cliques that was critical for improved client outcomes. Likewise, Banaszak-Holl, Allen, Mor, and Schott (1998) showed that a few central agencies serving the physically disabled provided the necessary link between disparate parts of the network; however, they found no evidence that performance, as measured by improved client outcomes, improved with these central links.

Performance in community health networks depends on how much information about patients or consumers is shared across organizational members and how well that information is integrated into changing organizational members' services. Early research on CHNs measured information-sharing as an overall network characteristic—for example, the level of network integration or centralization—and investigated whether network integration and structure affected the performance of all network members equally (as measured by improved service provision within member organizations). In doing so, researchers set a very high standard for network performance, in that the network may improve client or patient outcomes within some member provider organizations or may even more narrowly produce improvements among select clients or patients but may not necessarily improve care for the overall population or community served. Much of the past work has treated organizational members as equally contributing to the network's structure and in improving patient care (Alter and Hage, 1993). However, the differential abilities of organizations to contribute and transfer information, and the differential ways in which organizations learn and are able to integrate new information into service provision, suggest we need to differentiate between network members and examine how different levels of contribution and learning affect the performance of individual network participants and the overall network's performance.

Network Sustainment

Within the context of network performance, network sustainment will be defined as continuing participation of at least a subgroup of member organizations in group activities, although that sustained participation may not include all original network organizations and may not necessarily have any impact on patient or client outcomes. Although improving performance specifically as measured by client outcomes remains the ultimate goal of community health networks, such performance initially requires sustained participation from network members. Frequently, participation is sustained for a substantial period in anticipation of long-term benefits, and even then the benefits may be improvements in organizational processes rather than in health outcomes for individuals.

Network sustainment can be a difficult issue to define, never mind study, because not all network members need to remain within the network for it to be sustained. No research has examined which members are most important for network sustainment or what the critical volume of membership is for ensuring network sustainment. Equally important here, and the focus of our hypotheses, is an understanding of the reasons why individual organizational members choose to remain in a network and to maintain active participation in network activities.

There are many reasons why individual member organizations may choose to exit a community health network, including management problems, such as a lack of goal convergence; the domination of subnetwork objectives; free-ridership problems; and a lack of enthusiasm from those organizations that are different from the majority of network members (Doz, 1988). Partners may misinterpret one another's behavior (Borys and Jemison, 1989), or they may bring hidden objectives to the network, and the risk always remains that one party will abandon the network with the other partners' knowledge and expertise. Powell (1990) emphasizes that each point of contact in a network can be a source of conflict as well as concord. Partnership agreements must be renegotiated frequently to meet changing expectations (Dyer and Singh, 1998). Networks are also generally characterized by dependency and particularism. Network members may fear increasing dependence on network exchanges and that they may lose some of their ability to dictate their own future. Network members may also find that competitive pressures push them to leave the network. Finally, networks restrict access and thus foreclose opportunities for newcomers—either intentionally, or through barriers including unwritten rules, informal codes, or simply stable patterns of repeat trading that some network members may find oppressive (Powell, 1990).

Organizational members' motivation to participate and sustain network activity can be increased by resolving problems of network governance. Recent research on community health care networks has emphasized the importance of improving processes of governance, developing common missions, and minimizing conflict between members to ensure sustainment of the network (Alexander, Comfort, and Weiner, 1997; Mitchell and Shortell, 2000; Weiner and Alexander, 1998). Furthermore, community health networks, as collections of relatively diverse groups of stakeholders who have not necessarily interacted previously to achieve improved community health outcomes, must focus on aligning individual incentives with the network's common goal (Mitchell and Shortell, 2000).

At the same time, organizational members of a CHN will have different levels of motivation to participate in the network, and incentives to participate will work unevenly across the network. Key network incentives for individual organizations will include increases in reputation and social capital and the transfer of knowledge across the network. Sociologists view reputation as a key component of trust among exchange partners, and organizations benefit in their market position from linking to other organizations with strong reputations. Reputation provides an important incentive to the individual organization to join a network, because the reputations of the other network members may increase interest in the opportunity to work together, and, at the same time, can increase the social capital of network members who have weaker reputations. Subsequently, the reputation of both the network and other network members is also an important factor for participating organizations when choosing whether to continue to participate.

Knowledge transfer is another key incentive for drawing organizations into networks and sustaining interactions among network partners. Detailed knowledge does not transfer easily between organizations in the open market, given the substantial costs associated with measuring and valuing it (Capron and Mitchell, 1998). For example, networks may enhance the learning of new routines and practices of patient care, the sharing of knowledge about health problems, and discussion of complementarities in service provision. All of these changes represent processes of organizational learning, in which interactions among individuals from different organizations affect the routines and practices found within those organizations.

As we have already discussed, networks can provide a structure through which knowledge is transferred without increasing the costly hierarchical integration of widely diverse community health network members. A number of researchers studying the manufacturing sector (Anand and Khanna, 2000; Dyer and Singh, 1998; Dyer and Nobeaka, 2000) have found that networks are critical to developing interfirm knowledge-sharing routines and making relationship-specific investments appropriate to those routines. The benefits of organizational learning provide a strong incentive for organizational participation in the network over time. Network participants learn about other participants' practices and technologies— and, in CHNs, about each other's patients—by working together over time. This learning enables network participants to differentiate their products or services from nonnetwork participants. Consumers may ultimately benefit from the combined learning curve of network participants. Unfortunately, networks often develop to address time-limited or otherwise constrained service needs, and organizational learning oftentimes must extend beyond the needs of an immediate project to ensure more routine participation by organizational members (Starkey, Barnatt, and Tempest, 2000).

Learning and knowledge accumulation occur on at least two levels: at the level of the individual member organizations, and at the network level (Walker, Kogut, and Shan, 1997; Miner and Anderson, 1999; Starkey, Barnatt and Tempest, 2000). Learning at the level of individual network member organizations will not occur evenly across the network, nor will individual network organizations take advantage of network-level learning to the same degree. Nor is learning or knowledge steadily produced. We develop hypotheses here suggesting that both network structure and the characteristics of network members affect learning and performance at both the individual and organizational levels.

Hypotheses on Network Learning

Walker, Kogut, and Shan (1997) note that a common result of research on network structures is the finding that they tend to be neither uniformly dense nor uniformly sparse. In other words, networks are lumpy structures, with cliques of organizations interacting frequently and with much less interaction across cliques. For example, in biotech networks, R&D links are more common among cliques of firms working on a common problem (Barley, Freeman, and Hybels, 1992; Powell, Koput, and Smith-Doerr, 1996). Eventually, ideas developed in one clique are disseminated throughout the network through integrating links or core agencies. In this way, organizational members develop strong and weak ties that provide complementary sources of learning. Individual organizations have the opportunity to learn a great deal about the partners with whom they share a clique, as well as the opportunity to learn a little about organizations in other cliques. Without cliques, they have only the opportunity to learn a little about a lot of organizations. Coordinating organizations pool network knowledge, thus creating network-level learning superior to that present in a more evenly tied network.

HYPOTHESIS 1: *Integration across cliques, rather than integration across all network members, will be positively associated with learning at the network level.*

At the same time, if learning is to serve as an incentive for participation in the network, network learning must not diffuse outside the network. Indeed, many federally funded community networks have led to innovations that were rapidly shared across all service providers regardless of whether they were network members. For example, in the RWJ AIDS Health Services Program and in earlier projects serving the mentally ill, case manager systems were developed to help clients acquire needed services, and this improved method of service provision spread rapidly among all health care providers (Mor, Fleishman, Allen, and Piette, 1994). Nonmember organizations pay less to adopt such innovations once these ideas have spread outside the network because they do not need to invest in network activities. Member organizations may thus choose to drop their participation in the network if they see nonmember organizations rapidly adopting the innovative activities. At the same time, community health networks in particular face difficulties in preventing the diffusion of network learning to nonnetwork providers, given that the explicit mission of both individual member organizations and CHNs themselves is to improve community patient care, both inside and outside the formally defined community health network. Attempts must thus be made by the network to share or otherwise diffuse best practices and other forms of network learning, although in doing so, community health networks destroy the value of this learning as an incentive to network participation.

HYPOTHESIS 2: *Network sustainment will be negatively associated with the diffusion of network learning to nonmember organizations.*

Most of the research on community health networks, as well as on business alliances more generally, recognizes that individual organizations participate unevenly in network activities. In addition, as Weiner and Alexander (1998) found, network members may even have expectations that other members will dominate the network's activities. And while governance mechanisms may seek to even out participation, it can be generally expected that organizations will have differential capabilities to learn from the network, and, hence, some organizations will have stronger incentives to shape network structure and policies.

In particular, we would expect that member organizations differ in their capacity to learn from network activities. Central organizations, by their location, gather much of the information that moves through the network, even as it is disseminated to peripheral organizations. Indeed, central organizations often act as brokers in network exchanges (Banaszak-Holl, Allen, Mor, and Schott, 1998). To the extent that central organizations also gain strong reputations as community leaders in the network, they may have an easier time gaining access to information from other members of the network (Powell, Koput, Smith-Doerr, and Owen-Smith, 1999). Thus these central organizations have a clearer picture of the community health problems that are being addressed and of how new knowledge can be applied to existing health problems. Using that information will lead them to be leaders in integrating service delivery.

At the same time, large organizations, and particularly generalist organizations, will have an easier time gaining knowledge from network activities. Large organizations have excess resources that can be used to facilitate knowledge acquisition, including administrative capability for strategic planning and information gathering. At the same time, larger organizations may have divisional structures that allow individual units to develop their own strategic links to the network without requiring participation by central management. Weiner and Alexander (1998) provide an illustration of a governing decision in a CHN in which the small grassroots organization needed at least two weeks to make a decision that a larger institutional member of the network could decide in twenty-four hours. Part of the advantage of a large organization is that it need not slow production capability to invest energy in network learning activities.

Although size is a distinct advantage in improving knowledge acquisition, generalist strategies may also be an important intervening component in organizations' willingness to participate in network activities. Specialist organizations depend on their unique capabilities to produce a service to gain market advantage (Carroll and Swaminathan, 2000). At the same time, specialists may find that their services overlap completely with other network members (Baum, Calabrese, and Silverman, 2000) whereas generalists' capabilities will rarely be fully covered by other providers. For example, a small home health agency in a community network serving the disabled may find that the local health system provides many of the same services, whereas the hospital's services overlap only slightly with the home health provider's services. Hence, specialists may be particularly reluctant to share essential knowledge with potential market rivals.

HYPOTHESIS 3. *Large, generalist, and central members of the CHN will learn more from CHN participation than will small, specialist, or peripheral members of the CHN.*

It is difficult to understand why peripheral members of a community health network will sustain their participation as much as do central actors when they may not be acquiring new knowledge as rapidly or effectively. Hence, we argue that these members must have other incentives for sustaining participation or that they have other strategies for acquiring knowledge through the community network. First, peripheral members may benefit from gains in resources other than knowledge in the network, and indeed, studies have found that central organizations often diffuse monetary funds and patients outward in a community health network (Banaszak-Holl, Allen, Mor, and Schott, 1998).

Alternatively, peripheral members also benefit more through reputational effects in their participation with central members. Central members are often well-established players in the local health care community and hence have already developed reputations with other providers and with consumers (Banaszak-Holl, Allen, Mor, and Schott, 1998). In addition, central members of the network engage in frequent interaction with many of the other members of the network, which will serve to reinforce their reputation. Peripheral organizational members of the network interact relatively infrequently and with fewer other service providers, which can slow down their ability to gain a reputation for service quality. However, peripheral organizations can gain indirectly through the reputation of their interaction partners (Stuart and Podolny, 1996). Hence, we draw the following hypothesis:

HYPOTHESIS 4. *Peripheral members of the CHN will experience greater reputational benefits or actual resource transfers through network participation than will more central members of the CHN.*

The choice of a first-mover strategy (that is, r-strategy) may also affect an organization's ability to learn from the network and, subsequently, affect the extent to which the organization benefits from network participation. Business strategies are reflected in the organization's choice of resource investments and production technology and have an immense impact on future investments. R-strategists use innovation to gain a competitive advantage and often move rapidly into developing technological fields (Aldrich, 1999). R-strategists are willing to try innovative programs, such as those that develop CHNs. K-strategists, however, gain production knowledge through imitation of existing firms' practices and hence move late into developing markets. K-strategists are rarely likely to be among the early adopters of an innovation but often exploit business strategies that other firms have proven to be successful. At the time of this writing, many CHNs represent new ways to view the production of community health care services, and in that sense, they will attract r-strategists who are willing to try innovative approaches to developing services. Unfortunately, these network members will be less drawn to participate once the technologies for health care become more standard in the community, and they will be more likely to exit the network. Hence, we hypothesize that

HYPOTHESIS 5. *R-strategist members of the network will participate in developing CHN as long as the network sustains innovative learning but will be more likely to exit the CHN if the network shifts its focus away from innovative learning.*

Any particular r-strategist will face a choice when confronted with changes in organizational goals away from innovative learning.

The organization may seek to force changes in the network such that the network refocuses again on innovative change. Such a strategy will be more successful for organizations that have a central and controlling role in the community health network. However, even organizations that are influential in the network will find that systematic change in network goals and focus will be slow in coming and may never regain the "entrepreneurial" spirit that a network has when first formed (D'Aunno and Zuckerman, 1987). Hence, exit will be a common outcome for r-strategists.

Theoretically, business strategies are much more diverse than the r or k and generalist or specialist distinctions that we have used here. More research should explore the implications of organizational strategies for network participation, especially because competitive dynamics may be one of the foremost issues preventing more organizations from participating in developing community health services.

Organizations can learn from other organizations through vicarious processes of imitation without direct contact (Haunschild and Miner, 1997; Kraatz, 1995). Imitative learning requires fewer investments, as information on innovations is often taken from industry news or strategic assessments of the industry, and may have higher short-term returns than do innovation or exploration (Levinthal and March, 1993). Hence, many firms, and k-strategists in particular, will prefer to learn from the population instead of from the network, because direct learning occurring in the network is too costly. Imitation works better if one is imitating those similar to oneself, so networks wishing to encourage innovative rather than imitative learning should bring together more diverse firms.

HYPOTHESIS 6: *If network members learn through imitation only, there will be a high risk that members leave or do not actively participate in the network.*

Organizational learning is not a quick process, in part because organizations are not blank slates. Organizations already have established routines, for handling production processes and interacting with customers and suppliers, that gain inertia over time (Hannan and Freeman, 1984). In addition, because interorganizational learning increases with trust, well-established ties will be better conduits of knowledge transfer. Subsequently, we hypothesize that

HYPOTHESIS 7: *Individual learning in organizational members will increase with the age of and frequency of interaction within the CHN.*

Developing the Research Agenda

We have emphasized two important aspects of learning within CHNs necessary for network sustainment: (1) the network itself should develop higher levels of learning than does the local community of health care organizations, and (2) individual organizations, which will differ in their ability to acquire new knowledge in the network and to use that knowledge effectively, must be given appropriate incentives to maintain their participation. Empirically, these issues require intensive study not only of the ways in which network members cooperate but also of the substantive health problems they are addressing and the resources and knowledge they share. In addition, network members' contributions to network activities must be understood in the context of their own strategic position in the market and, hence, broader knowledge of each member's technological base and market position is needed.

Network-level learning is difficult to study directly, in that, similar to population-level learning, it represents a "systematic change in the nature and mix of routines as a result of the joint experience" of the member organizations (Miner and Haunschild, 1995). However, community health networks and partnerships have been found to be more effective at implementing programmatic changes that affect the routines used in health programs and services than at changing population health outcomes or behaviors (Roussos and Fawcett, 2000). This implies that successful network-level learning requires some cumulative change in the routines and procedures of the individual organizational members of the network. In other words, network participation must include substantial change in the operations of the individual organizational members and those changes must differentiate network members from nonnetwork members in the community if learning is to be defined as occurring at the "network" level.

Little evidence exists as to whether networks maintain exclusive control of their knowledge within local communities, and, hence, more research is needed on the comparison of programs offered within networks to programs or services common to non-network members. Although community health networks may be most effective in addressing population needs by disseminating programmatic changes within the community, further research is needed to determine whether by doing so, the networks make it more difficult to sustain participation over time.

A potential way to sustain networks while diffusing important health care processes to the community is to consider more carefully the mix of projects on which the CHN members collaborate. In their review of the literature on community health partnerships, Roussos and Fawcett (2000) found many programmatic benefits targeted to quickly changing how the community more generally handles health behaviors (for example, school nutrition programs; campaigns to add symbols to local restaurant menus for healthy food items; and public media campaigns to enhance awareness of nutritional, safety, or personal health issues such as smoking, cholesterol problems, and seat belt laws). However, network members may also work to develop joint capabilities and opportunities to collaborate that will not readily be diffused within the community (Gulati, 1995b). For example, CHNs can work together to offer greater access to immunization and preventive medicine programs through jointly developed service sites, they can build outreach programs that draw patients into the service sites of the CHN member organizations, and they can engage in joint lobbying for new resources.

Network studies have not focused their attention previously on how the types of services offered affects network growth and sustainment over time.

Learning that occurs within individual members of the CHN network may be more difficult to measure without better information on the characteristics of member organizations before network involvement. Collecting information on the prior characteristics of CHN members is critical, because evidence of learning processes is inferred from changes in organizational strategy, service provision, and performance of organizations (Mitchell, Baum, Banaszak-Holl, Berta, and Bowman, 2000). Also, although we expect that interactions within the network will affect many of the routines and practices of member organizations, they may not do so immediately—and frequently, the importance of network participation is only inferred when changes are observed during the period of network participation and for practices directly linked to network goals. Some of the ways in which individual member organizations can benefit from network participation include the direct sharing of technological knowledge and resources across members, the development of care standards or protocols, and, finally, the development of new services and processes within the network (Gulati, 1995b; Doz, Olk, and Ring, 2000).

Ironically, organizations often choose to join CHNs because they have the existing capability for a service, and believe they can, with minimal resource expenditures, extend use of that service. For example, many of the members of the AIDS demonstration sites in the RWJ project joined the network to provide case management to AIDS patients because they already had strong capabilities to provide case management through discharge planners or existing service coordinators (Mor, Fleishman, Allen, and Piette, 1994). These organizations have strong incentives for joining CHNs; however, they have fewer incentives for maintaining strong participation in the network, particularly if the potential benefits in improving those capabilities are achieved early and leave the organization with greater responsibility for providing services within the CHN. CHNs need to weigh the needs and interests of all members in building sustainable structures, and governance processes will play a critical role in balancing representation within the network. However, CHNs again should consider how the mix of service changes or substantial issues to be addressed will answer the learning needs of participating organizations.

Discussion and Conclusion

Our hypotheses link the business strategy of organizational members of CHNs to their ongoing participation in the CHN, which is ultimately critical for network sustainment. Business strategies are enduring characteristics of organizations that reflect deeply held missions, substantial resource investments, and often carefully defined market niches. Business strategies do not change quickly or dramatically in most organizations (Hannan and Freeman, 1977) and will have a substantial impact on managers' decisions of whether to join and sustain membership in a community health network.

In setting network sustainment in the context of the business strategy of network members, we are drawing on the phenomenal growth in the strategy literature on the importance of reputation and organizational learning for organizational behavior. This literature focuses on how organizations change and more generally make decisions based on an understanding of their own competitive strengths and weaknesses in addition to knowledge of environmental change. Competitive strengths and weaknesses are embedded within the routines and processes of the organization, and any structural or strategic changes that the organization makes must realistically lead to changes in the routines and processes that employees use. If CHNs are viewed as learning vehicles, network change might be better explained as the results of attempts to increase knowledge transfer, rather than as attempts to improve the efficiency of service production. In other words, networks—even while aiming at the improvement of client services—may develop more as structures meant to facilitate learning than as devices meant to improve client services.

The importance of routines and knowledge emphasizes the social aspects of market dynamics and the relative value of social capital over tangible assets. Organizations often learn new routines best through closer ties than those that develop through market exchange. Hence, the community health network offers excellent opportunities to communicate important knowledge of patients, their needs, and the services they use across organizational members. Organizational members, however, must be able to perceive the benefits of network membership in order to sustain participation. If the learning opportunities do not exist or lose their value, then members will seek opportunities elsewhere. Given that most CHN members are under severe cost and time constraints, network participation not only must be made valuable itself but also must be made valuable relative to other potential opportunities that CHN members may have.

Future growth of community health networks may also depend on how well the value of network participation can be demonstrated to the stakeholders of member organizations. As our economic world becomes more heavily dominated by knowledge industries, and with the growth of the Internet and information technologies, organizations have become more interested in managing and measuring their value of knowledge, routines, and nontangible assets. The development of cost accounting for nontangible assets helps members of CHNs analyze and evaluate the benefits of CHN membership.

In many health care organizations, the costs of CHN membership are not fully measured; these organizations contribute the time of existing employees or use existing technology and assets to contribute to CHN efforts. Likewise, the benefits of the CHN for individual organizational members have gone unmeasured. There is no literature that specifically examines the impact of network membership on the economic or financial performance of CHN members. In contrast, the literature on business networks provides substantial evidence that network participation is linked to firm-level economic and financial performance (Baum, Calabrese, and Silverman, 2000; Rowley, Behrens, and Krackhardt, 2000).

At the same time, health organizations may experience benefits of network membership through learning that organizational members do not readily attribute to network participation. Frequently, organizations may not evaluate how clinical processes or service provision have changed with CHN membership or may not consider what types of information CHN membership has contributed to strategic planning. The lack of accountability for network activities may be one reason that CHNs do not become central to the activities of member organizations. To the extent that CHN activities remain a hidden activity in the cost accounting of member organizations, they are more easily dropped when network participation becomes more expensive.

We have emphasized that member organizations in CHNs do gain benefits from CHN participation and, hence, these gains should be measurable. In fact, organizational learning should provide improvements in clinical care, knowledge of and accounting for patient needs, and the collaborative ties that contribute to inter-organizational alliances. However, to take into account these improvements, organizations need to evaluate their knowledge base before CHN membership and to consider CHN contributions to knowledge rather than just to improvements in outcomes. To do so, member organizations may need to shift the ways in which they evaluate the costs and benefits of CHN participation.

Likewise, networks themselves need to evaluate better the knowledge base developed through collaboration. CHNs have the major goal of contributing to improvements in the health of the local population, but this goal will be a disincentive for sustaining the network beyond immediate and costly improvements, as network members perceive that nonnetwork members of the community also adopt these strategies eventually. Subsequently, CHNs must blend goals for immediate and long-term improvements in care and for contributing to the community through unique capabilities limited to network participants. This conclusion parallels existing research on the governance of community health networks that has emphasized the importance of goal setting for CHN activity (Mitchell and Shortell, 2000).

Policymakers must allow for these and other requirements of network sustainment—as opposed to those of markets and hierarchies— when evaluating the effectiveness of community health networks. These network structures include those meant to facilitate learning and restrict diffusion of that learning outside the network. Our approach suggests that CHNs—even while targeting the improvement of client services—may develop first as structures meant to facilitate learning. Without learning and the restriction of learning diffusion, organizations have little incentive to continue participation in the network and thus little ability to take advantage of knowledge that might eventually improve care provision. Policymakers should thus evaluate CHNs in terms of both their ability to facilitate learning and their ability to provide better patient care. Such a dynamic approach recognizes the distinct structure and benefits of networks in relation to markets and hierarchies—and thus encourages network sustainment. Only through network sustainment can the eventual benefits of CHNs be realized.

8

· ·

Quality as an Organizational Problem

John R. Kimberly and Etienne Minvielle

The measurement and management of quality in health care in general, and in hospitals in particular, have become a national preoccupation, as continuing efforts to control costs in the sector have led to charges that quality is often sacrificed on the altar of cost control. The claim that managed care companies care more about their bottom line than about people is just the most visible sign of the underlying concern (for example, Randel, Pearson, Sabin, Hyams, and Emanuel, 2001).

We have argued elsewhere (Kimberly and Minvielle, 2000) that although quality has always been a focus of discussion, debate, and concern within the medical profession, its prominence in discussions and debates recently and more generally reflects both a concern that quality may slip in the face of efforts to "manage care" and a search on the part of payers for value in what they purchase. The former is fueled by a number of recent, highly publicized cases of alleged abuse by managed care organizations, while the latter is influenced by the development of capabilities—still primitive—permitting measurement and comparison of the clinical performance of both individual and institutional providers.

In this chapter, we argue that quality is an organizational problem; that is, that variation in quality is as much due to the way in which care is organized and coordinated as it is to the competence of individual care givers. Concepts from organization theory, and particularly from work done on the distinctive characteristics of the "professional bureaucracy," (Mintzberg, 1978) help illuminate the historical role of quality in health care organizations. But more recent developments in the quality movement suggest limitations to the model of the professional bureaucracy and actually suggest new organizational issues and opportunities, which in turn require new theorizing. The issue of quality illustrates the interplay between theory and practice. Organization theory, it turns out, has both influenced and been influenced by the evolution of quality as an organizational problem.

From the Reflection of Professional Bureaucracy to a Vehicle for Fundamental Change

Concern with quality has always occupied an important place at the core of health care organizations, be they hospitals, networks, or other settings in which care is provided. However, as soon as we look at how this concern gets translated concretely, the waters become muddied. What connection, for example, is there between research in evidence-based medicine and the creation of new ISO 9000 certifications that establish international quality standards? And how, under one rubric, do we justify concern with establishing rules and practices in hygiene to prevent nosocomial infections on the one hand and the creation of standards for ensuring that various types of surgical equipment meet certain technical functional specifications on the other?

So many different initiatives are being undertaken in the name of quality improvement that it is tempting to dismiss much of the activity as faddish in character. To do so, however, would be a mistake, for this diversity reveals an important characteristic of the quality movement. When rhetoric is put to one side, and patterns in the way these initiatives are developed are analyzed, including at whose instigation and for whose benefit, we see how the status of quality has been transformed as these initiatives have unfolded. Once principally derivative from the attributes of a professional bureaucracy, quality has become most recently a rallying point for fundamental reorganization of the hospital, reorganization centered on the patient's experience.

The History of Quality

It is common to associate the first phases in the history of quality with the theme of evaluation. The 1970s were first characterized by the recognition that there was variability in professional practice in health, and that these differences could not be accounted for by variability in the characteristics of patients, such as severity of illness or injury, or in the technical environment of the hospital. Wennberg and Guttenshon (1973) were pioneers, among others, in uncovering this variability. This finding, which was independent of clinical specialty and context of service delivery, led to the observation that two health care professionals confronted by the same clinical situation could behave quite differently. Under these conditions, reduction in this variability in clinical practice became a priority. Reduced variability, in turn, became an objective of quality initiatives, and the evaluation of professional practice became the principal vehicle for assessing quality.

Pressure from the media, employers, and activist consumer groups served as a further stimulus to evaluation of quality in hospitals, and greater transparency with respect both to outcomes and to internal hospital operations was demanded. We should note that when this pressure is exerted in a diffuse manner, physicians, because of their social and financial power and because of their involvement in new technology, are able to coopt evaluation efforts. We should also note that the 1980s witnessed the flowering of policies of rationalization in the world of health care, most notably the adoption of the diagnosis-related group (DRG) system of prospective payment by the federal government in 1983.

Although these policies were controversial, they all underscored the need for techniques and tools to measure and manage quality and spawned myriad efforts to quantify the different attributes of quality of care in the hospital setting.

In the academic world, the 1970s also witnessed the development of the concept of the hospital as a professional bureaucracy (for example, Heydebrand, 1973; Mintzberg, 1978). This conceptualization is relevant to understanding the evolution of quality initiatives. Each initiative can be seen as an effort by specific categories of actors in the hospital setting to appropriate quality and to frame the debate about quality issues in ways consistent with their own specific action spaces, beliefs, and interests. Physicians, nurses, and administrators all attempt to encapsulate quality within their own agendas and project its significance in ways that are consistent with their own interests.[1] As a consequence, taken together, quality initiatives may appear to be highly disparate and in some cases contradictory. However, when one conceptualizes the hospital as a professional bureaucracy, one can begin to understand the sources of and reasons for this variation: it is a reflection of the organizational context in which it is embedded.

To demonstrate, let us begin with that point in the evolution of quality characterized by, first, a concern with systematic evaluation and subsequently by a concern with quality assurance. The writing of Avedis Donabedian (1980b) is frequently cited as representing the first effort to create a framework for the evaluation of quality of care in the hospital. His now familiar framework argued for the evaluation of quality at three levels:

- The *structures* within which care is delivered, with specification of the human, financial, and material resources required

1. We do not mean to suggest that we see complete commonality of interests within categories. In fact, there is considerable variability among physicians, for example, based on specialty, age, and location of practice. However, we do see at a more macro level more commonality within than between categories.

- The *processes* of care, that is, all of the actions under-taken to provide care to the patient

- The *results* or *outcomes*, that is, changes in health status subsequent to care and the quality perceived by the patients.

As observers gave thought to these three levels and their impli-cations, a bias toward corrective action soon emerged, thus setting in motion movement in the direction of quality assurance. Two approaches characterized this movement. First, work rules based on conformity with preestablished standards or norms, and second, mechanisms for the review of undesirable incidents, such as falls, generally consisting of information systems permitting collection of data on frequency of such incidents. The 1970s witnessed much work in North America and Europe based on these methods, work characterized by two distinct orientations, one centered on profes-sional practices and the other concerning the operating policies of the hospital.

Professional Practices

Along with the evaluation of professional practices came an impor-tant consideration in the assessment of quality, concern with the best diagnostic and therapeutic strategy—in other words, concern for the technical mastery of care delivery. Depending on the coun-try, this evaluation was more or less championed by government agencies. In France, for example, it was government agencies that pushed this orientation at the end of the 1980s. In the United States, it was a mixture of public and private initiatives in the late 1970s and early 1980s that moved in this direction.

Clinical guidelines are the most obvious example of this orien-tation toward quality. They are defined as "a standardized and spe-cific description of the best approach for a given pathological condition, developed on the basis of an analysis of the scientific lit-erature and expert opinion" (Leape, 1990). Clinical guidelines thus deal with purely technical aspects of care. A variety of methods is used to synthesize the existing scientific knowledge on which they are based, including meta-analyses of the literature, consensus conferences, and surveys. Guidelines can also be classified on the basis of the statistical techniques used in the supporting research. This is the approach of evidence-based medicine. In both cases the underlying idea is that the behavior of professionals can and should be standardized in those areas of care in which enough is known to permit guidelines to be developed. Where enough is known about a given condition, in other words, professional practice ought to be similar across cases.

Operating Policies of the Hospital

The second orientation was aimed at actions relative to the functioning of the hospital and to quality as perceived by patients. Examples would be hospital policies regarding safety in the use of hospital equipment, policies on how patients are admitted, or surveys of patient satisfaction. Although these three examples are quite different, they are all based on a common principle: respect for general rules and regulations, either formulated by management, often in collaboration with clinicians having managerial responsibility, or derived from regulatory documents. These rules and regulations are not "guidelines"; rather, they are standards or norms which one hopes will be implemented consistently across different organizational units.

Professional practices and hospital policies together, emerging first from a concern with evaluating quality and subsequently from a concern with ensuring given levels of quality, created some important political dynamics within hospitals. Those who championed one approach or the other had their own reasons for doing so, reasons that were not necessarily widely shared. Thus, for any particular quality initiative, it was not obvious that there would be any extensive support beyond that of the advocates. The predictable result was varying degrees of "successful" implementation. Many initiatives failed to elicit and sustain real behavior change.

**Accreditation as a Force for Institutionalizing
Quality Assurance**

Accreditation has played a key role in the standardization of hospital *structures*, and has sought to influence *processes of care* and *results* as well. A defining feature of accreditation is the existence of agencies, external to the bodies being accredited, whose principal activity is to establish benchmarks against which each hospital seeking accreditation is regularly measured. These benchmarks represent a synthesis of clinical and administrative standards and norms that are derived from surveys of current practice. As such, theoretically, they represent the state of the art in work in both domains. At the same time, they institutionalize these practices, resulting in a sort of virtuous circle: the quality of a given activity is evaluated, corrective measures are put in place, and these measures are subsequently reviewed by agencies outside the hospital. In this way, quality is theoretically ensured.

As powerful as its accompanying incentives may be, accreditation alone cannot explain the degree of participation of various internal constituencies in quality initiatives. The participation of any single actor will depend largely on how the effort to evaluate or ensure quality, or both, affects the system of relationships and patterns of behavior in which he or she—be the actor a physician, a nurse, a manager, or other player—is enmeshed. The ultimate arbiter of successful implementation is "compatibility," that is, the extent to which the initiative and its behavioral requirements are aligned with the characteristics of a professional bureaucracy. The higher the compatibility, the greater the likelihood of successful implementation.

**How Quality Reinforces the Bureaucratic Character
of the Hospital**

Perrow's (1965) description of the extent to which hospitals are bureaucratic forms of organization is as relevant today as it was when it was first written. The objective of hospital bureaucracy is to internalize those norms that serve the client and that coordinate the work of professionals. Coordination is ensured by standards that determine in advance what should be done. The history of quality evaluation and of quality assurance is marked by this characteristic. Even though clinical and administrative orientations are concerned with different arenas for action, it is striking that they converge on this principle: the quality of a given action is a function of its conformity with guidelines or norms previously articulated, thus minimizing the risk of arbitrary action.

Classically, as described long ago by Weber (Gerth and Mills, 1958) this bureaucratization of behavior in the hospital is reinforced by a parallel constraint, the development of written procedures. Different slogans have accompanied quality assurance initiatives. "Write down what is done, and do what is written down"—this slogan emphasizes the importance of having a written record of what transpires, given the organizational risk that oral transmission of information inevitably engenders. Professionals are generally less enthusiastic about this constraint than are their administrative counterparts, and frequently complain about the number and types of paper forms they are required to fill out. The need for formal accountability, however, forces the development and proliferation of written procedures.

Quality as a Force for Maintaining Professional Autonomy

A professional bureaucracy differs markedly from a more "mechanistic" bureaucracy in both the sources and the objects of this need for standardization. In the case of a mechanistic bureaucracy, authority is vested in a position, whereas in a professional bureaucracy, authority derives from expertise and hence from processes of training and socialization in the context of peers practicing in the same knowledge domain (Becker and Gordon, 1966). Furthermore, in the case of the former, senior management typically creates and imposes standards on subordinates, whereas in the latter, standards are largely created externally.

Practice guidelines exemplify this distinction. With some variation from one country to the next, governmental initiatives have stimulated their development. In France, the reforms of 1991 and 1996 led to the creation of a national accrediting body, the Agence Nationale d'Accréditation et d'Evaluation en Santé (the National Agency for the Evaluation and Accreditation of Health Organizations). Similarly, national initiatives sought to impose clinical guidelines on physician practice patterns, but without much success. Ultimately, however, both physicians and nurses recognized the need to be directly involved in these initiatives, and the latter became progressively engaged in a vast process of standardization of practices, a fact that ironically reinforced the bureaucratic character of the professional settings in which they worked. This said, there are some further nuances that need to be acknowledged, to wit:

• The quest for standardization deriving from the evaluation of quality affected *practices* as well as *competencies* of professionals and their formal *qualifications*. A given level of qualification signifies a degree of theoretical competence that, however, is not always found in practice, and the actual degree of competence held by professionals does not always translate into the way they practice. Qualifications, competencies, and practices thus are distinct characteristics. Clinical practice guidelines attempt to blend the three, a way of "objectifying" a given level of qualification—a status achieved in view of initial training and reinforced through continuing education; a way of arraying competencies against the knowledge base contained in the guidelines; and a way of evaluating actual practice against standards through clinical audits. Thus, one might argue that the quality movement has stimulated a process of standardization of qualifications, of professional competencies, and of actual practice.

• With regard to Mintzberg's (1978) argument, in which standardization of qualifications is the principal mode of coordination of activities in a professional bureaucracy, the development of clinical practice guidelines represents a more differentiated view based on the state of scientific knowledge at a particular moment in time. This point is important: if the movement toward evaluation of quality and quality assurance gives new meaning to practices, competencies, and professional qualifications based on a more "scientific" view of medicine, it nevertheless changes nothing with respect to the principle of standardization. Standardization effectively serves to maintain existing ways of recognizing professional expertise and thus reinforces traditional patterns of work organization in the hospital sector.

• Overall, then, the process of standardization leads to the reproduction and perpetuation of habitual forms of legitimation, of socialization, and of training of professionals. Certain physicians quickly recognized opportunities to further their own interests in teaching and research in the hospital through the development of efforts to evaluate and ensure quality. Participation in the development of clinical practice guidelines or clinical research protocols demonstrating the efficacy of a particular practice gained physicians recognition in the scientific community, with opportunities to publish in prestigious journals or to present papers at important international conferences or both. Showing how their own work was at the leading edge of professional practice established them as experts and often allowed them to develop new kinds of training programs.

• At the same time, nurses saw in the evaluation of quality an opportunity to enhance their status. By demonstrating how important aspects of their work such as inhibiting nosocomial infections or reducing needle sticks can enhance quality, they have been able to appropriate parts of the movement for their own professional ends.

The behavior of physicians and nurses just described somewhat moderated a more general hostility in the professions to the diffusion of clinical practice guidelines. The situation is complex. Many professionals used quality as a vehicle for valorizing their own practices and competence, whereas others saw their autonomy threatened by the spread of guidelines. In both cases, they sought to gain control of the process of standardization. These efforts are evident at all levels: during the definition of the guidelines themselves, in the reliance on well-known experts in consensus conferences, in the diffusion of the guidelines with the influence of opinion leaders in the process to ensure local adoption, and finally in the priority given to self-evaluation by professionals of their own practices. At each level, peer control seems to be a key factor in the success of the diffusion process. The process unfolded in a way that was based on and reinforced usual exchanges among "experts," typically well-known university-based physicians, and other professionals. These processes of exchange correspond to what Mintzberg (1978) describes as the parameters of how organizations are conceived. They determine a way of organizing that is tied to the kinds of activity one finds in hospital departments—the operational centers of the structure of the hospital as a whole—and to the principles of cooperation that exist with other components of that structure. It is not surprising, therefore, to find the same principles reaffirmed in the context of the diffusion of guidelines.

The first of these organizational principles, as we have noted, concerns coordination of activities based on standardization of qualifications. A second calls for the preestablished character of "best practice" with reference to an external standard. The elaboration of guidelines contributes here in the sense that it emerges from dialogue among professionals outside the context of the hospital itself, most frequently in the context of medical societies or professional associations. Thus, the movement is associated more with what professionals see as being directly tied to their profession than to the particular establishments in which they work. In this way it is relatively independent of the organization itself. Finally, the third principle, no matter what the degree of standardization of qualifications, reaffirms the complexity of the physician's work, thus ensuring considerable latitude to the professional in the application of guidelines. This principle, which is central to Mintzberg's (1978) argument, needs to be refined further, as different conditions have differing levels of complexity and uncertainty associated with them and hence vary in the amount of standardization that can be applied.

This brings us to the heart of the debate between those who approve the development of guidelines for the "industrialization of medicine" and those who believe that each physician is an artist and that no two physicians will treat a given case in precisely the same fashion. The development of guidelines does not eliminate the control of professionals over their work; it can always be argued that a particular case has attributes that place it outside the parameters of the relevant guideline. And because it is physicians themselves who develop the guidelines, professional control is maintained. The distinction between "recommendation" and norm is key (Woolf, 1993); because of the continuously evolving nature of medical knowledge, it is necessary to maintain a certain degree of flexibility in the use of guidelines and to think of them as aids to medical decision making.

Viewed in this way, the movement for the evaluation and assurance of quality is grounded in the characteristics of professional bureaucracy. Certain of our observations, however, do not fit well with the model of the professional bureaucracy as put forth by Mintzberg. As the quality movement has evolved, standardization does not just concern levels of qualifications. The autonomy of professionals is diminished. And competence is no longer a synonym for experience. It is rather the continuous embodiment of scientific knowledge.

These reservations do not diminish the heuristic value of the model for interpreting the movement. The control of work by professionals is still very much in evidence. Consideration of evaluation and assurance of quality confirms the technical complexity of health care and the need for professionals to deliver it. This orientation, which helps to justify and maintain professional autonomy, coexists with increased administrative involvement in the management of logistics. As a consequence, the movement actually reinforces both parallel hierarchies in the hospital: the professional hierarchy, which goes from the bottom toward the top, and the managerial hierarchy, which goes from the top toward the bottom and which has more of the character of a mechanistic bureaucracy.

Beyond Evaluation and Assurance: The Emergence of Quality Management

Toward the end of the 1980s in the United States, approaches to the evaluation and assurance of quality were seriously questioned. In spite of demonstrable success in technical and logistical domains in the hospital, as well as in clinical practice, new criticisms emerged. Two principal arguments formed the basis of these criticisms: the failure to take organizational variables into account in approaches to quality, and the use of methods to improve quality that were too mechanistic in character.

Criticisms of Traditional Approaches

Berwick (1989) and Schumacher (1991) were the first to point out the limits of an approach that was exclusively oriented toward the analysis of professional practices. By focusing on diagnostic and therapeutic strategies only, the whole issue of implementation of the strategies was neglected at the same time that it was becoming more complex. Lomas (1990) pointed out that by considering quality solely as a function of medical expertise, the impact of others involved in the process was left out, as was the impact of the patients themselves, both of which are important determinants of the level of coordination of actions undertaken. These criticisms were drawn from approaches to quality in the world of industry, particularly the argument of Deming (1986), who held that 15 percent of the deficiencies in quality are related to questions of expertise and the remaining 85 percent to organizational problems. Furthermore, there was the recognition that a problem with quality is not simply a problem of a professional making a mistake but may well be a problem related to the way in which care is organized at the institutional level.

At the same time, Lomas (1990) and Laffel and Blumenthal (1989) criticized an approach to quality emphasizing conformity with standards, arguing that such an approach might confuse conformity with an ideal level of performance. There is no perfect correlation between conformity and performance on the one hand, and no guarantee that the level of performance achieved by conformity to the standard would be appropriate on the other. The risk in this approach is to develop "minimal standards which allow the delivery of care with minimal quality, in structures which respect minimal norms, to obtain results judged acceptable" (Berwick, 1989, p. 44)

The Emergence of Quality Management

In reaction to these criticisms a new movement emerged, variously called total quality management (TQM) or continuous quality improvement (CQI). For simplicity's sake we will use the term *quality management* to refer to both. This new movement was based on a number of principles:

- The first concerns the notion of quality improvement. Improvement results from continuous search for excellence in work.

- The second concerns the role of the patient. Quality is seen as the result of alignment between the service offered by the hospital and the needs of the user.

- The third principle gives organizational questions a central place in the search for quality. True management of quality requires management of the full range of ways of organizing work. The most extreme versions of TQM and CQI see quality as the central point around which the entire organization and its actions should be defined.

To meet these objectives, quality management requires a detailed description of activities within the hospital. Each activity is described as a process comprising different stages, each one of which may have dysfunctional attributes that may be detected using simple tools such as control diagrams or fish-bone diagrams or both. People coming from different departments that are involved in one way or another with the process being analyzed constitute working groups and use these tools in focused problem-solving sessions. The makeup of these working groups is a central point in quality management and resembles the principles used in defining the makeup of "quality circles." The ultimate objective of these groups is to reconstitute the entire process being analyzed and to give each member of the working group a better understanding of where improvements might be made. The tone of the work is unfailingly positive. Errors and dysfunctions represent opportunities for improvement, not mistakes to be sanctioned.

This diagnostic phase serves as a point of departure for change, change that is planned in the working groups and supported by the results of the diagnosis. By developing metrics that permit monitoring of progress, the working groups can assess the impact of the changes they suggest. Together the stages of diagnosis, action, and monitoring constitute the cycle of quality improvement.

A New Interpretation

There appears to be a significant gap between rhetoric and reality in the quality management phase of the evolving history of quality initiatives. Few studies have attempted to summarize the results of implementing TQM or CQI in hospitals; such evidence as there is suggests that the impact has been modest at best (for example, Loizeau, 1996; Shortell, O'Brien, and Carman, 1995). Despite the relative absence of empirical support for the impact of quality management, there continues to be an impressive number of highly diverse initiatives undertaken under the banner of quality improvement. It became institutionalized in the accreditation process in the United States in 1988 and has increasingly become part of the discourse of health policy in the industrialized world. In France, for example, where accreditation of hospitals became mandatory in 1996, externally stimulated efforts to improve quality represent an unprecedented intrusion into the internal affairs of both public and private hospitals.

Although much of the activity undertaken in the name of quality management may initially appear ineffective and somewhat faddish in character, closer examination reveals the seeds of profound changes. Far from being ephemeral, this movement toward quality management represents a significant departure from the idea of quality as reflecting the character of a professional bureaucracy. It substitutes new criteria for traditional ones: at the level of process, a focus on quality emphasizes the need to organize work around the patient and to reframe the role of the hospital in the context of a system of health services provided in multiple settings.

In the name of quality, certain principles embedded in the traditional model of the professional bureaucracy are called into question. The appropriate frame is no longer structural-functional, but derives from the ways in which collective action is organized. In identifying problems along the patient trajectory, effective organization is defined in terms of cooperative efforts in which physicians are certainly important actors, but in which they are part of a complex system including other important actors as well. Thus not only is the strategic issue of medical intervention important, but so is the issue of how the medical intervention is carried out—the logistical component of care. The latter is no longer viewed as a simple matter of logistics but as a complex systemic problem requiring cooperation among all parties. The role of the physician is to conceptualize the care required, while other health care personnel—rather than being simply followers of physicians' orders—become problem solvers who are necessarily closely linked in their work to physicians. This redefinition of the organization of work has several implications:

- First, the emphasis is on the work itself. As we noted earlier, Deming reframed the quality issue around the organization of work. Coordination of activity on the basis of standardization of qualifications or expert practices is supplemented by analysis of how work is organized. As part of this analysis, the concept of competence takes on new meaning. Competence is not simply demonstrated expertise but involves a whole range of know-how such as how one reacts to unanticipated events, the ability to anticipate dysfunctional work situations, or how one coordinates one's actions with others. Competence is thus based not only on medical knowledge, but also on organizational *savoir-faire*.

- The importance of the work unit also becomes relative. If the patient trajectory becomes the focus, interfaces between and among hospital services, and between these services and logistical services, become a primary concern.

- The specific way in which these aspects play out is a function of the kind of activity in the work unit and the role of the work unit in the organizational architecture of the hospital as a whole. But what becomes clear in this sort of analysis is that optimizing at the level of the work unit may mean suboptimizing at the level of the organization. Furthermore, if this architecture is highly decentralized, the link between the strategic apex and the work unit becomes modified. If the patient trajectory is the focus, intermediate levels of structure may be required to coordinate relations among work units or with other parts of the hospital structure. Similarly, because management of the patient trajectory is everyone's responsibility, an increasing amount of cross-functional interaction is required. This helps explain why both administrators and physicians sit on hospital quality committees and why we find directors of quality who are from the administrative component of the hospital. Nursing services are also represented. Physicians with managerial responsibility are in the thick of the action as well. So even if the results are not immediately evident, a new principle of multidisciplinary collaboration between professionals and administrators is emerging.

An Emerging Organizational Framework

The previous discussion suggests two alternative interpretations of the quality movement. In our attempt to be clear in our analysis, we have oversimplified things, particularly with respect to the chronological ordering in which we argued that the professional bureaucracy is being supplanted by a form of organization that places the patient trajectory at its center. The reality is more complex. The influence of the professional bureaucracy is still very strong in many establishments, and the newer form is still embryonic or consists mainly of slogans in many others. It stretches a point, therefore, to caricature the two as though they were both substantively and chronologically distinct, and our discussion presents a stylized version of the facts. But we do detect an evolution from a situation in which quality was translated and appropriated by logics unique to each category of actor in the hospital to one in which quality is seen as the responsibility of everyone and which is based on collective analysis of the patient trajectory.

Transversality, dysfunctions, and *cooperation* are all terms that have become part of the quality lexicon, and they have one thing in common. They all place the internal organization of hospitals at the center of analysis—improved quality is achieved through organizational change. A number of improvements have been made under this banner—better reception of patients, reorganization of the operating room, or improved dispensing of medicines—and their importance should not be underestimated. The hospital is nourished by these micro-innovations developed in daily work. But true quality management is more than this. The organization of work provides a framework for analysis that comprises all these improvements, but also includes more general considerations such as the system's rigidity and partitioning, the central position given to patients and their treatments, and the flows of information within the system. It is the integration of *all* these elements within a single framework that gives the focus on organization its added value. From this point of view, several benchmarks can be provided, with the help of theories and concepts from the management sciences.

To begin, we evoke a fundamental principle of management: an organizational response only has meaning in reference to an activity. Introducing more standardization or more autonomy does not have meaning in any absolute sense, but only in relation to the characteristics of an activity understood as a productive process. In this respect, taking care of patients can be characterized as a process in which the uniqueness of cases remains a basic datum. In order to symbolize this uniqueness, Corbin and Strauss (1988) speak of the patient trajectory. At the same time, these trajectories cannot be managed on a "craft" basis. Many patients are hospitalized simultaneously. Their length of stay also tends to be increasingly brief. The challenge confronting the modern hospital can best be described as that of mass customization, of managing uniqueness on a large scale (Minvielle, 1996).

This problem is not limited to hospitals and patient care. Many recent experiences in service industries and in manufacturing highlight the need to take aspects such as variety and responsiveness into account when developing production processes. Even if the determinants are different, studying the responses that were proposed is instructive. These responses disclose the rise to power of the notion of flexibility, a concept that is progressively becoming one of the major objectives of organizations in their experiments with higher levels of complexity.

The notion of flexibility must be understood here at the organizational level. Applying the principle of flexible organization in the context of the hospital implies two major orientations. First of all, the search for flexibility does not, perforce, contradict the need to maintain a certain degree of standardization. There is a tendency to invoke the Taylorist character of hospital organization when seeking to justify the need for greater flexibility in the work of professionals. This tendency both misinterprets the foundation of scientific management (Taylor, 1911) and introduces opposition precisely where the objective is to seek complementarity. Charns, Young, Daley, Khuri, and Henderson (2000), for example, have shown how the challenge of coordination is not to oppose "standardized procedures and control" versus "informal interactions and autonomy," but to know how to accommodate these two approaches in the same framework. The objective of flexible organization is therefore to find a balance between the development of standardization and programming on one hand and the development of autonomy and more informal practices on the other.

Second, this search for "flexibility" is played out in the context of an organization, which depends above all on the people within it. This fact has the effect of placing the concepts of know-how and organizational learning, both of which are highly people-dependent, at the core of the flexible organization (Nonaka, 1994; Argyris and Schön, 1978). As highlighted by Hatchuel and Weil (1992):

> [I]f the reduction of uncertainty or diversity is necessary, when they are there, there are not many alternatives to a sharing of know-how which enables each actor, not only to do what is asked of him, but also to be ready to respond to what has not been anticipated, and even better, to understand the consequences of this unforeseen event for his colleagues.

Several types of organizational know-how can thus be envisaged: the know-how associated with mastery of a task, the know-how associated with effective coordination of activities, the know-how associated with an effective response to unanticipated occurrences, the know-how associated with effective identification of organizational problems, and, finally, the know-how associated with effective empathy, which can be used by nursing staff in order to teach a patient how to be an actor in his or her own "trajectory." It is through their collective motivation that nursing professionals are able to engage effectively in an activity that lies outside any formal measures or explicit rules. The organizational framework emerging from these considerations constitutes the backdrop against which we develop a prospective view of the continued evolution of quality.

A Prospective Perspective on Incentives for Quality

Viewed prospectively, the search for quality presents, apart from any effects of ideas in vogue, the foundation for a new management philosophy. This new philosophy includes new forms of medical-administrative exchanges, new approaches to looking after patients, and even new forms of control. Understandably, this new philosophy begets numerous challenges at the organizational, managerial, methodological, and economic levels. Although each may require specific responses, they are also systemically connected. They are all parts of the same puzzle, and fit together along two axes. One axis is internal incentives. Improving quality depends both on practices of change management and on the use of reliable measurements. The other axis is external, and includes incentives geared toward using quality as a form of control.

Internal Incentives

There is, of course, no turnkey quality package that hospitals can buy in the marketplace—although myriad consulting firms would undoubtedly disagree. Rather, it is likely that many different experiments and experiences of the sort we describe elsewhere (Kimberly and Minvielle, 2000) will together create a foundation on which the next generation of quality initiatives will be built. There are no "quick fixes," and there will be continuing disillusionment as the various actors in the quality story realize that simply introducing the latest managerial innovation will not yield significant, lasting results (Jencks and Wilensky, 1992). Weaving quality into the fabric of organization requires a number of conditions: consensus on the diagnosis of problems, adaptation of approaches to management that have been successful in other settings to the idiosyncrasies of the hospital business, development of a sense of ownership on the part of those who are responsible for making the changes work, and investment in education and training for all concerned, to name only the most important. These factors together constitute a sort of point of departure for lasting organizational change and recall classical theories of change, elements of which have already been applied in the hospital sector and, more specifically, in efforts to introduce quality management (for example, Gillies and others, 2000). At the same time, there is a fundamental need to develop measures of quality in order to assess the impact of efforts that are undertaken.

Following this logic, the kind of organizational change required will be the development of measures of quality alongside new systems of relationships.

The Development of Measures of Quality

As disillusionment resulting from the relatively slow pace of change and relative lack of demonstrable results has proliferated, a certain skepticism about quality initiatives has emerged (Chassin, 1996). One way to counter this skepticism would be to develop empirical indicators of the impact of these initiatives. But, as we noted previously, a number of conditions are required for this to be possible. As Eddy (1998) has argued, a framework for attributing causality between actions undertaken to improve quality and measures themselves is absolutely essential. It is also essential that in associating actions and measurements a virtuous circle is created, one in which actions and measurements are mutually reinforced. Overemphasizing sanctions or controls linked to the measurement effort can be demotivating, particularly in the case of undesirable events (Grenier-Sennelier, Maillet-Gouret, Ribet-Reinhart, Jeny-Loeper, and Minvielle, 1998). This possibility is a reminder that every effort to measure performance has two facets, one that is prescriptive in nature and one that can lead to learning (Moisdon, 1997; Senge and Carstedt, 2001). Care needs to be taken to ensure that the weight given to prescription—in which decisions are made following better or worse results along with the assignment of responsibility—does not drive out or diminish the potential for learning from the measurement process. Finally, the development of routine measures of performance viewed from the perspective of the patient trajectory needs to be given high priority. Here much work needs to be done—the dimensions that should be included are clinical practices, coordination of care, and prevention of risk of infection, to name just a few. At the same time, experience suggests that there are a number of problems to be dealt with, including manageability, relevance, and validity of measures used. The ambition, however, ought to be to show that quality is no longer unmeasurable. Progress is, in fact, being made.

What Remains to be Done

Measuring quality assumes an ability *to circumscribe what needs to be included and to know how to array its various components*. This imperative may be surprising, given the number of books and articles that have been written on quality in health. Upon close examination, however, one finds multiple definitions of quality and various approaches to bounding the concept (Palmer, 1991). For example, the specificity of efforts to manage risk can lead to questions about whether risk management should be subsumed under the general heading of quality. On the other hand, measures of the utilization of resources—utilization review—are assimilated in measures of quality found in the National Library of Health Care Indicators.

In the same vein, if the classical distinction of the quality of structures, of processes, and of results is maintained, disentangling principles from which classification is possible can become quite complex. For example, waiting times are the result of a process; at the same time, they are something about which patients make judgments. Are waiting times then properly classified as an "objective" measure of quality or are they more properly classified as subjective measures, a function of how patients experience them?

These examples illustrate the numerous tradeoffs that are inevitably part of the evolving work on quality and that imperceptibly but measurably influence the character of that work. Together, the choices made influence the orientation given to the work and thus indirectly influence the actions taken by public authorities and professional bodies. By developing consensually validated measures of quality, the potential problem of appropriation by one group or another is reduced, although clearly not eliminated entirely. And while it is clear that the consumer's voice needs to be taken into account in efforts to measure quality, it is also clear that the subjective experience of the consumer is only one piece of the overall quality puzzle.

Improving the quality of the measurement tools is a second challenge. It is illusory to expect that the attributes of quality in health can ever be fully "instrumentalized," given their large number and the difficulty of measuring certain among them (Brook, McGlynn, and Cleary, 1996). Where measurement is possible, certain challenges need to be met. When an indicator is being constructed, the usual criteria of reproducibility, validity, reliability, context sensitivity, and flexibility need to be given priority. And when several indicators covering many dimensions of quality are being used together, other criteria such as their discriminant validity need to be used. It is also essential to be sensitive to the issue of causal inference among the measures and with respect to results. Particularly problematic are the relationships between measures of process and results. These are familiar problems to researchers, of course. We simply want to caution against relatively mindless approaches to measurement.

Once the measures are built, they need to be incorporated into the daily routines of the organizations they serve. The last phase, then, is one in which *initial experimentation is transformed into routine behavior*. Several factors will determine whether this transformation takes place successfully. First among these are cultural and managerial: the existence of opinion leaders among the health care professionals and in the management teams who can act as champions for the effort with their colleagues; the definition of a strategy for using the information generated; the incorporation of these efforts into the internal political agenda of the organization; and their reinforcement through the provision of appropriate incentives.

At the same time, many of the constraints will come from the way in which the collection and dissemination of data are managed. Experience has shown that what might appear to be technical factors actually pose delicate managerial challenges. The problem is not so much lack of relevant data in existing information systems, but rather how reliable the data are and how substantial are the costs to collect them on a regular basis. It is no exaggeration to say that these challenges have given birth to an entire industry in the United States, an industry whose export potential is significant.

The broad outlines of a prospective perspective on quality are thus discernible: objective rules for ranking, rigorous validation of measurement tools, and factors likely to lead to successful use on a routine basis. The path is not easy, and there are risks of failure. But the changes in mind-sets that are a prerequisite for success are already in evidence, so there is reason to be optimistic about internal incentives.

External Incentives

Whether it involves comparisons among health care organizations (a form of benchmarking), the allocation of resources, or planning based on indicators of the quality of patient care, there is a common concern: finding external incentives that take quality into account in the overall context of health policy. Current debates about quality in the context of managed care focus on how financial incentives on the insurance side may affect quality on the provider side. As insurers attempt to manage costs more strictly, quality, it is argued, may suffer. Berwick (1996), in fact, argued that payment mechanisms are only loosely coupled with quality. Quality is rarely seen as a criterion that might be used for resource allocation.

But what if it were? What if payment and quality were linked so that payment and improvements constituted a cycle with two distinct components—payment on the basis of a level of performance achieved and payment on the basis of corrective action taken to improve this level? There are obvious risks in moving in this direction. Introducing payment based on levels of quality might lead to gaming in the search for short-term results, with perverse effects arising from efforts to maximize payment in the short run (as in the case of DRGs). But this is not a reason not to go down this path. Payment weighted by quality represents the next logical phase in the evolution of how quality is taken into account in health care. As the recent Institute of Medicine report on quality suggests, "payment policies [must] be aligned to encourage and support quality improvement" (Hurtado, Swift, and Corrigan, 2001, p. 146). And as Coyle contends "Until payment policies reward quality improvement, providers will not place it at the core of their business strategy" (Coyle, 2001, p. 44).

By placing quality at the same level as efficiency or equity, its centrality in the structure and functioning of health care systems now and in the future is underscored. And as more experience is gained with managing quality as an organizational phenomenon, this idea will seem less and less radical.

Conclusion

Quality has become an important ingredient in the evaluation of health care systems, alongside cost and access. Efforts to assess and improve quality have led to an appreciation of its organizational character. And although quality and its dynamics are best understood historically as a reflection of the organization of the hospital as a professional bureaucracy, recent experience demonstrates that quality is, at least in part, a function of the modes of coordination developed and operative all the way along the patient trajectory.

There is an interesting interaction between efforts to measure and improve quality on the one hand and organization theory on the other. Among other things, organization theory brings to the analysis of quality an interpretation of the quality movement in two distinct phases. First, it highlights the influence of the organization of work on quality and underlines the significance of how information is collected and distributed within the hospital. Second, it emphasizes the interrelationship between the technical component of care and the clinical service component, and it calls attention to the link between professional expertise and organization in explaining variability in quality.

Efforts to measure and improve quality underline the importance for organization theory of the following:

- The patient (or product) trajectory and transversal relationships

- The way in which traditional forms of organization are being supplanted by new forms (for example, hospital versus network)

- The transition from weak forms of cooperation with a stronger sense of belonging (that is, forms that are hospital-based) to more robust forms of cooperation with a weaker sense of belonging and more ambiguous status differentials (such as forms that are network-based).

Although current efforts to measure and improve quality have the potential to change profoundly the way in which care is organized and delivered, the quality movement itself has not yet become fully institutionalized. When this happens, the search for quality can influence thinking across the entire spectrum of health, from the individual patient to policy at the level of national health systems. We believe that this search most likely will focus on three areas: how quality gets factored into the redefinition of performance at the hospital, network, and system levels; how quality improvement may be linked to payment; and what the role of prevention in the "production" of quality will be. Each of these represents opportunities for contributions from theory and from hands-on experience, and further interplay between theory and experience will undoubtedly continue to shape the evolution of the movement as a whole.

9

Trust

An Implicit Force in
Health Care Organization Theory

James L. Zazzali

A recent analysis of health care public opinion trends over the past several decades has demonstrated a decline in "the proportion of Americans reporting a great deal of confidence in the leaders of medicine," but that this decline " . . . has not affected Americans' high level of respect for practicing physicians" (Blendon and Benson, 2001, pp. 39–40). As for Americans' opinions of various types of health care organizations, results are mixed for hospitals, managed care companies, health insurance companies, and pharmaceutical companies, with hospitals coming out on top and managed care companies on the bottom. This evidence brings into question whether Americans trust their health care providers and the organizations that make up the various industries in the health sector. Further, many may be left wondering whether organizations in the health sector trust each other.

Unfortunately, there is a variety of reasons why consumer trust in health services organizations, leaders, and providers could falter, and why problems of trust between organizations may exist as well. There are reports about fraud and abuse on the part of health care organizations and providers; costs continue to spiral upward without concurrent increases in quality of care and service; new organizational forms that are unfamiliar to consumers (and, indeed, providers) are becoming more common; and the problems of the managed care industry, particularly with respect to access, continue to plague the sector. These factors, among others, have been associated with an increased level of attention being paid to trust by health services organizational researchers (Mechanic, 1998b). At the same time, this increased attention to trust has received consideration from mainstream organizational researchers (Bigley and Pearce, 1998; Rousseau, Sitkin, Burt, and Camerer, 1998; Sheppard and Sherman, 1998; Zucker, 1986), perhaps pointing to broader social phenomena of which the current manifestation in health services is only one part.

To see evidence of the increased level of attention being paid to trust, one need only turn to the literature, either in health services or within the nonsector-specific organizational journals. In 1994, there was a conference on the topic of trust from an organizational perspective at Stanford's Graduate School of Business; several books have been published on the topic in recent years (Annison and Wilford, 1998; Kramer and Tyler, 1996); in 1998 the Academy of Management Review devoted an entire issue to the topic; and individual articles about trust or related topics appeared at an increasing rate in the literature in the 1990s. For example, from 1990 to 1994, there were approximately 240 articles indexed in Medline, a computer-based bibliographical system, that contained the title word "trust," while there were approximately 690 from 1995 to mid-2002. However, in spite of this attention in the literature, it remains to be seen whether this topic will come to the fore as a major theoretical and empirical area of interest in the health sector or will merely be relegated to a secondary factor in the discussion of the various crises facing this sector.

This chapter has several goals with respect to examining the role of trust in health care organizational theory: (1) to understand what trust is and the various forms it may take; (2) to explicate how uncertainty in exchange relationships makes trust more desirable, yet can also make it more difficult to achieve; and (3) to describe how the failure of calculative and relational forms of trust in exchange relationships, particularly due to the role of uncertainty in these relationships, may be overcome by an influx of institutional forms of trust, an argument similar to that posed by Zucker (1986).

Definition of Trust

Trust has been an elusive term to define. Partial responsibility for the lack of a unified definition rests with the cacophony of voices that come from the many disciplines interested in trust, each cadre of social scientists equipped with its own glossary. Yet, this matter is complicated by the fact that trust is a multi- and interdisciplinary concept, with the discourse dominated by the intermingling voices from economic, psychological, and sociological perspectives. What is clear is that there are several different types of trust, and each discipline refers to them using distinct languages and terminologies that reflect the underlying beliefs about this concept, its functions, and its limitations. Furthermore, when examining trust, it is important to specify the level of analysis—whether one is referring to individuals trusting each other or organizations or to organizations trusting each other—as the level of analysis may inform the vocabulary used. Trust is not the only concept to suffer from the confusion that comes from a term being used in different ways by various social scientists. In the now classic collection of essays on neo-institutional organization theory (Powell and DiMaggio, 1991), there is a chapter dedicated to the terms *institution, institutional,* and *institutionalism,* as they have several meanings (Jepperson, 1991). Although at first this may appear to be a somewhat pedantic exercise, trust is such a concept in need of finer clarification.

It is not surprising then that there has been considerable effort over the past several years by organizational researchers to understand whether there is a common ground among these perspectives and to determine how sound the footing is. Some have taken on this task and argued that all definitions of trust encompass some sort of "willingness to be vulnerable" by a party engaged in an exchange (in other words, by the "trustor") (Rousseau, Sitkin, Burt, and

Camerer, 1998). Others have argued that this plurality of definitions is something that must be accepted, because the treatment of
trust should be expected to vary across particular situations. Further,
this group argues that limiting the definition of trust may result in
a meaningless construct that is difficult to operationalize across settings, or that trying to incorporate all perspectives into one's analysis of a particular situation would tax our limited cognitive abilities
(Bigley and Pearce, 1998). The "willingness to be vulnerable" seems
to accommodate many perspectives, but one should accept the
notion that discussions of trust should be grounded in the situa-
tional elements of the transactions that one is examining.

Interestingly, although there has been variation between many
social science perspectives on what trust is, there has been a fair
amount of agreement over what trust is with respect to how it
applies to the health sector. Perhaps this is due to the fact that many
of those writing about trust and health care come out of a sociological tradition. Many of the applications of trust to health care are
related to Zucker's (1986) notion of trust as a "set of expectations
shared by all those involved in an exchange" (p. 54) (although
Zucker was not specifically writing about health care).

In an application of trust to the case of the health sector,
Mechanic and Schlesinger (1996) propose a perspective similar to
Zucker's and state that trust "refers to the expectations of the public that those who serve them will perform their responsibilities in
a technically proficient way (competence), that they will assume
responsibility and not inappropriately defer to others (control), and
that they will make patients' welfare their highest priority (agency)"
(Mechanic and Schlesinger, 1996, p. 1693). Gray (1997) describes
how such "expectations" are present in the patient-physician relationship by stating that "Patients' willingness to accept medical
advice and services has rested on trust in physicians' technical competence and adherence to a fiduciary ethic that held that the physician's responsibility was to put the patient's interests above
self-interest" (p. 35). Other health services researchers develop sim-

ilar applications of trust in their work. Shortell, Waters, Clarke, and Budetti (1998) imply that historically physicians were thought to act in the best interests of their patients (that is, that physicians were good "agents" for their patients) and that this was needed because of the difference between the level of knowledge of patients and that of physicians as well as the degree of "psychological vulnerability" of patients. Sleeper, Wholey, Hamer, Schwartz, Inoferio, (1998) also imply a similar definition as to what trust is, and point to the same information asymmetries between patients and physicians. Thus, as it applies to the health sector, many see trust as being a set of expectations and often examine patients' expectations of their physicians.

Types of Trust

Many organizational theorists and researchers, writing about trust in general or about how it applies specifically to the health sector, use a variety of terms to define the different types of trust (see Table 9.1). In their search for a common ground, Rousseau, Sitkin, Burt, and Camerer (1998) outline four types of trust (one of which is a "straw man" and later discarded): deterrence-based trust, calculative trust, relational or affective trust, and institutional-based trust.

Deterrence-based trust, their straw man, enables "one party to believe that another will be trustworthy, because the costly sanctions in place for breach of trust exceed any potential benefits from opportunistic behavior" (p. 398). This would be analogous to the application of credible commitments and hostages from the transaction cost economics perspective (Williamson, 1983; 1984; 1996). Rousseau and colleagues ultimately reject deterrence-based trust as a form of trust because "[t]here is an apparent incompatibility between strict controls and positive expectations about the intentions of another party" (p. 399). Williamson (1996) also argues that one not refer to such sanctions as trust but rather as transaction-specific "safeguards." In fact, Williamson argues that the concept of

Table 9.1. Examples of Trust in the Social Sciences Literature.

Rousseau, Sitkin, Burt, and Camerer (1998)	Zucker (1986)	Williamson (1996)	Mechanic (1996)
Deterrence-based (costly sanctions)	Constitutive (tied to a particular sector or situation)	Calculativeness	Interpersonal
Calculative (reputation, certification)		Nearly Noncalculative or Personal	Social
Relational (repeated interactions)	Background Expectations (taken for granted)	Hyphenated or Institutional	
Institutional (social factors)			

trust not be used in reference to economic transactions: "Indeed, I maintain that trust is irrelevant to commercial exchange and the reference to trust in this connection promotes confusion" (p. 260). This type of "trust" has also been criticized for being "undersocialized" (Granovetter, 1985), for ignoring important social aspects of exchange relationships that others may consider sources of trust.

Calculative trust is based on "credible information" about the other party (that is, the "trustee"), often in the form of the other party's reputation or certification (Rousseau, Sitkin, Burt, and Camerer, 1998). Relational trust comes from "repeated interactions over time between trustor and trustee" and is related to the reliability of the trustee (Rousseau, Sitkin, Burt, and Camerer, 1998). Both calculative and relational trust are based on social interactions and are "constitutive" components of trust in Zucker's (1986) paradigm, in that they are related to a particular situation or sector. Furthermore, relational trust is analogous to Zucker's notion of "process" forms of trust production because it is tied to past exchanges or expectations. Institutional-based trust derives from both organizational and social factors, including organizational and societal norms, laws, and regulations, and would be a "background expectation" component of trust using Zucker's model. Within Rousseau and colleagues' topology, institutional-based trust may lead to calculative and relational trust (for example, if it is a norm that reputation matters, then reputation will matter).

Zucker (1986) is very much focused on this last form of trust and proposes an elaborate model outlining the development of social and organizational forms of institutional trust due to the deterioration of constitutive expectations of trust (in other words, calculative and relational trust) in American society. However, Granovetter (1985) has criticized institutional forms of trust as being "oversocialized," in that they place too much emphasis on the deterministic nature of social forces, whereas others have drawn attention to and criticized the control-like elements found in institutional trust (Rousseau, Sitkin, Burt, and Camerer, 1998; Shapiro, 1987).

To exemplify the tedious nature of how the notions of trust vary both across and within social science disciplines, one should consider that whether the described forms of trust actually constitute trust at all varies with the definition of trust that one employs. If one assumes that trust is a "willingness to be vulnerable," then all of the previously mentioned definitions are likely to be considered trust. However, if one assumes that trust is not only a willingness to be vulnerable but also relates to the "positive expectations of the intentions or behavior of another," as Rousseau, Sitkin, Burt, Camerer (1998) believe (and do many health services organizational researchers), then clearly one could see how deterrence-based trust would be discarded in favor of other forms.

Trust as an Implicit Force in Many Macro-Organizational Theories

Trust is generally thought to be relevant in exchange relationships or transactions, which is interesting because many of the major macro-organizational theories are also concerned with such relationships. However, trust does not figure prominently in these theories in a consistently overt fashion. Two transactional characteristics are relevant when examining the role of trust in such relationships: uncertainty and dependence-interdependence (Rousseau, Sitkin, Burt, and Camerer, 1998; Sheppard and Sherman, 1998). As the level of dependence-interdependence between transacting parties changes, the associated mechanisms of trust would also be expected to change (Sheppard and Sherman, 1998). Further, if all exchanges could be conducted under conditions of certainty, there would be no need for trust. Therefore, it is important to examine the level of dependence-interdependence between the parties who are engaged in exchange relationships and how uncertainty is present in such interactions. One might assert that the concepts of uncertainty and dependence-interdependence are what tie trust to the organizational theory literature, as these concepts figure prominently in agency theory (Eisenhardt, 1989; Jensen and Meckling, 1976), resource dependence theory (Pfeffer and Salancik, 1978), transaction cost economics (Williamson, 1996), and neo-institutional theorists' discussion of mimetic isomorphism under conditions of uncertainty (DiMaggio and Powell, 1991). However, as with many concepts that cut across multiple theoretical frameworks, the formulations of uncertainty and dependence-interdependence concerning trust do not necessarily coincide with previous treatments of these constructs in these theories of organization.

Agency theory, resource dependence theory, and transaction cost economics are, at a fundamental level, theories of exchange, and, to a certain extent, share a base set of principles or assumptions, particularly with respect to uncertainty. The sources of uncertainty in exchange relationships can be grouped into two categories. The first pertains to the potential for differing goals between transacting parties and recognizes that either party could act in its self-interest in trying to meet its own goals. These can also be described as goal incongruence and opportunistic behavior. The second set involves problems of information, in that each party may not have access to all of the information it needs and will not necessarily be able to process all of the information that it possesses accurately and reliably. These can be seen as information asymmetries and bounded rationality. Of course, these two sets can be related. For example, one party in an exchange may not share its goals or may misrepresent them, which presents an information asymmetry between the two parties, and in the case of misrepresentation, opportunism. In the following sections I present arguments that uncertainty can potentially be countered with some sources of trust, but also, paradoxically, can make some forms of trust more difficult to achieve.

It is important to note that the degree to which uncertainty and dependence-interdependence characterize exchange relationships in the health sector varies across the level of analysis to which one is referring. There are many types of parties engaging in health care transactions, and with the advent of relatively new organizational forms, transactions between some parties have only recently come into existence. There are transactions between patients and clinicians, between large purchasers of health care (such as employers, purchasing cooperatives, and the government) and health care organizations, between health care organizations and clinicians (either groups or individual clinicians) and others who work in these organizations, and between different types of health care organizations (such as HMOs, hospitals, pharmacies, laboratories, and radiology services). Much of the work on trust in the health sector has focused on the myriad relationships between patients, physicians, and managed care organizations. Agency theory has been particularly useful at more micro levels of analysis (in other words, patient-physician relations), although transaction cost economics and resource dependence theory are, perhaps, more applicable to the macro (that is, organizational) levels of analysis.

Opportunism and Goal Incongruence

Opportunistic behavior is prevalent in the health sector. On the demand side, patients have been found to engage in moral hazard when they consume health services (Manning and others, 1987). However, the public is often critical of managed care companies for their restrictions on coverage of benefits (Blendon and others, 1998), and managed care is often a target of distrust (Mechanic, 1997). On the supply side, there are reports of fraud or abuse on the part of individual providers or organizations. For example, individuals across the nation became aware of the controversial case of the dentist in Florida who had allegedly infected six of his patients with HIV. On a different but larger scale, the allegations that the then Columbia-HCA defrauded the federal government out of millions of dollars by filing fraudulent Medicare claims attracted much attention. Both of these cases were controversial, as the original evidence in the Florida case has been challenged (Barr, 1996), and in their settlement with the federal government, Columbia-HCA acknowledged no wrongdoing (Taylor, 2000).

The pharmaceutical industry has also come under attack for the rates at which firms provide access to new and experimental drugs and the price of brand-name medications. With regard to the price of anti-HIV medications in developing nations, Merck and what was Glaxo-Wellcome had been widely criticized for their previous pricing policies and had come under enormous pressure to lower the prices of these medications in developing markets. As a result, in the year 2001, Merck announced that it would cut the price of such medications 90 percent in these markets ("AIDS Drugs for Poor Nations," 2001). The widespread media attention that these examples have drawn points to the fact that the public is often acutely aware of the opportunistic behavior present in the health sector, particularly on the supply side. These examples would certainly be related to the problems of calculative and relational trust for those who interact with these entities.

Goal incongruence is another problem that permeates the health care industry, and is certainly linked to opportunistic behavior. Goal incongruence may be related to the degree to which each party is risk adverse, in that there could be potential differences in risk aversion between parties engaged in an exchange. On the other hand, it could be attributed to the multiplicity of organizational goals, as organizations are seen as having multiple and complex goals (Scott, 1992). Furthermore, the myriad principle-agent relationships that exist in the health sector add an additional dimension of complexity when one considers goal incongruence. For example, in the physician-patient relationship, the patient can be conceptualized as the principal and the physician as the agent (Eisenberg, 1986), and the broad goals of the patients and physicians overlap: patients want to get better and physicians want to heal. But there are additional goals of the physicians that the patients do not share, namely the physicians' interest in financial gains. Due to the advent of managed care and the decline of the fee-for-service market for many health services, these relationships have changed. Patients have largely been displaced or joined in their role as principal by their employers, for the employers are often negotiating contracts with health services organizations such as HMOs. Some argue that employers may instead be acting as agents for their employees (McLaughlin, 2001). Furthermore, the agency role of physicians has been complicated by the fact that they often occupy a second agency role for the health care organizations with which the employers are contracting (that is, physicians as so-called "double agents") (Shortell, Waters, Clarke, and Budetti, 1998). One could say that physicians have either been displaced or been joined in their role as agents by the health care organizations with which the employers are contracting.

This intrusion of organizations into the traditional principal-agent relationship between patients and physicians is complicated by the fact that this relatively new principal-agent relationship between health care organizations and physicians may be at odds with the goals of the patients (Mechanic and Schlesinger, 1996). Health care organizations that employ or contract with physicians are faced with the issue of how to structure these kinds of contracts. This can be seen as a problem of incentive alignment: what kinds of incentives do the health care organizations need to give the physicians to ensure that the physicians will behave "appropriately?" "Appropriate" behavior may mean delivering the best quality of care, or it may mean controlling costs, or both. Searching for the proper compensation packages for physicians (that is, for how to construct the right incentives for them to provide high quality of care at low costs) has been a challenging task (Robinson, 2001), with one author aptly commenting that it is "akin to the quest for baby bear's porridge in trying to get it just right" (Ogrod, 1997). Physician compensation arrangements are important because they have been found to be related to patients' trust in their physicians (Kao, Green, Zaslavsky, Koplan, and Cleary, 1998). Again, these sources of uncertainty make some forms of trust harder to achieve.

These are not the only principal-agent relationships of interest when considering goal incongruence. On a more macro level, large purchasers of health care also struggle with the question of how to structure the incentives of the health insurance companies they are contracting with to ensure that the insurers are "behaving appropriately." Employers, who negotiate the health insurance benefits for their employees, may want to minimize their share of the premiums while simultaneously obtaining high-quality services for their employees. Providers, such as large health plans, are faced with the challenge of creating value for the purchasers of their services (in other words, increasing the quality without inordinate increases in costs). For-profit organizations must meet the needs of the stockholders, which has prompted some to point out that, in the case of HMOs, those that are nonprofit may have an advantage over the for-profit organizations due to a lack of conflicting goals and interests between those who own the organization and those who purchase and consume its services (Lawrence, Mattingly, and Ludden,

1997), although the positive reputation effects of being a nonprofit HMO have yet to be fully realized (that is, calculative trust has not been established to its full potential).

Goal incongruence between patients and managed care organizations may be most visible when one considers the issue of access to care. Many Americans are not always satisfied with the limited access they have to certain procedures and technologies, and, perhaps more important, the lessening of a choice of physicians that they have been accustomed to over their lifetimes. It is not only the patients' goals and those of the managed care organizations that may be in conflict, as the problem also manifests itself with respect to those who work in the industry as well. Many physicians and physician groups are at odds with various organizational entities and have begun to unionize as a response to the challenges they face (Ellison, 2000).

Information Asymmetries and Bounded Rationality

The problems of information asymmetries and bounded rationality are numerous, and add an additional layer of uncertainty to exchange relationships. Clearly, the professionalization of those who provide health services provides for a major information asymmetry between patients and clinicians, as the professionals control a specialized body of knowledge that patients cannot access (although this is changing as patients become more informed). Furthermore, health care professionals are being challenged by the fact that they often do not have the actuarial abilities found in the large organizations with which they contract, and face difficulties deducing whether the "deal" contained in the contract they are being offered is a good one.

Similarly, both consumers and providers are faced with an incredibly daunting and complex public and private health care system in the United States. There are no standard benefits across health plans, laws governing the sector exist at both national and local levels and vary from state to state, benefits for public programs such as Medicaid vary from state to state, there is a diversity of clinicians who provide care, there is a diversity of organizational forms, and historically there have been far too few sound ways to judge the quality of the services that are being purchased or consumed. Even those individuals who study and teach classes in health services administration are often left in awe of the multiplicity of professional and organizational arrangements. These complexities have played an important role in the perpetuation of uncertainty in the exchanges in this sector.

Time is also a factor with respect to bounded rationality and information asymmetries. Time is important because time elapses between when a service is paid for, when one receives the service, and when one is able to judge the quality of the service. Consumers and purchasers expect that the providers will deliver a product or service according to certain specifications, making quality a factor. Unlike in the sale of a product, in the sale of a service the quality of the service often cannot be assessed until after it has been delivered. Products can be tested before a sale is made; however, a service cannot be judged in such a manner, and there is usually more variation in services than in products. In the health sector, this temporal factor in judging the quality of a service is complicated by how long one must wait until one judges the service. For example, if one chooses to judge the quality of care that a hospital delivers by looking at morbidity and mortality statistics, one must decide when to assess morbidity and mortality. At discharge? One month post-discharge? Two months? This challenge with assessing the quality of a product or service would certainly make calculative trust more difficult to achieve because of the bounded rationality of the consumers and the information asymmetries between the "experts" and the consumers as to the appropriate time period for making such an assessment.

The exchange relationships found in the health sector are complicated by these factors: a variety of principal-agent relationships; opportunistic behavior; poor information and limitations on the information-processing capabilities of the various parties; and the multiple, complex, and often competing goals of the organizations and parties that constitute and interact within this sector. These factors are important when examining trust in the health sector because they are quite prevalent. Taken either together or separately, not only do they account for increased levels of uncertainty in these relationships, but, as some have argued, they also account for the "erosion of trust" between patients, clinicians, and health services organizations (Mechanic, 1996). This is particularly true with respect to calculative and relational forms of trust. Furthermore, the agency and transaction costs may increase due to the uncertainty in these exchange relationships. However, the role of trust in principle-agent relationships and transactions in general is paramount, in that it has the opportunity to decrease the agency or transaction costs. Thus we are faced with somewhat of a paradox: uncertainty in exchange relationships may make some forms of trust harder to achieve, but also makes trust more desirable, in that trust not only may mitigate uncertainty but may also decrease the agency and transaction costs for those involved.

Interorganizational Linkages as Trust-Building and Trust-Deteriorating Mechanisms

Resource dependence theory (RDT) and transaction cost economics (TCE) are both concerned with exchange relationships and the formation of interorganizational structures. In the case of RDT, theorists study how organizations can increase the probability of obtaining vital resources; in the case of TCE, how organizations govern their transactions to decrease transaction costs. Theories of interorganizational linkages, such as RDT and TCE, are very much about trust. For example, mergers may be seen as a way of dealing with exchange relationships in which trust has proven to be problematic. Resource dependence theorists explain the development of interorganizational relationships such as joint ventures, cartels, and interlocking directorates as a way for organizations to ensure the attainment of vital and scarce resources and to minimize the control of external organizations over them (Pfeffer and Salancik, 1978). What is implied and left largely unsaid is that such arrangements may also facilitate trust between these organizations.

In the case of vertical integration, Zucker (1986) indicated this in her early work on trust: "When trust has been disrupted, vertical integration is one way of producing it" (p. 93). This may be true for the organizations engaged in exchanges, as within the typology developed previously one can see how vertical integration may solve some of the problems of uncertainty at the organizational level and potentially decrease agency and transactions costs, although this is certainly open to empirical assessment. However, in the case of the health sector, this may not hold for the patient or consumer of the services of such organizations. In fact, the increased levels of vertical integration have created new organizational arrangements and forms that are often foreign to patients, and, ironically, may lead to a deterioration of trust between the patients and these organizations or the health care providers who are affiliated with them. Thus organizational arrangements meant to build trust at one level of exchange may concurrently raise issues of trust on another. Without trust, exchanges among these parties are likely to be costly for some of those involved because they either will have to engage in increased levels of monitoring, haggling, or enforcement to ensure that the agent is acting appropriately, or potentially accept the outcomes of opportunistic behavior.

Legitimacy Building as Trust Building

Neo-institutional theory may provide a way of understanding some methods for dealing with the current problems of trust in the health sector. Many of the proposed solutions to the dilemmas we now face with respect to the problems of trust in these exchange relationships (that is, trust-building exercises on the part of health services organizations) can be seen as attempts at legitimacy building. Zucker (1986) formulated a rather compelling thesis that changing social conditions led to decreases in the forms of trust that previously had existed and permeated exchange relationships ("process" and "characteristic" forms of trust), and that this void was filled by increases in "institutional" sources of trust. We are currently at a point in history in which there may indeed be another void forming. Zucker (1986) also claimed to have "no hidden structural/functional agenda," meaning that she did not believe that "disruption of trust automatically leads to its replacement" (p. 54). If one rejects structural functionalism, then it is possible that nothing would fill the void as current forms of trust are eroded. If, however, one does believe that something will fill the void, structural functionalist or not, then the question is: what follows?

Some have argued that health services organizations, particularly managed care organizations (MCOs), are actively engaging in trust-building exercises (Mechanic, 1998c; Mechanic and Rosenthal, 1999). In their study, Mechanic and Rosenthal (1999) report that the top three "trust building" exercises reported by MCOs were specific efforts to improve patient satisfaction (reported by 94 percent of respondents); use of focus groups to ascertain public or client concerns (79 percent); and mediation for dispute resolution (75 percent). Whether these actions alone would constitute building calculative and relational trust between MCOs and the patients they serve is open to debate. However, as these organizational behaviors become institutionalized as norms among MCOs, it may be that these organizations will gain legitimacy by adhering to such norms (Meyer and Rowan, 1977). Therefore, organizations could potentially gain legitimacy by measuring patient satisfaction, even if such activities were actually "decoupled" from the "technical core" of the organization.

Strong arguments have been made that the legitimacy-seeking behaviors of MCOs is an indicator of their "trustworthiness" (Flood, 1998; Sleeper, Wholey, Hamer, Schwartz, and Inoferio, 1998), thus pointing to the importance of institutional-based trust in addressing some of the challenges facing MCOs. Simply put, health care organizations and those who work for and in them can potentially gain legitimacy and build institutional trust by adhering to the prevailing norms and expectations that govern organizational behavior. To expand upon this point, consider the quality-of-care assessment movement and how it exemplifies the potential importance of institutional-based trust for the health sector. Certainly calculative trust is important, as reputation effects and certification of the trustee are ways of mitigating some of the possibilities for opportunistic behavior and serve as what I would call "entry level" markers of quality: HMOs and hospitals are accredited and professionals are licensed and board certified. Elements of relational trust clearly exist in health care as well, as patients are more likely to go back to clinicians with whom they have experienced a good outcome. However, the effects of reputation and entry-level indicators such as accreditation and certification are limited, and the ability of patients to judge adequately the technical clinical quality of care that a particular organization or provider delivers is likely to be weak at best. Even with these elements of calculative and relational trust in place, it is questionable whether they really operate to any effective degree. One could argue that they are not enough to guarantee that the quality of care and service will meet the needs of the patients. This parallels the situation described by Zucker (1986) with respect to the failure of constitutive expectations of trust (in other words, calculative and relational trust).

Zucker argued that in the period of 1840 through 1920 institutional forms of trust surfaced and buttressed the various exchange relationships in American society, and ultimately, calculative and relational forms of trust. The question then becomes whether we will observe the same phenomenon in the health sector. Will the failure or inadequacy of calculative and relational forms of trust be supplanted by institutional forms of trust? Or will we abandon trust altogether and rely on deterrence-based mechanisms in these exchanges (as per Williamson)? To a certain extent we have seen a situation parallel to the one described by Zucker. A cadre of professionals are equipped with the expertise for evaluating the quality of various health services organizations, and the activities of these professionals are starting to become institutionalized. This is not too dissimilar from the development of and expansion in the use of civil servants that Zucker described. For example, the National Committee for Quality Assurance (NCQA) has developed the Health Plan Employer Data and Information Set (HEDIS), which allows for a rather sophisticated organizational assessment of MCOs. Such assessments can be used to compile "report cards," comparing MCOs across various dimensions of performance measures, and these report cards clearly mitigate some of the information-processing limitations of the purchasers and consumers of health services. As such practices become more widespread and institutionalized, this may allow for calculative and relational trust to resurface. Other forms of institutional-based trust include new laws and regulatory actions that govern the behavior of health services organizations. The "Patients' Bill of Rights" and the host of condition-specific measures mandating certain benefits (for example, actions against so-called "drive-through deliveries") are specific examples, although some see such interventions as "substitutes" for trust, not as forms of institutional trust (Mechanic, 1998a).

Conclusion

The topic of trust has received increasing attention in recent years, both within and outside of the health services literature. There is a fair amount of variation in the nomenclature used to describe trust. Much of this variation stems from the multi- and interdisciplinary attention given to this concept, resulting in different types of social scientists using their respective lexicons to describe seemingly similar concepts. However, part of the confusion also stems from the fact that the concept of trust operates at different levels of analysis, with different sets of actors. Many perspectives reflect the notion that trust is indicative of the trustor's "willingness to be vulnerable" (Rousseau, Sitkin, Burt, and Camerer, 1998). The health services organizational literature has coalesced around a definition encompassing the notion that trust involves sets of expectations, often pertaining to patients' expectations of physicians or health services organizations.

Dependence-interdependence and uncertainty categorize the relationship between the trustor and the trustee, and sources of uncertainty include opportunism on the part of the trustee, the bounded rationality of the trustor, and goal incongruities and information asymmetries between the two. In the health sector, the myriad principle-agent relationships that exist add an additional layer of complexity in understanding how trust operates in this sector. Paradoxically, the same factors that some forms of trust may mitigate, thereby reducing the agency and transaction costs of exchanges, may also make the achievement of other forms of trust more difficult. In an era in which calculative and relational forms of trust have been "eroded," institutional forms of trust may be likely to arise.

10

Health Care Organizations as
Complex Adaptive Systems

James W. Begun, Brenda Zimmerman,
and Kevin J. Dooley

It is not surprising that the word "system" slips easily into the vernacular of those working in and studying health care organizations, in statements such as "local health care systems are the forerunners of regional systems," "the U.S. health care system is in crisis," or "health systems are consolidating and integrating." Although many types of "systems" exist, people most commonly invoke the "machine" metaphor when thinking about organizational systems (Morgan, 1997). It is appealing to think of health care organizations, singly and in concert, as receiving inputs, transforming them, and producing outputs, such as improved health. This machine metaphor leads to a belief about how the "system" can be studied: examine its parts separately and understand their mechanics. The machine metaphor also leads to beliefs about how the "system" can be improved: if the system is not working as planned, then identify the broken part and replace it. If the system is too costly, then work toward economies of scale. If the system is not working in a coordinated fashion, then tighten the interconnections between parts of the system.

Any model of an organization or an organizational system is in fact an approximation, a simplification of reality. Yet these models are of utmost importance as they shape the way people believe the system works and hence constrain the possible ways people think that research can be conducted and that the system can be improved. For example, in light of increasing pressures to cut costs, health care organizations have engaged in a flurry of activity involving mergers, acquisitions, and other forms of structural change. Economies of scales are invoked as input demands are spread over a smaller base of overhead and fixed costs. Using the machine metaphor, the belief is that one can increase the "input" stream without having to increase the size of the machine proportionally.

Yet thinking of and operating organizational systems as machines have not led to effective organizational research and practice. For example, researchers and commentators both conclude that "[i]ntegrated delivery systems clearly have not performed up to our expectations" (Johnson, 2000, p. 4); and "[c]ontrolling health care costs continues to perplex providers, as payers exert pressure and new models seem less promising" (Anonymous, 1999). These sentiments are frequently echoed in the arenas of quality improvement, patient safety, and access to care. Linkage, coordination, standardization, rationalization, and vertical and horizontal integration have failed to advance health care delivery to acceptable levels of satisfaction for both internal and external stakeholders. The health care "system" continues to defy control—it is a "machine" that appears to have a mind of its own.

We argue that improvement of health care organizations individually and collectively, and research on those organizations, will be best facilitated by comprehensive application of the metaphor of the system as a living organism, rather than that of the system as a machine. Such a metaphor is conveyed by the science of complex adaptive systems (CASs), which reformulates systems theory in a way that produces a "model" of the organization more closely related to reality. Whereas traditional systems theory (for example, Senge, 1990) has its roots in explaining the behavior of "dead" systems (complicated electromechanical systems), complex systems science is concerned with explaining how "living" systems work. This offers a transformational leap from the crude understanding of systems that developed in the 1960s and formed the basis of a science of organizational systems. The messy, open systems of complexity science are immensely different from the closed, well-behaved systems that were the original focus of systems science. Although health care organizations have continued to apply systems science of the 1960s and 1970s, systems science has made transformational changes in its understanding of systems. These new insights have yet to be reflected substantially in the practice of health care organizations and the research activities of those studying health care organizations.

In this chapter, we outline the development of complexity science and its major precepts as they apply to organizations. We discuss areas of application to health care, focusing attention on managing complicated relationships among organizations and the stimulation of change and innovation. The goal of this chapter is to describe what it means to conceptualize health care organizations (and aggregates of organizations) as complex adaptive systems, rather than as traditional "dead" systems. Implications for researchers are emphasized.

Complex Adaptive Systems

Complex adaptive systems are omnipresent. Examples include stock markets, human bodies, organs and cells, trees, and hospitals. *Complex* implies diversity—a wide variety of elements. *Adaptive* suggests the capacity to alter or change—the ability to learn from experience. A *system* is a set of connected or interdependent things. In a CAS, the "things" are independent agents. An agent may be a person, a molecule, or a species or an organization, among many other things. These agents' actions are based on local or surrounding knowledge and conditions. A central body, master neuron, or CEO does not control the agent's individual moves. A CAS has a densely connected web of interacting agents, each operating from its own schema or local knowledge.

All CASs share some features. We describe four that are relevant to organizational theory applications. CASs are dynamic, massively entangled, emergent, and robust (Eoyang and Berkas, 1999; Marion and Bacon, 2000).

First, CASs are characterized by their dynamic state. The large number of agents in the CAS, the connections among the agents, and the influence of external forces all combine to result in constant and discontinuous change in the CAS.

Second, relationships in CASs are complicated and enmeshed, or highly entangled. Many CASs are composed of large numbers of interdependent parts and influenced by a large number of interdependent forces. In addition to being numerous and interdependent, parts and variables, and their relationships, can be nonlinear and discontinuous. Small changes in variables can have small impacts at some times, and large impacts under other conditions. Conversely, the effects of large changes in variables can vary from negligible to large, depending on the state of other variables.

In their interactions, the agents of a CAS both alter other agents and are altered by other agents. Feedback loops among agents can generate change or stability in the system, depending on the relationships among the agents. In the case of feedback loops that generate change, two systems that initially are quite similar may develop significant differences over time. Even the same system, after the passage of time, may bear little resemblance to its previous configuration. Because the context for each CAS is unique, and each CAS is context-dependent, each CAS is unique.

Third, CASs exhibit emergent, or self-organizing behavior. As stated by Marion and Bacon (2000, p. 75):

> [C]omplexly structured, non-additive behavior emerges
> out of interactive networks. . . . [I]nteractive agents unite
> in an ordered state of sorts, and the behavior of the re-
> sulting whole is more than the sum of individual behav-
> iors. Ordered states . . . [arise] . . . when a unit adapts its

individual behaviors to accommodate the behaviors of units with which it interacts. Poincare observed this phenomenon mathematically among colliding particles, which impart some of their resonance to each other, leading to a degree of synchronized resonance. Interacting people and organizations tend similarly to adjust their behaviors and worldviews to accommodate others with whom they interact. Networks with complex chains of interaction allow large systems to correlate, or self-order.

Applied to human systems, these findings will be quite familiar to sociologists and social psychologists. Humans adjust their interaction based on characteristics of the other parties to the interaction. Extensive communication among large networks of humans can create self-ordering structures, such as norms, and spread them.

Fourth, a CAS may be sensitive to certain small changes in initial conditions. An apparently trivial difference in the beginning state of the system may result in enormously different outcomes. This phenomenon is sometimes called the "butterfly effect," based on the metaphor derived by meteorologist Edward Lorenz that a difference as seemingly insignificant as a butterfly flapping its wings in Brazil can change the predicted weather in Texas from a sunny day to a tornado. However, this sensitivity has to do with the exact path that the complex system follows into the future, rather than its general pattern. CASs, including the weather, tend to maintain generally bounded behavior, regardless of small changes in initial conditions. The paths of such systems are sometimes described as attractors.

As a result, CASs are robust, or fit. They exhibit the ability to alter themselves in response to feedback. Complex systems possess a range of coupling patterns, from tight to loose (Marion and Bacon, 2000). These different patterns help organizations survive a variety of environmental conditions. Loosely coupled structures cushion and moderate response to strong shock. More tightly coupled structures tend to identify and implement quickly to a response. Although adaptive in the moment, such a response may turn maladaptive as the environment shifts. As a whole, the complex structures provide multiple and creative paths for action. If one pattern of interdependency in a network is disrupted, other units can respond due to their interdependence with the disrupted unit. Robust response means that the complex system can effectively adapt to a wide range of environmental changes, giving it "amazing resilience" (Marion and Bacon, 2000).

Growth of Complexity Science

Complexity science, the study of complex adaptive systems, does not consist of a single theory but rather encompasses a collective of theories and constructs that have conceptual integrity among themselves. Complexity science is highly multi- and interdisciplinary, and its proponents include biologists, chemists, anthropologists, economists, sociologists, physicists, and many others in a quest to answer some fundamental questions about living, changeable systems.

Social scientists came to know about and be interested in complexity through a variety of avenues. Perhaps the most important early event was the formulation of chaos theory (Gleick, 1987). Chaos theory presented two propositions that were attractive to social scientists:

- Small, seemingly inconsequential events, perturbations, or changes can potentially lead to profound, large scale change

- That which appears to be random may in fact have an underlying orderliness to it

In addition, the word *chaos* itself was something that in a vernacular sense resonated with current reality.

Organization scholars, and in particular organizational change and development researchers, became interested in how chaos explained the way in which organizations changed, or more important, how they could be changed, using concepts such as self-organization, emergence, and bifurcation (Prigogine and Stengers, 1984). Whereas the concept of chaos had its roots in physics, concepts of self-organization and emergence drew more from the living sciences of biology and chemistry. Much intellectual focus was switched away from chaos, which described a particular type of behavior found in complex systems, to the more basic question of how such complex systems work in the first place. Complexity science today includes contributions from the theoretical areas of artificial intelligence and agent-based systems (for example, Axelrod and Cohen, 1999), game theory, evolutionary theory (especially neo-Darwinist ideas, including punctuated equilibrium), cellular automata, and computational biology. Books by Waldrop (1992) and Lewin (1992), both titled *Complexity*, solidified this disciplinary hodgepodge under a single semantic umbrella. The biologist and physician Stuart A. Kauffman's (1993; 1995) work provided much of the theoretical basis for the "adaptive" component of complex adaptive systems.

Table 10.1 summarizes some key, broad differences between complexity science and the science of linear, stable systems. Complexity science emphasizes indeterminism rather than determinism, variation rather than averages, and local control rather than global control. Nonlinear rather than linear relationships are the norm, and a metaphor of "morphogenesis" is preferred to a metaphor of "assembly."

The natural and physical science foundations of complexity science produce both strengths and weaknesses for organizational researchers (Begun, 1994), and the diffusion of complexity science into academic research is occurring at a slow rate. One reason for the slow diffusion of complexity science is the fact that it exists

Table 10.1. Complexity Science Versus Established Science.

Complexity Science	Established Science
Holism	Reductionism
Indeterminism	Determinism
Relationships among entities	Discrete entities

Nonlinear relationships
  critical mass thresholds
	Linear relationships
	  marginal increases

Quantum physics
  influence through iterative
    nonlinear feedback
  expect novel and probabilistic world
	Newtonian physics
	  influence as direct result of force
	    from one object to another
	  expect predictable world

Understanding; sensitivity analysis	Prediction
Focus on variation	Focus on averages
Local control	Global control
Behavior emerges from bottom up	Behavior specified from top down
Metaphor of morphogenesis	Metaphor of assembly

Source: Adapted from Dent, 1999, Table 1.

among, not within, traditional scientific disciplines. Academics accustomed to functioning with bounded theories within bounded disciplines resist embracing new cross-disciplinary perspectives, as has been the case throughout the history of science (Kuhn, 1962). The mathematical elegance and sophistication of much of physical science research is a problem for some social scientists, either because of philosophical differences (social systems cannot be modeled, physical systems can) or because of a lack of training in the methods, leading to an inability to trust or interpret the material. The natural science foundations are a source of attraction for others, particularly those with biological backgrounds, including clinicians, who may be more comfortable extrapolating from natural science. Many of the applications of complexity science to social systems are metaphorical, again a source of attraction to some and aversion for others.

Another reason for slow diffusion is that complexity science is relatively new and is still struggling for legitimacy and institutionalization. Appropriate questions about its relevance to human organizational systems, as opposed to biological and physical systems, remain. As with any body of new ideas, there is a danger that complexity science will be overgeneralized, overextended, exploited, and abused by those enamored of everything new. Certainly this process is under way with complexity science and organizations (Maguire and McKelvey, 1999), and it is important to recognize and thwart those tendencies. Goldstein (2000), for example, notes how a "bias for believing that self-organization and emergence are nothing but advantageous for a complex system can be seen in organizational applications," including his own. Atchison (1999, p. 50), commenting on the interpretation of change processes in health care from a complexity perspective, expresses concern about "the current enthusiasm of anything labeled 'complexity science.'" Underneath the hype, however, is a signification and permanent leap in scientific knowledge anchored in the physical and natural sciences.

Applications of Complexity Science to Health Care Organizations

Social phenomena, including organizations, became the subject of investigations using methods and metaphors from chaos and complexity theory early in the 1990s (Eve, Horsfall, and Lee, 1997; Goldstein, 1994; Kiel and Elliott, 1997; Priesmeyer, 1992; Stacey, 1992; Wheatley, 1992). A growing number of researchers continued to explore extensions of complexity science to the study of organizations, signaled by special issues of the journals *Complexity* (in 1998) and *Organization Science* (in 1999), and by the new journal *Emergence* (new in 1999), which is solely dedicated to organizational applications. Applications of complexity science to organizational processes such as change and innovation are becoming more common in mainstream outlets as well (for example, Lichtenstein, 2000;

Van de Ven, Polley, Garud, and Venkataraman, 1999). Also, a large number of books purporting to establish business advantage to those organizations that adopt complexity approaches have appeared (for example, Lewin and Regine, 2000; Kelly and Allison, 1999). The business models inspired by complexity science generally consist of simulations or agent-based models ("agents" are the central actors in abstract models of CASs) using such tools as genetic algorithms and artificial neural networks to address production-scheduling issues, predict complex outcomes (such as financial market movements), and explore advanced artificial intelligence applications (Wakefield, 2001).

Comprehensive reviews of organizational applications and extensions, both theoretical and empirical, of complexity science are available elsewhere (Anderson, 1999; Lissak, 1999; Marion, 1999; Stacey, 1999). Extensions of complexity science to health care organizational theory began to emerge in the scholarly literature in the mid-1990s. A series in quality management in health care, for example, examined clinical pathways as nonlinear, evolving systems, and provided associated tools (Sharp and Priesmeyer, 1995; Priesmeyer and Sharp, 1995; Priesmeyer, Sharp, Wammack, and Mabrey, 1996). Marion and Bacon (2000) used complexity science to interpret the fitness of three eldercare organizations, emphasizing the larger networks in which the organizations were embedded. Begun and Luke (2001) analyzed organizational arrangements in local health care markets in 1995 as a function of initial conditions in local systems at the precipice of change in the early 1980s. Arndt and Bigelow (2000) speculated on potential applications of complexity science in health management research. Dooley and Plsek (2001) used models of complex natural processes to interpret the generation of medication errors in hospitals and concluded that the recommendations embedded in the Institute of Medicine report (Kohn, Corrigan, and Donaldson, 2000) do not go nearly far enough in terms of their ability to generate significant organizational learning and thus improvement. Begun and White

(1999) extended the metaphor of complex adaptive systems to the nursing profession, noting particularly its inertial patterns and resistance to change.

Contemplating the implications of complexity science for the practice of health care management and leadership, Zimmerman, Lindberg, and Plsek (1998) contributed a primer on complexity science, with nine management principles for leadership and management in health care organizations. McDaniel (1997) and McDaniel and Driebe (2001) construed the leadership imperatives of health care executives from the perspectives of quantum and chaos theory, and applied complexity science to the process of management in health care delivery.

In sum, over the past decade the literature demonstrates a diffusion of complexity science applications, from social systems in general, to organizational systems, and now to health care organizations. It can be expected that such applications to health care will continue to draw increased attention as more researchers are exposed to the science. To help develop such efforts, we next explore how complexity researchers might approach two specific research topics in health care management.

Key Differences Between a Complexity Science Perspective and Established Perspectives

In this section we identify key differences between established theoretical perspectives commonly used in health management research and the complexity science perspective. Established perspectives in health care organization research include those that commonly are found in textbooks, are taught in doctoral programs in health administration, and are used commonly in the health care management research literature. A partial laundry list would include the following: resource dependence, transaction cost, agency, structural contingency, population ecology, institutional, and the "hybrid" strategic management perspective. The established perspectives share a number of common traits, summarized in Table 10.2. Due to some variation within the established perspectives, in Table 10.2 we restrict judgments about such differences to three established theories: structural contingency, transaction cost, and institutional theory. These three theories have been used in a recent journal issue to characterize the nature of change in health care organizations and markets (Stiles, Mick, and Wise, 2001; Wells, 2001; Young, Parker, and Charns, 2001).

First, we examine the time orientation of the perspectives. Established theories are based on a view of the future as relatively knowable. Researchers should be able to specify models that allow for reasonable prediction. The complexity perspective assumes the converse, that the future is relatively unknowable. Emergent properties cannot be predicted from a system's individual parts due to the multiple nonlinear interactions and feedback loops among the parts. Historical patterns are an acute source of information in some established perspectives, particularly institutional theory, wherein the role of history is to inform the future. Other established theories, particularly those derived from economics, are largely ahistorical. Complexity science validates the relevance of history to the state of every existing system, although the degree to which systems are history-dependent can vary from none to extensive. Importantly, the high relevance of history in the complexity perspective does not remove the expectation that novelty, and transformational change, can emerge in a CAS at any given time. History is highly relevant, but not necessarily deterministic. This, again, reinforces the irrelevance of the prediction of details, or paths (versus patterns), as a goal of research on CASs.

Second, the CAS perspective entails different assumptions about the unit and levels of analysis (spatial framing). Established perspectives typically identify an organization, which we label a "reified organization," as the domain of study. Reification involves the assignment of material reality to an abstract concept. The assumption that the legal entity known as an organization is the most useful unit of

Table 10.2. Comparison of Established Perspectives and the Complexity Science Perspective.

	Established Perspectives	Complexity Science Perspective
Temporal Framing		
View of the Future	Relatively knowable	Relatively unknowable
Relevance of History	None (transaction cost) to high (institutional); when high, history is deterministic	High, but history may or may not be deterministic
Spatial Framing		
Domain of Study	Reified organization in the environment	Relationships among individuals, subsystems, systems
View of the Environment	Outside the organization; evolves separately from the organization	Part of the domain of study; coevolves with the organization
Levels of Analysis	Single to few, relatively independent	Multitude of nested levels
Construct Framing		
Strategy	Relatively designed	Relatively emergent
Structure	Equilibrium; relatively centralized	Nonequilibrium; relatively decentralized
Purpose of Organizational Relationships	Efficiency, fit, institutional conformity (legitimation)	Learning; cocreation of meaning
Key Information for the Organization	External environmental intelligence	Functioning of relationships
Information Processor	Reified organization	Individuals; complex systems of individuals

analysis is challenged by complexity science. The complexity perspective gives analytic priority to the relationships embedded inside, outside, and around entities within the bounded, reified organization itself. Accordingly, the environment is a construct that has little meaning to the complexity researcher; rather, relationships among organizational entities and environmental entities are the domain of interest. Coevolution of these relationships characterizes change better than the separate evolution of "the organization" and "the environment." Kauffman's (1995) depiction of systems seeking peaks on constantly changing rugged landscapes, and transforming those landscapes and themselves in the process, is a complexity-inspired analogue to the traditional organization-environment relationship. A final difference in spatial framing between the established and complexity perspectives is the tendency of established perspectives to focus on one or a few levels of relatively independent analysis. Complexity science notes the embeddedness of all systems within larger ones, and the need to analyze relationships across levels of systems.

Finally, several differences between "what is studied" by established perspectives versus by complexity science can be further refined. Key constructs are framed differently. On one hand, according to established perspectives the strategy of an organization is relatively designed by the reified organization. The strategy of a complex adaptive system, on the other hand, is relatively emergent. Strategy changes unpredictably over time, based on learning from relationship coevolution. Structures concommitantly are relatively flexible, and there is no "equilibrium" structure. Relationships coevolve for the purposes of learning and the creation of meaningful systems. In contrast, established perspectives assume a reified organization pursuing external environmental intelligence to fit the organization to the environment better or to optimize its economic efficiency within the environment.

We argue that the complexity perspective's operating assumptions are better equipped than established perspectives to yield useful research questions on complex adaptive systems. However, conducting research from a complexity perspective requires corresponding methods of research that are far from well-developed.

Consequences of Complexity Science for Research Methods

As might be expected, application of new theories often may require the use of new and different research methods. Novel discoveries and paradigms typically emerge through the efforts of "explorers" (Rogers, 1995); explorers typically represent a minute fraction of the research population. In complexity science, these explorers primarily have come from physics, biology, and mathematics, and have included few social scientists. Explorers are not necessarily overly concerned about context or application. As their novel ideas gain exposure, diffusion proceeds to the "pioneers." Pioneers bring the ideas across disciplinary boundaries and seek connections between theory and practice. They are open to learning from the explorers, in an interdisciplinary way. Pioneers may be thought of as generalists, and may in fact often lack the specialized skills (or interest) to pursue the intricate details of implementing the ideas into singular domains. Researchers investigating the interaction between complexity and social science currently fall into this category. For complexity science to have an impact on a particular theory domain, it must be adopted by a majority of researchers and practitioners considered "settlers." Settlers perform the equally important duty of "normal science" (Kuhn, 1962). This group places great emphasis on domain context. They are interested in optimizing an idea to its specific domain application. They tend to learn and communicate strictly within their own domain.

Note that it is the pioneering group that is probably most challenged with respect to research methodologies. These new concepts may be difficult to import into the domain, especially when the existing paradigm (collective schema) of the settlers is in opposition.

The pioneers must adhere to the rigor expected by the nature of the scientific order and yet be careful not to get caught in the trap of using the wrong methods to study new phenomena. Pioneers indeed have to invent new research methods alongside their research hypotheses.

The vast majority of research on health care organizations can be classified as "positivistic," which dictates that hypotheses be stated and then subjected to falsification (Popper, 1959, p. 41). Experiments, whether planned or ad hoc (such as empirical surveys or case studies), are the essence of such refutation. Some proponents of complexity science contend that striving to fit within the positivistic research framework threatens the transformational nature and potential contributions of complexity science (Stacey, Griffin, and Shaw, 2000).

For complexity science to be applied in a positivistic framework, it must be capable of generating testable hypotheses. This is difficult for a new discipline, as definitions for basic constructs such as emergence and self-organization are fluid and not well agreed upon. Even the concept of "chaos" suffers from a dichotomy of meaning (Dooley and Van de Ven, 1999). Further, these constructs must be operationalized into measurement instruments. Currently, perceptual scales for measuring these constructs do not exist, and if measured at all, they are observed via secondary sources. For example, "organizational complexity" may be observed by counting the number of different functional roles present in the organizational chart (Dooley, 2002a).

Causal links in the proposed theory must be tested. However, empirical tests of most theories in the social sciences, including health care organizational theories, assume linearity and unidirectional causation. The statistical methodologies available to test other model forms are grossly inadequate. Consider a simple theory linking motivation and performance. It is generally agreed upon that this relationship is bidirectional, as individual theories support the causal links in both directions (Gallistel, 1990). How could that bidirectionality be proven, though? At the very least, to address bidirectional causality, longitudinal data would have to be planned and collected. Elaborate time series methods would have to be used. Real social systems pose a problem to even this strategy, however. Model parameters are likely to be time varying, a challenge for any statistical methodology. The time lag—the delay between cause and effect—is also likely to be dynamic. Clearly, modeling approaches need to be further developed to test multicausal social systems. One may even conclude that such deductive inquiries are no longer valid.

Qualitative research methods may serve researchers well in disentangling dynamic, complicated, emergent systems. To date, many applications of complexity science to organization have involved multimethod case studies over time. One methodological tool that complexity science does have in abundance is a rich set of poetic metaphors: the strange attractor, the butterfly effect, self-organized criticality, fractals, and so on. It is not surprising to see this new language give rise to new creative ideas, and be used to sell "older" ideas in new ways. Metaphors allow the understanding of one concept (or phenomena) in terms of another (Lakoff and Johnson, 1980). They are artificial symbols to assist thought (Turbayne, 1962) and provide "windows into the soul of the social system" (Burke, 1992). Hallyn (1990, pp. 28–29) captures the different uses of metaphor when used in a research context:

> A metaphor does not always have the same status. . . .
> I shall differentiate a discursive status (valid in the case
> that aims to enlighten or convince), a methodological
> status (implying a heuristic function), and a theoretical
> status (linked to a vision of the world that poses a priori
> the existence of a real analogy). It is clear that only the
> two latter types belong in a poetics of the hypothesis. A
> metaphor is discursive when it is applied to persuasion

and exposition. The theoretical status applies especially to . . . "absolute" metaphors, which are the "first elements of philosophical language, irreducible to the realm of logical terminology."

Much of the current social science research concerning complexity is based on discursive metaphors, for example, claiming that leadership is a "strange attractor." (A strange attractor is the pattern of a pathway, in visual form, produced by graphing the behavior of certain systems.) This type of research should be expected from the pioneers, who may be less concerned with methodological rigor than with the richness of concept these new ideas bring; discursive metaphors can play a powerful role in spurring creativity. Proper discursive use of metaphors still requires proper understanding of the underlying science. Health organization researchers may be in a good position with regard to this requirement, as many have backgrounds in systems theory or biology, good backgrounds from which to develop knowledge of complexity science.

Simulation may be an especially productive means by which to pursue the application of complexity science to health care research questions (Dooley, 2002b). Simulations fall into three broad categories: simulations involving human interaction only, simulations whereby the human interacts with a computer, and simulations involving a completely computerized medium. In all cases, the theorist has a complex system in mind and wants to explore what might happen when system variables are systematically introduced. System simulations are thus prepared to capture the relevant system behaviors and control extraneous variables whenever possible, and just as important, to provide results in a manageable amount of time. The validity of the simulation depends on the assumptions made to simplify the simulation and on the rules chosen to embody action, sense making, and decision making within the simulation.

A Complexity Science Perspective on Integration and Innovation in Health Care Organizations

To make the comparison between a complexity science perspective and established perspectives more concrete, we examine two domains of health management research and practice that could particularly benefit from a complexity science perspective. The domains are (1) innovation in health care delivery, and (2) structure and performance of integrated delivery systems. The two research domains are not mutually exclusive, but each has a distinctive tradition of theory and empirical research.

Researchers and practitioners in both of these research arenas are deeply affected by the complexity of health care delivery. It is commonly espoused that "[t]he health care field is complex, perhaps the most complex of any area of the economy" (Morrison, 2000, p. xvii). Complexity is reflected in the number, variety, and fragmentation of producers involved in the delivery of health care: potential patients (who are consumers of prevention), actual patients, professionals, provider organizations, buyer organizations (including large employers who purchase on behalf of employees), insurers or payers, and suppliers. Glouberman and Mintzberg (2001a; 2001b) more abstractly conceptualize extensive differentiation in the health care sector into four "worlds," of cure, care, control, and community. Deep-seated differentiation, in turn, leads to inability to diagnose and design effective interventions for innovation and improvement that rely on coordination and control. This feature of health care delivery complicates decisions about how to structure integrated delivery systems and the ability to predict their performance. Too, complexity affects the ability of the health care systems to generate diversity and innovation, particularly innovation that is transformational.

Researchers can approach innovation and integration in health care from a variety of established theories or perspectives. In the following discussion, we again use institutional theory, transaction cost theory, and structural contingency theory to represent established perspectives. Complexity science offers a different and potentially more powerful alternative. To frame and bound the discussion of the complexity perspective, we explore research implications of the characterization of complexity science previously given in Table 10.2. Research implications of each characteristic of complexity science are denoted in Table 10.3.

Innovation in Health Care Delivery

Innovation in health care delivery is significant in magnitude and impact. For example, it is estimated that the total U.S. research and development spending for both the National Institutes of Health and research-based pharmaceutical companies was $34.9 billion in 1999 (Henny, 2000). Many of these innovations have had significant, positive consequences on individual and public health. For example, the DISCERN medical error warning system, a computer-based system that examines a patient's prescriptions for adverse drug interactions, is estimated to have saved numerous lives, and $5.3 million in health care costs, within Banner Health Systems' three Phoenix-based hospitals (Snyder, 2001). Innovative new services are not isolated to specific medical procedures and systems, but extend also into the domain of both integrated health systems and the conduct of public health.

Within the public health arena, much innovation effort has been focused on HIV/AIDS. The Joint United Nations Programme on HIV/AIDS and the World Health Organization estimate that, worldwide, some 5.3 million people were newly infected with HIV in 2000, 36.1 million are living with HIV/AIDS, and 21.8 million have died since the beginning of the epidemic (UNAIDS/WHO, 2000a; 2000b). AIDS is especially prevalent in developing countries; Africa has three-fourths of the AIDS-infected population. The general public health in such countries is significantly affected. For example, it is projected that life expectancy in Zimbabwe will be

Table 10.3. Research Implications of the Complexity Science
Perspective.

	Complexity Science Perspective	Implications for Research
Temporal Framing		
View of the Future	Relatively unknowable	Patterns may repeat, but without predictive power; anticipate surprise; study emergence
Relevance of History	High, but history may or may not be deterministic	Requisite to study history (versus cross-sectional only); conduct longitudinal analysis
Spatial Framing		
Domain of Study	Relationships among individuals, subsystems, systems	Study patterns of interaction among agents
View of the Environment	Part of the domain of study; coevolves with the organization	Study coevolution of organization and environment
Levels of Analysis	Multitude of nested levels	View issue from multiple, nested levels of systems
Construct Framing		
Strategy	Relatively emergent	Study changes in strategy and conditions that facilitate change
Structure	Nonequilibrium; relatively decentralized	Assess flexibility of structures; simple rules; minimum specs
Purpose of Organizational Relationships	Learning; cocreation of meaning	Assess degrees of coparticipation, learning, sharing
Key Information for the Organization	Functioning of relationships	Study quality of relationships
Information Processor	Individuals; complex systems of individuals	Study individuals and coalitions, versus reified organization

reduced from sixty-three years in 1985 to thirty-five years in 2010 (Bonnel, 2000). The epidemic also has severe economic consequences. For example, in South Africa, AIDS is expected to reduce gross domestic product by 17 percent by 2010 (UNAIDS/WHO, 2000a; 2000b).

According to the U.S. Centers for Disease Control and Prevention (CDC), various HIV prevention efforts in the United States through the 1990s have reduced HIV seroprevalence by 50 percent within the vulnerable community, by 40 percent within New York City injection drug users, and by 75 percent for babies contracting AIDS from their mothers (Centers for Disease Control and Prevention, 2001). The CDC has broad-based goals of preventing AIDS through decreasing new infections; increasing knowledge of serostatus; increasing the linkages among prevention, care, and treatment; and strengthening monitoring, capacity, and evaluation.

Strategies for the prevention of AIDS generally fall into three categories: access, counseling, and social strategies (Auerbach and Coates, 2000). Prevention has increased as people gain access to condoms (Centers for Disease Control and Prevention, 1998) and sterile needles (Des Jarlais and others, 2000). Counseling strategies to deal with high-risk behavior have been successful, including in developing countries (Auerbach and Coates, 2000). Social strategies raise peer interaction to a community level through education and awareness programs (Latkin, Madell, Vlahov, Oziemkowska, and Celentano, 1996).

General theories of innovation suggest that new approaches to HIV/AIDS prevention should not be formalized or centralized (Damanpour, 1996). Formalization involves specified rules, roles, and procedures; creates an environment of risk aversion and attention to efficiency; and is negatively associated with innovation. Centralization involves the extent to which organizational members have freedom to act on their own accord. Highly centralized systems will tend to stifle creativity, as innovation ideas need to travel up and down an organizational hierarchy before they can be acted upon. In the case of HIV/AIDS, this may suggest numerous, parallel innovation efforts, unhampered by formal government oversight.

The innovation literature also stresses the need for the system to have the absorptive capacity to take innovation inputs and create useful outcomes (Fiol, 1996). This absorptive capacity may be dependent upon prior accumulation of knowledge (Cohen and Levinthal, 1990), the ability of different role players to interact effectively (Souder and Moenhart, 1992), and the structure of social networks within the adopting system (Rogers, 1995). Within developing countries struggling with HIV/AIDS, novel means for diffusing knowledge about protection and care may benefit from a "social" absorptive capacity, in that previous public health innovations have had to struggle with the lack of a mass-media-infused culture and to invent creative ways to diffuse ideas and spur adoption (Rogers, 1995).

We next present and discuss a case example of one social system that has faced and addressed AIDS treatment in innovative ways. Then, we discuss the case as the subject of research based on established perspectives and the complexity science perspective.

Brazil AIDS Case

In 1997, the World Bank reported that an estimated 30 million people had contracted the human immunodeficiency virus (HIV), and 90 percent of those were in developing countries (World Bank, 1997). AIDS in developing countries is often assumed to be an intractable problem, based on five key assumptions:

- The impact of today's interventions (and prevention efforts) will take a generation or two to play out.

- The cost of the antiretroviral drug cocktails is out of reach for poor countries.

- Treatment is a luxury poor countries cannot afford, and they opt to focus almost exclusively on prevention.

- Uneducated, illiterate patients cannot manage their own complicated drug therapies.

- Meaningful solutions require sophisticated, integrated national health care systems.

Brazil's approach to AIDS challenged all of these assumptions and reversed the spread of AIDS. Brazil's efforts really began in earnest in the early 1990s. By 1994, organizations in Brazil were producing their first generic antiretroviral drugs. Within five years, Brazil's efforts had made a major impact on reducing the spread of the HIV virus. In the 1980s, Brazil was held out as an example of one of the countries worst hit by AIDS, yet today, Brazil is touted as a model for developing countries fighting AIDS, despite the fact that its annual per capita income is less than $5,000 (Downie, 2001). In the 1980s, Brazil's AIDS problem was more severe than South Africa's (Darlington, 2000). Today, South Africa's HIV infection rate is 25 percent, whereas Brazil's is 0.6 percent (UNAIDS/WHO, 2000a). In 1992, the World Bank predicted that Brazil would have 1.2 million AIDS cases by 2000, but the actual count was closer to 0.5 million.

The government of Brazil gives free drugs to AIDS patients. Brazil uses the controversial clause of the World Trade Organization that allows countries to violate patent laws in cases of national emergency (American Medical Association, 2001). Brazil argued that the AIDS epidemic is or could become a national emergency. Estimates of the resulting cost reduction vary, and costs are being further reduced as more and more of the drugs are produced in generic form. At a minimum, the cost of the drug therapy per patient per year is 65 percent lower than the $12,000 cost in the United States. Some estimate that it could be further lowered to be 90 percent less than the U.S. cost (Darlington, 2000).

The question implicitly posed in Brazil was not "how can we provide treatment when the drug costs are so high?" but "how can we reduce costs so that we can provide treatment to all who need it?"

Organizations in Brazil chose to use treatment as part of the prevention strategy. When people know they can get treatment, they are more willing to come in to hospitals, clinics, or certain nongovernmental organizations (NGOs) for tests (Rosenberg, 2001). The situation is not deemed to be hopeless. While patients are there for treatments or tests, they also get information and spread the prevention ideas. Today the bulk of the spending is on treatment, yet the prevention goals are being met. The question implicitly posed was not "with our limited resources, should we focus more on prevention or treatment?" but "how can we achieve our prevention goals while treating all of those currently infected?"

Nurses and other health care workers teach patients how to take the drugs. They use whatever methods they can to communicate the drug routine to their patients. They draw pictures of the sun or the moon to denote different times of day. They draw pictures of food on the labels of the pill bottles for those that need to be consumed with food. In addition, they help the poorest patients link up with NGOs, churches, and other organizations that offer free food. In spite of the high illiteracy rate in Sao Paolo, Brazil, the adherence rate for the drug regime is at the same level as in San Diego. In both cities, 70 percent of patients achieve an 80 percent adherence rate (Rosenberg, 2001).

Rather than being defeated by the overwhelming challenge, participants in the effective system considered such questions as "What methods of communication will work to convey the drug therapy routine to a patient—even a homeless, illiterate patient?" and "If food is an issue, how can we ensure greater compliance with the routine by linking with charities that can provide food at the right times of day?"

Brazil had an established infrastructure of hospitals, clinics, and public health services. However, it was a very patchy, irregular system (Rosenberg, 2001). There were huge differences in the services available across the country and to different segments of the population. Brazil's AIDS efforts have recognized and strengthened existing connections to do the treatment and prevention work necessary to grapple with AIDS. The efforts have used over six hundred existing NGOs and community-level care organizations to reach the country's poor. The country now has 133 testing and counseling centers. Health care clinicians work alongside NGOs and other organizations to provide the full range of services needed. "It is a well-organized, well-formulated program that works because the government has managed to integrate the whole society—especially NGOs" (Buckley, 2000).

Established Perspectives on Innovation

As a relatively innovative advance in the delivery of health services, the Brazil AIDS case provides a provocative research setting for health organization theorists. Established theoretical perspectives would point researchers in particular directions. Transaction cost theory, for instance, would lead the researcher to address such issues as the costs of information exchange between collaborators: What intraorganizational costs were avoided by the government through use of existing networks of NGOs, churches, and health care clinics? How were the costs of service reduced for the individual health care organizations and NGOs through collaborating on this national agenda? How is the information flow less expensive in Brazil? What needed to happen to reduce those information exchange costs?

A structural contingency perspective would give priority to assessing the fit between organizational forms and their environment. In particular, did the information-processing capabilities of the organizations and the network of organizations match the degree of uncertainty in the environment? Did the Brazilian organizational forms have the requisite variety, given the uncertainty in the environment? Was there sufficient flexibility in the organizational forms to handle the rapidly evolving environment? Was the optimal level of provider integration achieved via the network of organizations handling Brazil's AIDS crisis, given their reciprocal interdependencies?

Finally, researchers applying institutional theory would investigate current and past institutional structures (for example government policy, tax laws, professional norms, societal values) that both enabled and constrained governmental and societal reaction to HIV/AIDS. Institutional theory would study processes whereby the "new" treatment and prevention systems may or may not become permanent. The perspective would suggest studying the strength of the three different forms of institutional effect—imitative, normative, and coercive—on the diffusion of the new practices (DiMaggio and Powell, 1983).

Complexity Science Perspective

The complexity science perspective would lead researchers to be less "surprised" by Brazil's achievements in HIV/AIDS prevention and treatment. While recognizing the overwhelming forces supporting the "old" system, the perspective would lead one to investigate the sources of novelty—the tiny differences that made a big difference in producing the "new" system, contrasted with the forces that allow systems to get stuck in suboptimal solutions and interventions (Kauffman, 1995). How were the histories of the entities in Brazil and the traditions of Brazilian culture used to generate rather than constrain the emergence of new patterns? What were the transforming exchanges, containers, and differences that enabled self-organized solutions to occur (Olson and Eoyang, 2001)? To what extent were "wicked questions" that are crucial in breaking the pattern from previous attractor patterns raised and addressed (Zimmerman, 1991; 1993; Zimmerman, Lindberg, and Plsek, 1998)? What were the far-from-equilibrium conditions that induced Brazil's reactions to HIV/AIDS (Goldstein, 1994)?

There is a wide variety in the systems operating at all levels within the Brazil AIDS system. What are the patterns of interaction that repeat at all scales? Where is there scalar invariance indicating an equation or simple rule of interaction that repeats at micro, meso, and macro levels (for example, a rule that "poor people can be responsible for their own health")? And do the dynamics of actions taken for HIV/AIDS prevention and care indicate that the innovation system is being driven by few or many factors? Are these factors acting independently or interdependently (Dooley and Van de Ven, 1999)?

As novelty in complex systems arises without a "big plan," the complexity perspective would suggest that the network of providers dealing with HIV/AIDS prevention and care emerged from multiple and parallel experiments, not from under any organization's control (Choi and Dooley, 2000). To what extent was the network built by combining existing, separate entities, and to what extent were minimum specifications used (Zimmerman, Lindberg, and Plsek, 1998)?

Complex systems operate through relationships among agents of the system. What were the qualities of the relationships among agents in the system (Goodwin, 1994)? One could examine a variety of relationships, including caregiver-patient relationships, government-NGO relationships, relationships of patients to their disease, and information feedback and feedforward loops. At the micro level, relationships are formed by conversation. How reflective is the discursive content of conversations between workers and patients of the larger cultural system regarding HIV/AIDS prevention and care (Corman, Kuhn, McPhee, and Dooley, 2002)? How are the organizational forms informing and being formed by their AIDS work (as opposed to, how are they adapting to their environment [Zimmerman, 1993])?

While all of the perspectives generate interesting and useful research questions, complexity science broadens the scope and significantly changes the direction of research questions that one might ask about the Brazil AIDS case. Relative to temporal framing of the research (see Table 10.3), complexity science offers more optimism about the possibility for radical change, and more effectively directs researchers to the potential sources of novelty in the system. Longitudinal analysis is implicit in the research method.

Relative to spatial framing, the complexity perspective draws the researcher to study relationships among the entities within and across existing systems in Brazil, rather than only within and among "reified" health care delivery organizations. Specific analysis of the quality, emergence, and outcomes of relationships among individuals, groups of individuals, and organizations is explicit in the complexity approach.

Next we review a second area of research and an associated case, to further illustrate research consequences of the complexity perspective.

Structure and Performance of Integrated Delivery Systems

Vertical and horizontal integration have been favored strategies of business organizations, under certain conditions, throughout history. Waves of consolidation (horizontal expansion and integration) and incorporation of buyer and supplier organizations by a focal organization (vertical integration) occur periodically in sectors of the business economy. Pressures for integration, such as increased competition and regulations to control cost and quality, have led health care organizations to embrace higher levels of integration since the 1970s. Initially, researchers employed theory to argue that integrated systems, under the right conditions, would lead to reduced costs and increased quality of services. In the 1980s, vertical integration was viewed as the most promising strategy for positioning health care delivery organizations for the future. The exemplary integrated delivery system (IDS) would combine physicians, hospitals, long-term care facilities, and a payment mechanism under one organizational entity. This exemplar was presented in the literature as the "ideal" structure for health services delivery (Shortell, Gillies, Anderson, and Erickson, 1996).

In the 1990s, researchers made useful discoveries about the difficulty of both implementing vertical integration and delivering on its promises. Studies concluded that many of the allegedly integrated systems in fact demonstrated few characteristics of "systemness"

(Shortell, Gillies, Anderson, Erickson, and Mitchell, 2000). Case-study-based reviews of integrated systems demonstrated the considerable diversity within the organizational form "IDS" and resulted in more realistic depictions of the "unfolding" of IDSs over time (Young and McCarthy, 1999). Researchers empirically sorted the population of IDSs into five clusters of systems and four clusters of networks, with wide variation within the set of IDSs (Bazzolli, Shortell, Dubbs, Chan, and Kralovec, 1999). Attention shifted to the "network" form of IDSs (Savage and Roboski, 2001) and the possibilities of "virtual" integration (Coffey, Fenner, and Stogis, 1997). The promises of integrated delivery were unfilled, leading to a research symposium in 2001 on the theme, "The Failure of Integrated Delivery Systems" (Friedman and Goes, 2001).

One such IDS that weathered trials and tribulations in the 1990s was Allina Health System, based in Minneapolis-St. Paul. Its recent history is summarized in the following case study.

Allina Health System Case

Allina Health System was created by the July, 1994, merger of HealthSpan, a large hospital and physician system in Minneapolis-St. Paul, with Medica, a health plan with 900,000 covered enrollees. Both Medica and HealthSpan had formally existed for only a short time previous to the merger, but their roots were deep in the community. For example, Medica's 1991 initial partners included Hennepin County Medical Society's managed health plan that had begun as an IPA (independent practice association) in 1975. The roots of Allina's hospital system can be traced back to 1857 (Grazman and Van de Ven, 1996).

The Allina Health System combination was hailed as "The first time since Kaiser (Permanente) that the triumvirate of Doctors, Hospitals, and Insurance have been put together in one place" (Grazman and Van de Ven, 1996, p. 1). Allina Health System had $1.8 billion in 1994 revenues and was the second largest employer in Minnesota after Northwest Airlines. Its strategic rationale was the belief that a full vertical merger was necessary to create a unified health promotion strategy, a large capital pool, and stability of long-term planning and investment in such areas as information technology and preventive care. Unlike a joint venture or loose affiliation, the merger promised the alignment of incentives, the ability to bear large-scale risk, the accountability for the health of a population, and the authority to sign contracts with one organizational entity (Young and McCarthy, 1999). The state of Minnesota and a powerful business coalition, the Business Health Care Action Group, were instrumental in spurring consolidation and integration in the Minneapolis-St. Paul market.

Allina was structured with an executive office at its head and three divisions: Delivery Services, which included three metropolitan and several nonmetropolitan hospitals, home health, and other diversified services; Professional Services, which included fifty-five physician group practices employing four hundred physicians as well as contracts with some eighty-seven hundred other providers; and Health Plans. A president's council brought together leadership from the three operating groups. As a key part of its vision, Allina strived to be recognized as an innovator in community health improvement. Success in this arena was demonstrated by the 1999 McGaw Prize for Excellence in Community Service awarded by the American Hospital Association.

In its early history, Allina focused on creating a consistent corporate identity across its markets and a highly integrated, economically efficient organization. Internal management attention was devoted to performance measurement systems, including patient satisfaction measurement, major investment in coordinating its information system, and a corporatewide financial control system. Several physician group practices were purchased, and the difficulties of aligning physicians with the health plan and hospitals proved to be a continuing challenge (Bunderson, Lofstrom, and Van de Ven, 1998).

By the year 2000, Allina had grown to include eighteen hospitals and to generate gross revenues of $2.9 billion (Galloro, 2001b), but trouble was on the horizon. The Minnesota Attorney General began an investigation into the expenditures of Medica, alleging that Medica engaged in lavish spending on image consultants, executive salaries and perks, and corporate entertaining, and that Medica subsidized similar expenditures in other divisions of Allina. After several months of continuing negative publicity in the local and national press, Allina in 2001 agreed to split off Medica as an independent not-for-profit organization. The Medica and Allina boards were replaced by boards appointed with approval of the Attorney General, and several top executives in Allina and Medica were replaced. The actions soiled the reputation of "one of the country's most prominent not-for-profit healthcare systems" (Galloro, 2001a). The new leadership of Medica immediately announced a 20 percent staff layoff (Howatt, 2001), and new Allina leadership denounced the criticized expenditures as surprising and inappropriate (Marcotty and Burcum, 2001).

Established Perspectives on Integrated Delivery Systems

Lessons from Allina's merger and de-merger with Medica can be interpreted from any number of established theoretical perspectives. In analyzing the Allina experience, a contingency perspective would direct attention to inadequacies in the organizational form chosen by Allina in 1994. That form, the fully vertically and horizontally integrated system, was predicated on an elusive future in which capitation would rein. Success of the form required that Allina-affiliated physicians and Medica enrollees would cooperate with integration by using only Allina hospitals. In fact, only about 25 percent overlap was attained between Medica members and Allina hospitals, compared to the 75 percent estimated as necessary to "reap the benefits of integration" (Galloro, 2001b). From the structural contingency perspective, Allina's problems arose from a strategic choice by Allina's top leadership that may have been reasonable for the environment anticipated in 1994 but which did not emerge as expected.

Transaction cost theorists postulate that loose coupling, via contract, in many cases is more efficient than the more tightly coupled IDS exemplar (Mick, 1990). A transaction cost theory approach would focus on the efficiency of full integration of the health plan and of physicians within a hospital system, and would explore the possibility that expected efficiencies never materialized. As a result, for example, there was little evidence of cost savings that Allina could offer to offset external criticism of its internal spending practices.

Institutional theorists have hypothesized that the IDS movement was largely a mimetic response to pressures for industry conformity (Mohr, 1992). Accordingly, an institutional theory perspective might suggest that the culture of the Twin Cities and Minnesota promoted "progressive" experimentation in health care delivery and collective solutions to social problems, but that a key element of culture—the community responsibility of nonprofit enterprise—was neglected by Allina in its drive for legitimacy in the eyes of employers and health care industry peers. Allina was an early adopter of structural innovation in the health care industry but failed to cultivate other important sources of stability and legitimacy.

As with the Brazil AIDS case, established perspectives provide useful ideas for research on the topic. A complexity science perspective builds on, extends, and deepens understanding of the Allina case.

Complexity Science Perspective

As noted in discussion of the Brazil AIDS case, the complexity perspective's "view of the future" would equip the researcher to interpret the unfolding of Allina not as a major surprise or a failure but as more of a natural unfolding of learning about complex relationships. The histories of the entities or agents in the multiple systems would no doubt be relevant to understanding the differences between Allina's hospital, physician, and health plan divisions that created tensions. Mapping the multiple, nested systems covered by the Allina Health System rubric would be a major undertaking, with consumers, hospitals, health plans, physicians, the local community, and the state among the major interacting units. Failures at one level (for example, Allina Health System) may be successes at another level (for example, consumers, state).

After identifying the key relationships among individuals and coalitions in Allina's internal subsystems and between those individuals and coalitions and external organizations or systems, the complexity researcher would want to understand the quality of each of the relationships. How much participation was there from all parties in the key relationships? In particular, to what extent did physicians and consumers influence the direction of the hospitals and the health plan? Through what entities did the health plan relate to the community? What interests were represented in top management and in setting Allina's and Medica's strategic vision?

A central theme of conventional wisdom on IDS formation is the need to establish a shared mission. Established perspectives generally argue that successful change occurs when people are persuaded to hold the same beliefs. Equilibrium and harmony are equated with success. As argued by Stacey, Griffin, and Shaw (2000, p. 5), however, "the very difference managers seek so strenuously to remove is the source of spontaneous, potentially creative change. . . . Managers may be struggling to change their organizations in ways which ensure that they stay the same." In this sense, a complexity perspective might speculate that the Allina story, and many other stories of "failed" integration, derive from overstructuration and overcontrol in an uncertain and dynamic environment. The overcontrol results in the stifling, rather than generation, of innovative efforts at creating value for consumers (Zimmerman and Dooley, 2002).

The focus of analysis in complexity research shifts from the externally imposed designs or intents of designers of systems to how things really unfold in systems. Traditional systems thinking has created a vicious cycle of (1) design a system, and (2) when the system does not act as predicted, redesign the system. The assumption is that leaders can control the evolution of complex systems by intentions and clear thinking. Complexity science leads one to ask different questions. For example, when an intended design does not play out as predicted, how do things continue to function? Stacey, Griffin, and Shaw (2000, p. 59) refer to this as the potential to "get things done anyway." How do patients continue to get care, and clinicians provide care, despite the machinations of formal organizations? Complexity science focuses on how this "anyway" behavior unfolds through everyday interactions and in spite of the fact that leaders continue to focus on the systems that attempt to secure predicted changes.

The original decision to merge Medica and HealthSpan in 1994 could represent bold experimentation by risk-taking executives, and its "failure" could be reinterpreted as a case of successful learning on the part of the organization, albeit at the expense of damage to the careers of several organizational leaders. Researchers from a complexity perspective would be interested in how Allina's structure and strategy coevolved with other forces. To what extent were individuals and coalitions in Allina resilient and able to "learn"? To what extent was Allina trapped by the histories of its component subsystems? In what ways was the emergence of novelty encouraged or discouraged? Why were "wicked questions" challenging extravagant expenditures not raised and fully debated internally?

Applied to the structure and performance of IDSs more generally, complexity science would argue that integration is more effective, and expectations more realistic, when the complex nature of the "integrated" entity is recognized and addressed from the start. Integration of complex entities is more effective if they are allowed to "e-merge" rather than if they are "merged" (Zimmerman and Dooley, 2002). Linenkugel's (2001, p. 8) conclusion that "if you've seen one merger, you've seen one merger" reflects the growing acceptance of the complex nature of integration in health care, as does renewed focus on the process, rather than the structure, of integration (Burns, Walston, and others, 2001).

Conclusion

In considering the experience of health care organizations and the growth of complexity science in the past two decades, two points stand out. First, health care organizations are a rich field for the study of complex adaptive systems. To date, organizational researchers using complexity science have looked toward the "Santa Fe" school, scholars in evolutionary biology and physics and mathematics, for their inspiration. Although the study of the emergence of order in (for instance) ant colonies may provide useful insights, the most complex systems are social systems, and health care organizations are the most complex within that subdomain. If one believes that a science is "pushed" and progresses by studying its most complex problems and situations, then complexity science needs to coevolve its next set of theories with a vigorous examination of health and health care management issues.

Second, complexity science should be well-represented among the perspectives available to health organization researchers interested in furthering contributions to science and to practice. A more realistic view of the future would be one in which surprise is anticipated rather than shunned, the focus is on patterns of interaction rather than on reified structures, and new concepts are continually developed to study the emergence of novelty and the success of distributed control. These combined would produce a powerful addition to the theoretical complement of the health organization theorist.

11

Strategy in an
Institutional Environment

*Lessons Learned from the 1990s
"Revolution" in Health Care*

Roice D. Luke and Stephen L. Walston

U nprecedented change gripped the health care industry in the
1990s, leading to significant restructuring of both systems and
markets. But perhaps of equal importance was the change that did
not occur—the restructuring that fell short of universally embraced
expectations held by executives, clinicians, policy analysts, and academics in the first half of the decade. Among a number of predictions, it has been expected that vertical integration, horizontal
combinations, and system integration all would spread across the
industry, as hospital and physician competitors positioned themselves to compete as local systems of delivery in the increasingly
aggressive managed care environment. Such expectations were
widely chronicled by opinion leaders and think tanks (American
Hospital Association, 1990; 1992; Brown, 1996; Catholic Health
Association, 1992; Conrad and Shortell, 1996; Shortell, Gillies,
Anderson, Mitchell, and Morgan, 1993). The Health Care Advisory Board, for example, which in the 1990s became a major oracle
for advising health providers on strategy, predicted that markets
nationally would be dominated by fully integrated systems (The
Advisory Board, 1993).

Indeed, in that period the number of local hospital combinations—which in most markets provide the foundation for forming

integrated systems—did expand rapidly in number. The percentage of acute care general hospitals in clusters of two or more per market more than doubled throughout the 1990s, rising from 24 percent of urban hospitals in 1989 to 53 percent in 2001 (Williamson Institute, 2001). And the number of such clusters also nearly doubled, increasing from 250 local systems to 459 in 2001. This represents a significant shift toward consolidation in local markets within the hospital industry. It is notable that all categories of hospitals engaged in the consolidation movement, including Catholic hospitals and systems, public hospitals, teaching hospitals, and even nearby rural hospitals in many cases.

Overall, however, the financial achievements of the local hospital combinations have been underwhelming (Bazzoli, Dynan, Burns, and Lindrooth, 2000; Clement, and others, 1997; Lin and Wan, 1999; McCue, Clement, and Luke, 1999), although most of the research on this is fairly preliminary. Current studies are needed to examine the local clusters now that they have had time to mature and refine their interorganizational relationships and management systems.

The results of physician-practice consolidation are widely believed to have fallen far short of expectations generated in the early 1990s. Undoubtedly, the most dramatic failure occurred in the attempts by physician practice management companies (PPMCs) to acquire physician practices on regional and national bases. Many such companies rose and then fell within short periods of time (Reinhardt, 2000). In 1996 and 1997, PPMCs were still being promoted as a significant means by which physician costs could be reduced and doctors' clout in markets improved (Schonfeld, 1997). By 1998, the three major national firms—PhyCor, MedPartners, and FPA Medical Management—had collapsed, as did many others. Physician-based HMOs also fell short of expectations, as the much acclaimed group- and staff-model HMOs lost ground relative to the upsurge in the more loosely structured model types (Interstudy, 2001).

The picture is somewhat less clear on the hospital side of physician consolidation. In pursuit of their integrative strategies, hospitals acquired physician practices in the 1990s at an unprecedented rate. In a 1999 survey of systems and networks conducted by the American Hospital Association (AHA), 29 percent of the "systems" listed one or more "outpatient" facilities (most of which were composed of physician practices) within their systems (27 percent of the so-called "networks" reported outpatient facilities in their networks) (American Hospital Association, 2000a). An even higher level of hospital participation in physician organizations is indicated in the AHA's 1999 Annual Survey (2000b). Fully 35 percent of hospitals reported that they were engaged in one or more of seven forms of physician practice management or ownership (45 percent of the hospitals reported that either they or their systems were so engaged). Many of these reported arrangements, however, involved participation in physician-hospital organizations (PHOs), independent practice associations (IPAs), and other partnership-type arrangements. Despite the many examples of failure, the most notable of which was the demise of Philadelphia's Allegheny health system (Burns, Cacciamani, Clement, and Aquino, 2000), many hospitals and systems have retained their physician practices. Some appear to be making progress toward the ideal of the integrated system. However, the percentages just discussed very possibly overstate the degree to which hospitals actually control physician practices.

Most important, few full-blown integrated delivery systems (IDSs)—in which physicians, hospitals, other providers, and managed care products are tightly joined within single systems (Coddington, Moore, and Fischer, 1994)—emerged out of the restructuring of the 1990s. Many individual hospitals and systems claim to be IDSs (Friedman and Goes, 2001; Luke and Begun, 2001), the term having become fashionable in the industry. However, most self-identified IDSs fall very far from full integration. They lack the kinds of horizontal, vertical, or tight ownership arrangements one might expect of an integrated system.

The divergent outcomes of the 1990s restructuring, particularly the twists and turns in vision, theory, and paradigm, call out for interpretation and explanation. The U.S. health care industry has just completed one of the most costly and far-reaching natural experiments in its history. It needs to be determined what the restructuring (or the lack of it) indicates about health care systems and markets in the current decade.

Conceptual Frameworks

Scholars have sought for years to identify appropriate conceptual frameworks that could explain organizational behavior in health care. Three of the most prominent among these are industrial organization economics, transaction cost economics, and resource dependency. On the one hand, each of these provides a singular rationale or motive for why organizations might enter into more complex structural arrangements. On the other hand, their predictions for organizational restructuring are often similar. As summarized in Figure 11.1, each would predict the creation of vertically or horizontally integrated forms, or both, in response to market and other important environmental threats.

In addition to the three frameworks mentioned, institutional theory has been used to explain some of the seemingly irrational behaviors of organizations. By emphasizing the role played by sociopolitical dynamics, this framework provides a basis for understanding organizational restructuring that might not be fully grounded in sound economic and organizational logic.

Although each of the frameworks conceptualizes general organizational responses to environmental stimuli, no one of them should be expected to explain adequately the specific behaviors of organizations within specific industries, especially within an industry as distinctive and complex as is health care. Further, when looking at behavior from a strategic perspective—the view taken in this chapter—the search for a single rationale to explain behavior may

Figure 11.1. Four Conceptual Frameworks.

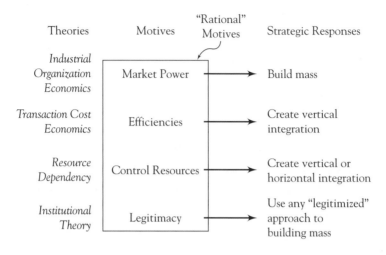

in fact be inappropriate. Strategy analysis is conducted by firms within a contingency framework, the objective of which is to obtain competitive advantage, conditioned upon whatever market or environmental threats are perceived to be present at a given point in time (Luke, Begun, and Walston, 2000). In effect, strategic decisions are made within a classic SWOT (strengths, weaknesses, opportunities, and threats) analytical framework, which conceptualizes strategy as the outcome of an analytical process in which a variety of motivating rationales and determinants are considered simultaneously (Andrews, 1971). We argue that no one explanatory construction is sufficiently robust to explain the behaviors exhibited in the 1990s within the health care industry, a conclusion that is fully consistent with a strategy-analytical perspective.

By extension, we also suggest that the 1990s restructuring cannot adequately be understood without giving careful consideration to the distinctiveness of the industry itself and the unprecedented environmental pressures of that period. We are dealing not just with a specific industry but with one that is highly unique in its economic and sociological underpinnings (Starr, 1982). And looking at the

1990s, we are observing an unusually turbulent period, when considered from a historical perspective (Morrison, 2000; Zelman, 1996).

The 1990s in health care was a time in which a sharply increased emphasis on strategic rationality ran directly into conflict with many long-established institutional constraints. As a result, traditional structures and assumptions were severely tested, as many health care organizations considered for the very first time a number of important strategic options. In sum, given the uniqueness of the health care industry as well as its relative inexperience in responding to market forces, we suggest that institutional theory might well account for many of the distinctive strategic responses observed among health care organizations in the past decade. We are not suggesting that the theoretical "baby" of economic rationality be thrown out with the bath. We are suggesting, however, that the major theoretical perspectives be reexamined, integrated, and altered as needed, taking into consideration our understanding of the events of the 1990s and the uniquenesses of this industry.

We suggest that an integrated model is needed, one that joins the various explanatory frameworks into a single strategy choice framework, and we make our own attempt at this. But first, we introduce and comment on the primary conceptual perspectives.

Industrial Organization

In his highly influential book *Competitive Strategy* (1980), Porter filled in an important analytical gap in the strategy literature. He did this by applying the tools of industrial organization (IO) economics—which traditionally focuses on policy and on the determinants of market efficiency (Scherer and Ross, 1990)—directly to the analysis of strategic decision making by individual firms. Porter translated key concepts from IO economics into terms that could be used in analyzing competitor behaviors and markets.

IO economics has long held that market structure influences conduct within markets and that together these two determine overall market performance (Bain and Qualls, 1987; Rumelt, 1974).

Porter pointed out that this same construction of determinants holds when analyzing individual firm decision making and strategic performance. In his "five forces" model, shown in Figure 11.2, he reasoned that strategy is the product of firms reacting to five specific market or power threats.

Of the five, threats from direct competitors are the most important in terms of consequences for individual firm strategy. To the threat of rivals are added four external threats, which are arrayed in the figure along both vertical (buyers and sellers) and horizontal (threats of entry and of substitution) axes. Porter identified a number of other, more specific strategic and structural factors that, although not explicitly included in the figure, nevertheless influence the intensity of rivalry and barriers to entry. These include, for example, the impacts of high fixed costs, presence of overcapacity, market growth, and switching costs. We note that when all such factors are incorporated into a strategic decision-making model, the task of reducing strategic explanation to singular theoretical arguments becomes all the more challenging.

Porter also provided an extensive analysis of how changes in levels of threat and power translate into specific strategic responses.

Figure 11.2. The Porter Model.

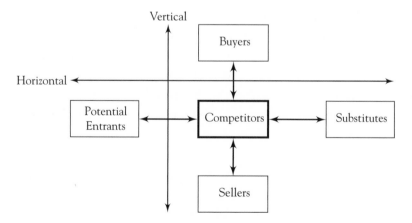

Source: Adapted from Porter, 1980, p. 4.

Unfortunately, in conceptualizing strategy, Porter narrowed his focus to the strategy of "positioning" (1996), which specifically has to do with projecting distinctive value to consumers—that is, projecting low cost, high quality, high service, high accessibility, and other distinctive market positions. Although positioning clearly represents an important approach to achieving competitive advantage, it captures only one of the many strategic options available to competitors. Others include, in particular, a variety of power strategies—for example, the pursuit of horizontal, vertical, and other forms of organizational reconfigurations (Luke, Begun, and Walston, 2000). Porter did, however, explore power strategies as well as many other approaches to gaining competitive advantage (1980). He did not, though, explicitly identify these as strategic options and, as a result, constructed a much-too-limited definition of strategy.

Because of Porter's particular emphasis on positioning, Mintzberg (1990; 1998) labeled the ideas he brought to the field the "positioning school." More appropriately, this school would be labeled the "market structure school," as Porter's primary contribution was to bring to the analysis of strategy the intellectual frameworks and analytical tools of IO economics.

There is no doubt that a number of the forces identified in the Porter model were very important in health care during the 1990s. These included, in particular, the rapid penetration of managed care in health care markets; anticipated growth in the aggressiveness and size of business coalitions; increased willingness by state and federal governments to use market forces to bring health care prices and costs under control; destabilizing effects of threatened substitutions (for example, ambulatory surgery displacing traditional surgery performed within hospitals); consolidation of hospitals into powerful local hospital systems; and the threat of physician consolidation, which challenged the market power of the forming hospital systems. All such changes and more can be fitted within the Porter model and used to assess individual firm strategic responses.

Transaction Cost Economics

The transaction cost economics (TCE) perspective also fits very well the conditions prevalent in the 1990s. It posits that organizational structures exist to economize on the costs of exchanging goods and services in a market environment. Transaction costs are incurred when undertaking any kind of exchange, whether to obtain inputs or to dispose of outputs. They include costs of monitoring, information gathering, administrative support, and negotiations and compromise. These costs rise with transaction frequency, the idiosyncrasy of the exchange, and, overall, the degree of uncertainty in a market or environment.

Vertical integration, which internalizes buyers and sellers within the same organizations, is a logical strategic response to rising transaction costs (Williamson, 1975; 1986; Ouchi, 1977). Accordingly, some have in recent years advanced TCE as a rationale for vertical integration among health care organizations (Conrad and Dowling, 1990; Mick and Conrad, 1988). Given the increased intensity and complexity of exchange between doctors and hospitals and the increasing possibility of losing physicians to competing organizations, as often occurred in the 1990s, TCE could explain why hospitals seek to acquire admitting and referring physician practices. Under heightened uncertainty and the possibility of greater opportunistic behavior, TCE might also explain why providers and managed care companies would turn to vertical integration as a means by which to manage more efficiently exchanges between them.

One possible explanation, however, for why vertical integration failed to take hold in the 1990s in health care may be a misreading of the sources of uncertainty in the environment. The rationale for vertical integration varies by whether the uncertainty stems from the input or the output sides of markets. If the uncertainty is on the input side (supply and production), it might well provide justification for vertical integration. Uncertainty on the input side points to strategies that focus on reducing transaction costs by controlling and smoothing production. Uncertainty on the output side (product demand), however, ties directly to the control of revenues, to the complexity in transactions as well as unpredictability in revenue flows (Williamson, 1981). TCE addresses costs of exchange more than risks inherent in unpredictable revenues. Facing the latter, organizations are likely to pursue organizational flexibility to cope with the unpredictability of demand, a move that, obviously, is incompatible with vertical integration (Harrigan, 1985; Mick, 1990). As a corollary, it is well known that rational planning (the formality of which is analogous to vertical structuring) is generally less effective under conditions of demand uncertainty (Mintzberg, 1994). However, as Mick argued (1990), vertical integration might still be justified under conditions of demand uncertainty, especially if by so integrating, the combined entities gain market power or other advantages. These arguments, however, are more compatible with the reasoning of industrial organization or resource dependency than of TCE.

From the perspective of providers in the 1990s, the initial and primary threats came from managed care, which, of course, is on the demand side. The increased penetration of managed care products did result in considerably increased complexities of exchange as well as important threats in revenue flows. Possibly more important, the growing power and aggressiveness of managed care companies pointed more directly to vertical structuring on the part of provider systems than did the uncertainties in revenue flows.

Resource Dependency

Resource dependency proposes that organizations survive to the extent that they effectively manage their environmental demands or, more specifically, acquire and maintain essential resources (Pfeffer and Salancik, 1978). Environmental constraints facilitate the choice and decision-making processes, and they minimize the impacts organizational leaders can have on organizational performance. Under resource dependency, therefore, leaders may serve highly symbolic roles. Past actions provide guideposts to managers as they manipulate the environment and attempt to match constraints with organizational operations and structures.

Importantly, complex organizations will exist so long as they are capable of eliciting necessary resource contributions through viable coalitions of support. Resource dependency thus suggests that managing the exchanges and relationships with interdependent organizations may be more important to survival than managing production efficiencies. Resource dependency thus differs from TCE by emphasizing strategic more than operational reasons for organizational restructuring. Vertical and horizontal integration, as discussed previously, are thus to be viewed as strategic mechanisms organizations might need to cope with interdependencies more than to facilitate better management of internal processes or the costs of exchange. Vertical integration ensures direct control over critical sources of exchange, and horizontal integration enables organizations to increase relative power, thereby countervailing threats from buyers in the vertical channel.

Early in the 1990s, providers expected that exclusive contracts would be given to those systems that generated low costs and offered low prices in market negotiations, provided a comprehensive mix of services, and arranged full geographic coverage within given markets. To win those contracts, they were expected to pursue both vertical and horizontal integration at the local market level. Their strategic options included horizontal integration among hospitals or among physicians beyond local markets to countervail the threats from other rivals or powerful buyers. Such strategic responses are fully compatible with the resource dependency perspective.

All of these reasons—to build market power (IO), to reduce the costs of exchange (TCE), and to control resources (resource dependency), as well as others—are likely to have played a role in shaping the strategic decisions of health care organizations in the 1990s. In some market environments, say in highly oligopolistic market structures (which characterized most urban hospital markets), providers might have emphasized horizontal strategies, given significant threats coming from rivals. Competitors that enjoyed more monopolistic positions, for example, as was (and is) the case in most nonurban markets, might focus more on strategies that reduce entry or substitution threats and ensure that patients do not migrate to the urban areas. In such situations, vertical integration might be the strategy of choice, as it would facilitate a more complete coordination of the full range of provider services, thereby deterring incursions by distant rivals and encouraging patients to obtain their care at home. In some markets, providers anticipating increased penetration of managed care companies might choose to integrate forward as an entry-deterring strategy (which could, for example, explain hospital strategies in Philadelphia and Minneapolis). Further, smaller rivals operating within oligopolistic markets, when confronted by much larger, dominating competitors, might adopt niching strategies by specializing or seeking out "safe" geographical areas within their broader markets where little competitive threat would be expected. Then, of course, competitors might conclude that a variety of viable threats exists, and thereby adopt strategies that position them best to cope with the uncertainties of market pressures.

It should be clear that a great variety of determinants of strategy exists. It follows that each of the major theoretical approaches could explain some, but not all of the strategic behaviors that occurred among health care players in the turbulent market environment of the 1990s. Moreover, the mix and relative importance of determinants at one point in time might be very different in another. Such is the view one might take when considering events from a strategic perspective.

Institutional Theory

Finally we come to institutional theory, which involves the mechanisms "by which social processes, obligations or actualities take on a rule-like status in social thought and action" (Meyer and Rowan, 1977, p. 341). Institutional theory suggests that the patterns of organizational formation may be shaped as much by myth and irrationality as by the rational objectives of organizational leaders (Scott, 1998). This view thus contrasts dramatically with the previous three perspectives.

Myths that generate formal organizational structure have two key properties: (1) they contain rationalized and impersonal prescriptions that imbue social actions with technical and rational meaning (as expressed in institutional rules), and (2) they are highly institutionalized and thus fall beyond the discretion of individuals or organizations. Given the latter property, institutional myths are taken for granted as being legitimate, apart from their actual effect on organizational outcomes. In health care, importantly, such myths are often established and reinforced through licensing, certifying, and schooling, as well as by other broad social mechanisms. The myths occur readily when there is causal ambiguity between organizational processes and the standards used to evaluate outputs, which is often the case in health care.

As the rules for engagement are based on myths, legitimacy is asserted based on mere suppositions of rational effectiveness. Institutional acceptance of suppositions becomes more important than empirical support. Ultimately, structures and programs become industry standards, as more and more members join in. This leads to a "bandwagon" effect, in which benefits and promise are adduced without there being a clear understanding of actual outcomes. As rules become more widely accepted, organizations look increasingly alike. This isomorphism often causes (1) an incorporation of inefficient elements, (2) the employment of external or ceremonial criteria to define structural elements, and (3) the dependence on externally justified strategies that presumably decrease uncertainty and increase an organization's survival. Institutionalization thus makes formal organizational structures similar and more complex than might otherwise be the case (DiMaggio and Powell, 1983).

Scott (1998) suggested that health care is especially susceptible to institutional pressures of the kind experienced in the turbulent period of the 1990s. Throughout that decade, hospitals consistently and universally adopted "faddish" structures and programs, most of which produced expectations unlikely to be fulfilled. These included the variety of organizational forms and strategies already discussed as well as the pursuit of "hot" management techniques, such as total quality management (TQM) and reengineering (Walston, Kimberly, and Burns, 1996). Institutional influences also delimited much of the range of strategic experimentation in the recent decade. And because institutional thought may have frequently trumped rational analyses of individual situations, failed expectations and actual failures in strategy may have been the inevitable result.

It should be pointed out that arguments other than institutional could explain the many copycat behaviors observed in the previous decade. Imitation of rival approaches for achieving competitive advantage, for example, is well recognized in the literature as a rational and often effective competitive tactic (Ghemawat, 2000). Further, the simultaneous movement by many competitors in the same strategic directions, as occurred in the 1990s, could be attributed to distinctive market conditions faced by all. For example, one could argue that individual hospitals had little option other than to seek partners within their own local markets, that is, to consolidate horizontally with hospital rivals and integrate vertically with physicians, all at the local level.

Integrated Model

Institutional constructs both prescribe the range of acceptable actions and act as barriers to strategic improvisation, thus closing out choices that otherwise might provide competitive advantage. This dual function—legitimizing and constraining—was clearly very important in the 1990s.

When combined, the rational and institutional arguments explain much of the strategic behaviors observed in the 1990s. Therefore, rather than give priority to one or the other, we choose to integrate them into a single framework. Figure 11.3 incorporates the four major explanations of organizational restructuring within a "legitimized-strategy" model. As indicated, the three "rational" arguments are comingled within the strategic choice process. They form the analytical core within a strategy framework. The institutional influence is placed outside this core, emphasizing its more general and often implicit role in shaping strategic choice. In the figure, institutional forces are conceived as creating barriers, which effectively restrict strategy options to those that might be considered legitimate. We define institutional barriers as *intervening influences that shape and reshape strategic decisions consistent with institutional norms.* In effect, institutional barriers reduce the range of options and even highlight particular choices that might be deemed "acceptable" or "desirable" at a given point in time. Use of the term *barriers* aligns the institutional influences conceptually with other important market barriers (that is, entry, exit, and mobility).

Institutional barriers as such have not been addressed in health care literature. This is possibly because in health care they came most clearly into view during the period of the 1990s. Institutional barriers, it would appear, can lie dormant until activated by strategic initiative or pressure. Undoubtedly, the strategic activism of the 1990s stimulated a concomitant rise in institutional restraint. As a result, the many attempts to restructure health care organizations ran head-on into the powerful institutional traditions that have for so long protected the autonomy and constrained the behaviors of health professionals and organizations.

Institutional mechanisms are the channel through which the considerable distinctiveness of the health care industry expresses itself in strategic decision making. Although many distinguishing

Figure 11.3. The Constrained-Strategy Model.

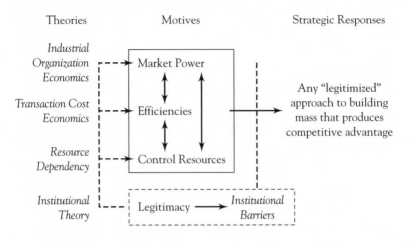

characteristics of the industry have been identified (Boulding, 1966; Donabedian, 1973; Luke and Begun, 1987), the focus here is on those features that are likely to have affected, and continue to affect, strategic decision making. Many of the distinctive features of the industry are deeply grounded in the moral context of health care and are embedded in the roles, rules, and procedures of health professionals and organizations. Institutional barriers both shielded and constrained the strategic responses of religious-based and, more generally, not–for-profit institutions. They preserved a cloak of operational autonomy for physicians, even after the physicians' medical practices had been acquired by hospital systems of physician practice management companies. They checked the spread of for-profit hospital systems, limiting efforts to form national systems and complicating efforts to acquire selected hospitals and other businesses. They frustrated the formation of vertical models that appeared to offer considerable advantages in terms of efficiencies and market power. And, in general, they preserved a higher degree of market fragmentation in the industry than might have been the case had market forces and strategic options not been constrained.

An interesting example of a highly legitimized idea that swept the industry in the 1990s was the so-called "market stages model" (APM/University HealthSystem Consortium, 1995). Initially a consulting contrivance, the stages model immediately filled a critical void in our understanding of the unprecedented turbulence in health care markets. It advanced guideposts that could be used to assess which strategies might most appropriately be pursued by health organizations, given the particular stage at which a given market might be. The construct spread rapidly throughout the industry. And it was not uncommon for persons to claim as a kind of badge of honor that their markets had moved into more "advanced" stages along the continuum provided by the model. Despite widespread institutional backing, the stages model enjoyed little empirical support (Burns, Bazzoli, Dynan, and Wholey, 1997). And by the end of the decade it effectively fell out of favor—in institutional terms, it lost its legitimacy as a market construct.

Many other legitimized ideas caught hold in the last decade. One of the most prominent, the integrated delivery system, received critically important moral justification by the professional associations that first proposed the concept (American Hospital Association, 1990; 1992; Catholic Health Association, 1992). Most especially, it was conceived as the ideal model for achieving efficiencies while at the same time improving quality (for example, see Conrad and Shortell, 1996). It was seen as the vehicle through which the many loose interconnections characteristic of the health care "system" might finally be formalized and internalized. And, significantly, it was viewed as a mechanism that could reach out to whole communities and, in the process, enhance their health outcomes and overall well-being. As with the stages model, however, the articulated virtues of this institutional construct enjoyed limited empirical support, despite the many claims on its behalf.

We would note that the efficiency arguments for the IDS model can be traced to the well-documented early successes of

Kaiser and other noted HMOs (Miller and Luft, 1993). Unfortunately, the research on HMOs did not specifically identify operational integration—the core idea underpinning the IDS—as the central contributor to earlier HMO successes. Nor did the research assess group and staff model HMOs in the context of intense market competition, such as was observed in the 1990s. And it did not consider the problems inherent in integrating around a hospital base, as was implicit in the IDS concept (Walston, Kimberly, and Burns, 1996). It appears that the rationale and findings supporting fully integrated HMOs were simply assumed to apply not only to hospital-based IDSs but to highly competitive markets as well.

Institutional Barriers

Given the consequential role that we believe institutional barriers played in constraining strategy in this industry, we explore further some of the important sources of institutional constraint. Specifically, we highlight four such sources:

- Professional model and autonomy expectations

- Physician-hospital interdependencies

- Mission-strategy conflicts

- Multilayered policy oversight

Professional Model and Autonomy Expectations

Professional communities and their established associations have proliferated in health care. They represent some of the most stable and important institutional structures in the industry (Freidson, 1970a; Stevens, 1989). Among many of their functions, they devise means by which their services might be distinguished from those provided by other professional types. And they create principles and norms to guide both service delivery and deportment. Most important, they reinforce the legitimacy of provider groups and delivery organizations.

As is well recognized, the professions enjoy varying but overall high levels of autonomy, which both protects them from control by outside entities and grants to them power to influence the immediate environments within which they work (Freidson, 1975). This includes shaping the conditions under which health care organizations are able to pursue their strategies in a competitive environment (Begun and Lippincott, 1993). The upshot of all of this is that professions and their associations erect and often enforce a wide variety of institutionalized constraints that are likely to affect significantly the strategic behaviors of their members.

The demise of the physician practice management companies is a case in point. These ran directly into the constraints of converting historically autonomous physician practices into common businesses to be managed distantly by corporate entities. Their problems have been attributed to financial causes (Reinhardt, 2000). But at the heart of the many financial miscalculations were the challenges inherent in organizing and managing physicians who retained high expectations of autonomy in both the clinical and administrative zones of work.

The struggle to integrate the diversity of health care professionals into local systems is another case in point. Health care has long been characterized as a "system," recognizing the significant degree to which existing organizations and individual providers were and are interdependent. Because the levels and pathways of interdependency are numerous and complex, one might expect, for example, taking a transaction cost economics (TCE) perspective, that the various delivery components would long ago have been internalized into formal delivery arrangements. However, as is well known, despite longstanding pressures, providers have consistently and successfully resisted integration into formal systems. Historically, myriad informal cooperative arrangements have provided the system connections and, at the same time, preserved well-established autonomies. Thus, even in the turbulent environment of the 1990s, health care organizations encountered serious difficulties in formalizing the informal.

It is not surprising, therefore, that as the industry began to consolidate in the 1990s (especially at the local level, where systemness enjoys its greatest potential), many health care organizations gravitated to the less-committing option of loose coupling. It is clear that they saw in this weaker organizational form the possibility of achieving strategic objectives with little sacrifice in autonomies. Even where more formal, owned arrangements were adopted, established power bases of individual participants were commonly left in place, producing in effect yet another variation on loose structuring. As a result, efforts to coordinate strategic agenda among the joined organizational members, whether owned or more loosely structured, were often countered by strong resistances to change.

Loose arrangements varied widely in legal form both within and across sectors in the health care industry. They ranged from hospital partnerships, physician hospital organizations (PHOs), independent practitioner associations (IPAs), foundations, so-called "group practices without walls," hospital "operational mergers," and many other permutations of loose arrangements. As might be expected, these were widely heralded and generally legitimized in the institutional environment. But few produced the kinds of bureaucratic mechanisms needed for bold strategic initiative, including moving toward true system integration, eliminating duplicated and excess service and management capacities, joint contracting, and multimarket expansion. Many of these arrangements were little more than structural artifices that met institutional expectations and protected traditional autonomies and power centers.

The 1997 merger between the Stanford University health system and the University of California health system provides an excellent example of the resistive power possessed by professional workers (Van Etten, 1999). This full merger, which brought two very prestigious academic medical centers together, was unable to eliminate long-standing power centers deeply embedded within the schools, their associated academic and clinical departments, professional groupings, and the hospitals themselves. Thus, with rapidly declining financial circumstances exacerbated by considerable structural complications, it did not take long for the two sides to recognize that the inherent institutional barriers could not be overcome. The merger was disbanded two years later in 1999. Similar patterns can be observed in other high-profile divestitures, including the widely publicized breakup of the Allegheny Health System in Philadelphia and the separation of Allina's providers and managed care services in Minneapolis.

It is true that by the early 1990s, loose organizational arrangements had received much acclaim in other industries and in the management literature (Kanter, 1994; Powell, 1990). However, health care organizations applied loose structures in the 1990s at a far higher level of strategic importance than was typical in other industries (Luke, Begun, and Pointer, 1989). In the latter, partnering companies tended to use loose structures to achieve very specific, typically marginal objectives, leaving the overall strategic agendas of the collaborating organizations essentially untouched. In health care, by contrast, especially in the 1990s, many partners banked their futures on the strategic combinations. And they attempted this without creating the kinds of bureaucratic structures generally needed to bring together disparate organizations. Significantly, many of the local combinations joined partners that had for years been direct and often very aggressive competitors with one another, thereby adding mistrust to weak alignments and autonomy constraints. In selected cases, they joined players that were embedded in powerful religious and other ownership structures (discussed more further on), thereby adding conflicting values and objectives to the problems of sustaining integration. With all of this, many combinations have consistently compromised on structural arrangements, despite the high strategic purposes such arrangements were intended to fulfill.

However, coming out of the 1990s, most horizontal hospital combinations are still holding together, despite weakened environmental pressures for consolidation. And post-1990s anecdotal evidence suggests that the hospital systems are gravitating toward tighter arrangements, as the hospital partners seek to overcome the significant challenges inherent in coordinating strategic agenda within loose structures. It is clear that horizontal arrangements are relatively easier to accomplish, especially if not overly confounded by issues involving affiliated health professionals. The point is this: because of long-held expectations of professional autonomy, health care organizations in the 1990s readily entertained structural compromises that were essentially incompatible with the strategic demands placed upon them (Luke, Begun, and Pointer, 1989). With experience, however, they might find ways to overcome some of the institutional constraints they encountered initially.

Physician-Hospital Interdependencies

Joint or simultaneous physician-hospital engagements in strategy are also complicated by the great diversity of operational, clinical, and strategic interrelationships that exist between the two. Physicians function as employees, suppliers, buyers, and partners for hospitals, often all at the same time. It is true that the specifics of these diverse interrelationships might vary across physicians, specialties, hospital types, and localities. Nevertheless, physicians and hospitals across the board depend heavily on one another to carry out the everyday work in which they are engaged. It would be a mistake, therefore, not to consider their interrelationships explicitly when analyzing the strategic behaviors of hospitals and physicians.

From a market perspective, their interdependencies can usefully be differentiated by whether or not they are inherently competitive or cooperative. We explore competitive interdependencies under two topics—direct competitors and substitutes—and cooperative interdependencies under four—bidirectional vertical, joint producers, complementors, and shared regulatory environment. Standing alone, no one of these should be considered significant. But in combination, they add up to a major source of institutionalized constraint to the strategic maneuvering of both physicians and hospitals. We discuss each of these sources of constraint below.

Competitive

Direct competitors. Physicians and hospitals compete with one another in a number of arenas, most especially in the provision of ancillary services. They can compete with one another regardless of whether the physicians are or are not members of a given hospital's medical staff. In the 1990s, many hospitals saw the need strategically to expand their service offerings to compete in the new managed care environment. In so doing, it was not uncommon for them to come into direct conflict with physicians who themselves had already implemented such services or were planning (or hoping) to do so. Generally, the hospitals were better positioned to expand in this way. They had the capital and the managerial resources needed to engage in costly service expansions. Nevertheless, medical staff members often exercised their leverage to force the hospitals to compromise on planned investment strategies. Likewise, hospitals did the same to physicians who took the initiative to compete directly against them, relying upon their considerable resource and market power.

The relative balance of power between physicians and hospitals, however, may have been altered as a result of the significant consolidation that took place in the hospital sector. Physicians lost ground because they entered into many consolidation ventures that then failed. Hospitals, by contrast, significantly strengthened their local market positions by successfully entering into local market combinations and, in some cases, into regional and national systems.

All such moves added measurably to their already significant advantage in market power relative to physicians. The added strength gained by hospitals may thus have tipped the delicate balance of power in the ongoing struggle for control between physicians and hospitals. This could have significant implications for the ways in which the two ultimately interrelate in the future.

Substitutes. Rivalries between physicians and hospitals in the 1990s also took the form of substitution threats. Services offered by physicians sometimes displaced existing or new hospital technologies and services. For example, many hospitals hired certified nurse anesthetists (CRNAs) to provide anesthesia for surgery in lieu of using anesthesiologists. Also, podiatrists, nurse midwives, and others gained privileges in hospitals, a domain that traditionally had been the unchallenged realm of physicians. Similarly, physicians provided services that displaced those historically offered exclusively by hospitals. These included, for example, offering complicated surgical, radiological, and laboratory procedures on an ambulatory basis. As with direct competition, substitutes entangle the strategic decision making of both physicians and hospitals.

Cooperative

Bidirectional vertical. Physicians both buy from and sell to hospitals, a relationship that, while vertical, is effectively bidirectional. Primary care physicians send referrals to hospital-based specialist physicians and directly to hospitals for the acquisition of ancillary services needed by their patients. Looking in the opposite direction, hospitals "acquire" the services of physicians who treat patients within their walls. Primary care physicians follow up with and may visit their patients during their hospital stays and consult with specialists about their care.

It is true that some of these relationships may not involve buying and selling per se. In most cases, no financial exchange is transacted between physicians and hospitals. Because insurance companies provide the financing, a contractual or production relationship as opposed to market exchange might better characterize such relationships. Financial exchange can take place between them when, say, physicians rent office space from buildings owned by hospitals. Also, from the perspective of service production, services and patients do flow vertically between them. And because the flows go both ways, we characterize this aspect of their relationship as bidirectional vertical. The important point is that this interdependency, founded in highly institutionalized role relationships, constitutes an important constraint on the degree to which each can act independently in strategic decision making.

Joint producers. Closely related to the bidirectional vertical concept is the concept of physicians as joint producers of services with hospitals, a relationship that has long been recognized (Smith, 1955). Acting as outside contractors, physicians direct the clinical processes within hospitals and they perform some of the important services. The simultaneity of production conducted by hospitals and physicians, in combination with their loose structural arrangements, establishes this as one of the most distinctive, institutionalized arrangements to exist in any industry. From a transaction costs perspective, were such joint production conducted within other industries, the workers would likely be internalized as employees by the organizations that owned and managed the production capacity. The fact that physicians have remained independent over the years highlights the enduring strength of their professional power.

Complementors. Complementary relationships (see Brandenburger and Nalebuff, 1996, for the strategic significance of complementarity) between physicians and hospitals have always been important. It was not until managed competition became the driving logic for health care organization and financing, however, that their mutual complementarity took on real strategic significance. As mentioned earlier, a prevalent assumption in the early 1990s was that managed care companies would prefer to contract with fully integrated health care delivery systems. Thus systems that covered the local geographical territory and offered the full complement of services required to service the beneficiaries of managed care organizations (MCOs) would, it was assumed, be preferred. MCOs would enter into comprehensive and exclusive contracts with such systems. A direct consequence of this assumption was that hospitals across the country attempted to develop full-service capacities, which was to include physician practices. As we now know, the expected pattern of contracting failed to materialize and, partly as a result, the acquisition of physician practices as a strategic move by hospitals slowed and in some cases came undone.

Nevertheless, the two remain highly interdependent when facing a market environment. Hospitals can hardly advertise their distinctive capabilities without referencing the strength of their medical staffs. Hospital and hospital system Websites, for example, are replete with references to their affiliated physicians. It is clear that in this increasingly market-oriented environment, hospitals and physicians must face the consumers jointly.

Complementarity between physicians and hospitals also exists with regard to upstream relationships in the supply channel. For example, physicians and hospitals rely on many of the same distributors to supply medical-surgical supplies and pharmaceuticals. Assumptions of complementarity, for example, played a part in McKesson's (a major pharmaceutical distributor) acquisition of General Medical (the leading distributor to physicians and the third largest distributor to hospitals) in the 1990s. McKesson had hoped to supply medical-surgical and pharmaceutical supplies jointly to both physicians and hospitals, thinking there were important distribution economies in doing so. Whether McKesson was right in its judgment has yet to be determined.

The continuing, albeit slow, formation of integrated systems has increased the shared interest between physicians and hospitals to engage collaboratively in the management of both supply and demand channels. This will likely be reinforced by the emergence of e-business, which increases the potential for shared communications, advertising, financing, and distribution between hospitals and physicians and their constituencies.

Shared regulatory environment. The power of physician-hospital complementarity extends well beyond traditional market relationships. It covers their relationships with the legal and regulatory communities as well. Increasingly, malpractice suits name multiple members of the delivery system, including hospitals and physicians. Likewise, the effort of regulatory bodies that set reimbursement levels for both hospitals and physicians has added to the interdependency over time. Fiscal constraints often force funding agencies such as Medicare and Medicaid to set reimbursement from one relatively fixed pot of money. Such actions pit provider groups against each other, as they fight for their share of the funds. With the continuing consolidation of the industry, the shared interest in the regulatory and financing environments is likely to increase further in the future.

In the end, it is the confluence of both competitive and cooperative relationships between physicians and hospitals that creates such significant institutional constraints to independent strategic decision making. In some markets or with some organizations the relationships might tend to be more competitive and in others more cooperative. If a market is made up of many large physician group practices, such as is the case in the Los Angeles basin or in many large western and midwestern markets, the groups, given their individual economic strength, might more likely engage nearby hospitals as competitors. In markets in which they are less well organized, physicians might be less willing to direct major competitive ventures against hospitals. The growing asymmetry of power that increasingly favors hospitals may well lead physician groups to engage in cooperative ventures with hospitals. This could generate a renewed interest in foundations, PHOs, IPAs, MSOs, or other hybrid organizational forms.

The central point is this: physicians and hospitals interact in a complex world of institutionalized interdependencies. This does not mean that they cannot act independently of one another, but that the relationships between them are of such consequence that they function as institutional screens through which important strategic decisions are filtered before enactment. Given the ongoing shifting in the balance of power between them, the institutionalized barriers to action might come down somewhat, though they seem unlikely ever to disappear. The inherent legitimacy of physicians is well-rooted in tradition, the power of knowledge, and the criticality of their work. Market forces and organizational restructuring are thus likely to erode their positions of power only on the margin— at least, so the history of their interrelationships informs us (Freidson, 1975).

Mission-Strategy Conflicts

Much of the health care industry is deeply embedded, both formally and informally, within community and religious institutional frameworks. Virtually all hospitals view themselves as "community" providers. And throughout the past century, a substantial percentage of hospitals identified themselves as church-related. Many carry faith-related names, even when they are no longer controlled by religious organizations. With all of the consolidation and organizational restructuring of the past ten to twenty years, the formal religious interconnections for many individual hospitals have either been eliminated or greatly attenuated. Many hospitals, for example, though listed in the American Hospital Association database as "church operated," are clearly members of health systems that are not operated, owned, or controlled by a church. Then, again, the 1990s produced a number of nonchurch hospitals that are now run, if not owned, by faith-based organizations.

Some of the new systems also combine hospitals across religious faiths or ownership types (for example, the combination of Catholic and Seventh Day Adventist systems in Denver, forming Centura Health). Given the strength of the institutionalized expectations, it is surprising that so many still appear to be holding together. Not all have survived, of course. The breakup of the Daughters of Charity-Baptist merger in Jacksonville is especially interesting, given the important role played by unreconciled institutionalized conflicts. The merger joined two religious-based organizations within a structurally compromised "operational" merger. By preserving certain powers of the original owners, critical structural fractures were put in place that ultimately would give way when the circumstances of the markets changed. The two partners had initially come together to ward off anticipated threats from managed care, Columbia/HCA (now HCA), and other powerful not-for-profit hospital rivals. When these market threats failed to materialize to the degree expected, residual internal conflicts, combined with a weak structure, led to the demise of the merger in 1999.

Rough estimates can be made of the numbers of church-affiliated institutions. By the beginning of the new century, approximately 12 percent of acute care general hospitals were Catholic and another four percent were other-church affiliated, out of approximately five thousand of such hospitals nationwide (Williamson Institute, 2001). The vast majority of church-affiliated hospitals are members of multihospital systems (87 percent). Over the past couple of decades, the numbers of church-affiliated hospitals declined steadily, especially for non-Catholic religious groups. The Catholic numbers have actually remained amazingly steady in recent decades, which reflects the strong institutional hold religious orders and other Catholic organizational entities have on their hospital systems (White, 2000). The many recombinations of Catholic systems into larger, hybrid multihospital systems (such as Catholic Health Partners and Catholic Health Initiatives) has jumbled specific ownership connections traditionally tied to religious orders. Despite this, the Catholic identity of these new organizations remains strong, even considering the increasing degree to which lay administrators and boards control these organizations.

Aside from formal linkages, religious as well as community values have permeated much of the health care industry and continue to do so. So long as there is death and suffering in health institutions, this will likely remain the case. From a strategic point of view, religious and community traditions are very much intermingled in the overall missions of most health care organizations. The term *community hospital* conveys more than mere location or the population served. It references a long tradition of highly institutionalized values that have shaped the conduct of health care organizations and individual professional workers for a very long time. Important and wideranging debates over public policy are rarely able to distance themselves from the many well-established religious-community traditions in health care.

For example, the debates over whether hospitals should remain not-for-profit, patients should have a "bill of rights," indigent patients should be given access to care, or certain clinical procedures should or should not be performed all have deep religious and moral bases that constrain and shape policy as well as strategy decisions. Likewise, battles over whether a hospital should allow itself to be acquired by a for-profit company, whether a local hospital system should compete on price with another local system, or simply whether a not-for-profit hospital system should expand beyond its current size are often waged on moral grounds, which themselves have strong religious and community underpinnings.

Community roots play an important role in constraining geographic expansion beyond local boundaries. Multimarket moves have been restricted for the most part to the small number of for-profit corporations and to Catholic systems. For the latter, of course, the multihospital structure was dictated by religious institutional development, not by market rationality. And the for-profits have been driven by the objectives of individual investors and developers. A few well-advanced not-for-profit systems have attempted to grow beyond local boundaries in the 1990s, but these are either exceptions (such as Sutter Health) or had engaged in multimarket expansion before the 1990s (for example, Intermountain Health Care). The 1990s move by the Mayo Clinic to both Florida and Arizona provides a dramatic exception for locally based not-for-profit hospitals, despite the benefits multimarket expansion strategies potentially could produce.

Not-for-profit systems, which represent nearly 80 percent of all multihospital systems and just over half of the system hospitals, generally have tended to avoid movement across local market boundaries in pursuit of system growth (Williamson Institute, 2001). Sixty percent of these systems are single-market companies—they are located in either one metropolitan statistical area or, in the case of a small number of them, in a few rural areas all in a single state—and this despite all of the strategic maneuvering of the past decade. This compares to 19 and 20 percent of for-profit and Catholic systems, respectively, that are located in single markets. Also, 88 percent of not-for-profit systems are concentrated within single states, which compares to 34 and 35 percent for for-profit and Catholic systems, respectively (Williamson Institute, 2001).

Local system formation was actually the predominant strategy pursued by hospital systems in the 1990s, a period in which only a few firms, mostly for-profit and Catholic hospital companies, pursued, or continued to pursue, multimarket strategies. It is clear that the local markets had become the focus of competitive strategy for most hospitals unaccustomed to aggressive multimarket strategic behavior. Movement into new geographies would force them to confront well-established, highly institutionalized webs of provider interconnections and community commitments and to cast aside preexisting territorial understandings and expectations.

Overall, the need to satisfy organizational and institutional goals and missions weighs heavily on most health care organizations, even those that are for-profit. All hospitals and hospital systems are challenged to balance the public interest with the private interest. Pressures from boards, professional organizations, and governmental entities encourage hospitals to cooperate and seek to rationalize services to serve their publics better, while, at the same time, they are driven to meet the bottom line.

Multilayered Policy Oversight

The complexity of the formal institutional environment also has increased in recent decades, especially since passage of Medicare in the mid-1960s. This has produced a complex array of entities that constrain and shape the strategic moves of health care organizations. Ranging from statutory legal barriers to restrictions created by voluntary accrediting agencies, these often circumscribe some of the most important strategic actions taken by health care organizations (such as mergers, acquisitions, and new market entries). A number of key legislative acts focusing on payments under Medicare, for example, played key roles in shaping strategy in the 1990s. These included the Tax Equity and Fiscal Responsibility Act (TEFRA) of 1982, the hospital inpatient prospective payment system (PPS) in 1983, the physician resource-based relative value scale (RBRVS) in 1992, and the Balanced Budget Act (BBA) of 1997. Other restraints affecting health care strategy included certificate-of-need laws, antidiscrimination laws, laws and regulations relating to the corporate reorganizations, the formation of charitable trusts, and charitable solicitations. There were also antitrust, fraud, and abuse statutes, including the Federal Anti-kickback Statute, Federal Stark I and II laws, and state anti-self-referral laws.

A more recent institutional barrier to integration focuses on the use of health care information, namely the Health Insurance Portability and Accountability Act of 1996 (HIPAA). Finally, in some states, corporate practice of medicine laws restrict the purchase and ownership of physician practices by hospitals and other entities. Indeed, a case could be made that the institutional reach of legal-regulatory structures in health care goes well beyond that commonly found in most other industries. It is true that this cloak of formalized restraint could be viewed itself as a consequence of a more fundamental institutional structure. Whether it is an outgrowth or at the core of the institutional environment, there can be no doubt that this multilayering of policy oversight weighs heavily on the strategy-making processes of health care organizations.

Summary and Discussion

We have argued that a wide variety of institutional factors greatly shaped choices and limited the degree to which health care organizations pursued "rational" strategies in the past decade. Such forces appear to have generated a bewildering array of unusual, sometimes unworkable organizational arrangements within health care. Many loose structures were undoubtedly designed to accommodate well-established institutional constraints rooted in both the public and private sectors of the industry, more than to produce competitive advantage per se.

The existing organizational theories help to identify a variety of motivations for strategic decision making in health care. Industrial organization, transaction cost economics, resource dependency, and other explanatory frameworks all provide alternative lenses through which the major organizational alternatives in strategy might be viewed. By providing rational bases for organizational actions, they help to explain many of the strategic moves pursued by health care competitors in the turbulent 1990s. They do not explain the strategic moves that are not pursued or that do not work out as might have been expected. Nor do they singly provide sufficient explanation of what are often very complex strategic patterns of strategic decision making.

Underlying each of the theoretical perspectives is the assumption that for the most part health care markets and organizations will act in ways that are consistent with their economic well-being. As a result of the strong institutional constraints, many health care organizations, however, have had little experience with economic rationality. And given the precipitous shift in the 1990s toward a market environment, it is reasonable to expect that economic rationality will continue to be sacrificed.

Mintzberg (1978) appropriately identified the learning processes through which strategic decisions typically pass, whereby highly rationalized strategic choices are reconsidered, modified, and often toned down as they move from concept to implementation. The gambit of compromises that can be made in strategic decisions, given their importance to organizations, can be very great. We suggest in this chapter that the pathways through which the grand strategies of health care organizations must pass are riddled as much by the sands of economic, organizational, and market realities as by the often insurmountable terrain of institutional values and constraints.

Institutional constraints can be very entrenched and thus appear to be immutable. History would suggest that such is the case in health care. Yet, the economic forces that raged through the industry in the 1990s left their imprint. The structures of some sectors within the industry were dramatically altered, especially those in the hospital and managed care sectors. Managed care became the dominant vehicle for organizing payment, much consolidation occurred, and market forces appear now to be widely accepted as a part of the new economic "reality." However, the landscape is littered with models for combining hospitals and physicians, both horizontally and vertically. Some of these survived the 1990s, others did not.

Nevertheless, the pressures that brought about change in the first place—cost increases, growing numbers of uninsured, and concerns over integration and quality—although temporarily ameliorated in the mid-1990s, remain with us. And it is not obvious how the new market conditions of the current decade will affect the institutional environment, let alone health organizational strategy. Whether or not institutional forces will continue to play powerful roles in strategic decision making in health care, now that the industry has experienced such widespread change, cannot easily be determined. It is likely, however, that the now much larger and more powerful health care organizations, especially as represented in local hospital systems, may serve as important counterbalances to some of the institutional constraints. However, as the power of some of the institutional constraints is diminished, that of others will remain tenacious, and their impacts might even be greater over time.

Institutional structures, given their overarching importance in health care, deserve added conceptual and, if possible, empirical assessment. What is clear is that we need a better understanding of the relationships between institutional and economic forces in this industry. For without this, we risk misspecifying our organizational and economic models and, possibly more important, misinforming policy makers and practitioners who are in the throes of making critical strategic decisions.

12

· ·

Research and Policy Implications

Stephen S. Mick and Mindy E. Wyttenbach

In this closing chapter, we synthesize elements of theorizing from across this volume. Arising from this synthesis are avenues for research exploration at both the theoretical and empirical levels. In an effort to advance scholarship and analysis of health care organizations, we suggest several broad areas of further inquiry that are based on our own reading of this volume's authors. Readers are invited to determine their own as well.

Institutional Forces and Markets

A good portion of this book can be described as an exploration of the dynamics and consequences of the confrontation between institutional and market forces. The purposeful use of market forces began timidly, but hopefully, in the 1970s, through such devices as the HMO Act of 1973, a Nixon-era cost-containment policy initiative that intended to create a subsidized competitive alternative to the private practice of medicine and to demonstrate the theoretical efficiencies of organized and coordinated group medical practice. Through the combined efforts of the TEFRA of 1982 and the enactment of the PPS system in 1983, hospitals experienced a transition throughout that decade of an inpatient payment system for Medicare that was supposed to induce caregiving efficiencies through economic incentives. Simultaneously throughout this period, the Employee Retirement Income Security Act opened a new world of alternative financing and delivery possibilities by allowing employers to self-fund their employee health insurance programs and to break the stranglehold that fully funded but highly regulated insurance entities held on purchasers of group health insurance policies. All of this intertwined with the development and growth of various managed care approaches to care, most of which attempted to capture the putative efficiencies that market discipline could now induce.

In the 1990s, the federal Health Security Act tried but failed to create a national system of regional and state competition between purchasers and providers of health care. This system was also supposed to harness the power of market competition through managed care entities, not only to effect cost containment and enhance quality but also, through the projected savings such a scheme was to offer, to extend health insurance coverage to many millions of uninsured Americans. The failure of this initiative was a lost battle only, not a lost war, because the private sector embraced managed care completely, such that by the end of the decade, most working Americans and most Americans covered by Medicaid were enrolled in one form of health plan or other. For a brief moment in the mid-1990s, the triumph of market forces appeared complete as the growth in costs in the United States was flat for the first time in anyone's memory.

Then, toward the end of the decade, and quickly, cost increases began anew. Insurers, including health plans, started to seek price increases in an effort to improve profitability after a period of aggressive market share growth with deferred insurance premium increases. Hospital consolidation launched a new era of concern about antitrust behavior, as local market after local market witnessed the growth of a handful of dominant horizontally integrated hospital systems. These consolidated systems, now freer of market pressures to compete successfully, sought greater reimbursement from insurers; this in turn fueled cost increases. Many organizational arrangements and experiments proved not only difficult to sustain (for example, health system ownership of physician practices) but also more expensive to manage because of elevated transaction costs, as in the case of integrated delivery systems. Aggressive managed care practices to control physician and patient behavior were abandoned.

In short, nearly three decades' worth of steady movement in both public and private arenas to harness the power of market forces has, in the early 2000s, come under scrutiny. Many of the chapters of this volume have wrestled with what theoretical insights there might be to understand this apparent backsliding from a reliance on well-operating markets as the lynchpin of American health policy.

The background is set in Scott's chapter, in which readers are exposed to a broad overview of the changing health care environment in the San Francisco Bay Area from the post-World War II era to the 1990s. There the author outlined the increasing complexity and competitiveness among health care organizations, as well as the evolution of various organizational forms in a dynamic interplay of environment or market and organizational entities. Part of what he documents is the "erosion" of physician autonomy and the challenge of managerial strategy and control over the historically sacred terrain of medical practice. These changes are directly attributable to managers' actions as agents of market-oriented doctrines.

The central research question that emerges from this evolution is whether "managerial logics," to use Scott's term, have actually prevailed to the extent predicted. Have the recent managed care backlash and attendant phenomena such as the relaxation of managerial control devices, the flight of health plans and systems from owning physician practices, and the unraveling of efforts to form highly integrated delivery systems belied the triumph of managerial hegemony in health care delivery? The experience of many managed care organizations in California that attempted to require the use of hospitalists (hospital-based physicians who manage patient care on inpatient floors) for plan beneficiaries in the mid-1990s is instructive. The severe opposition from nonhospitalist physicians has slowed this promising approach to patient care and relegated it to a more experimental marginal status. Despite some clinically-based arguments by antagonists of the hospitalist approach to patient care, it is the institutional logic that has mattered, because good-to-excellent clinical care has been provided through hospitalist-like systems throughout the world. In fact, institutional norms and values favor hospitalist care in countries such as France, countries that spend nowhere near what the United States does for inpatient services and do not have a discernible difference in quality.

Other chapters have proposed a broader array of possibilities or have elaborated on more specific outcomes stemming from the interaction of market versus institutional forces. The fourfold typology of hypothetical interrelationships between market forces and institutional pressures outlined by Alexander and D'Aunno provides a template suggesting that there are various ways that institutional forces and market attributes can relate to each other. White's chapter on Catholic health systems proposes that allegiance to institutional norms probably is being eroded by the press of market forces, although he also suggests that the values traditionally inherent in Catholic health care organizations are being abandoned at a very slow pace and with extreme reluctance. White's argument could well be extended to a host of other health care organizations, including academic health centers and their mission of teaching and research, a mission that has been heavily challenged by market pressures from managed care plans and from nonteaching hospital systems that are under no compunction to recognize and accommodate themselves to teaching and research missions. And in the Luke and Walston chapter, there is a well-developed argument that insists that without a thorough understanding of the power of institutional forces, much of the turmoil of the 1990s health care system will simply be misunderstood and misinterpreted.

Wholey and Burns's focus on markets as systems of exchange relations that emphasize economic transactions not only conjures up a variety of fresh ways to think of the interaction of organizations in markets but also connects with other authors of this volume who have wrestled more directly with the institutional versus market view of health care organizations' operating and strategic environments. This is because the emphasis on relations among actors and the focus on the exchanges themselves allow that the normative and value-laden elements of exchange enter into any consideration of organizations and economic transactions. This perspective transcends the strict theoretical allegiance that economists hold toward definitions of markets and their operations, including the less than optimal functioning of markets under conditions of "market failure." Market failure is generally attributed to a handful of conditions, alone or in combination, such as too few purchasers of services (monopsony), too few sellers of services (monopoly), uneducated publics or publics not allowed to exercise choice, producers not incurring the full costs of production, consumers not incurring the full expense of what they obtain, and the like. The power of these forces cannot be gainsaid; however, the origin of these conditions leading to market failure often remains mysterious. A focus on interactions and exchanges promises to elucidate processes that make health care markets work in ways that need a noneconomic rationale to understand. For example, why are publics uneducated or why do they make uninformed choices? Can one assume it is because people are inherently stupid and ignorant? Or can one seek a more productive explanation through the lens of social factors such as would be generated through networks of acquaintances, for example, transmission of local cultural traditions or exposure to normative criteria of choice, such as the result of effective advertising by a health plan?

The same may be said of the typical way health care organization theorists view organizations and their markets. There is often a tendency to think of health plans, hospitals, nursing homes, and the like as entities that are somehow bounded apart from the environments in which they exist. This perspective leads to scholarship that is self-limiting in its ability to go beyond the idea of markets and organizations as simply context and entity interacting, reacting, preempting, and the like. The idea of markets as exchange systems allows the notion in our studies of organizations as semipermeable membranes, populated and enmeshed in exchanges in a bewildering array of combinations, with varying intensity and frequency.

As Wholey and Burns argue, there are weighty policy consequences that emerge from the juxtaposition of "relational strength," the force of social integration and networks, and publics acting as monadic decision makers expressing market choice. Their argument is that greater choice is associated with lower relational strength. But the inherent emotional vulnerability of many conditions of illness will lead to increased bonding between patient and physician, that is, greater relationship strength. Under circumstances like this, what is the power of "choice" and "information"? Illness, on the other hand, may increase patient-physician relational strength and thereby decrease the usefulness of choice. The impact on quality of care is therefore an open question, and this is a major area for theoretical work and empirical investigation.

A second general issue is the power that relational exchanges confer to providers of health care, a power that lies in contrast to the power of open, free market exchanges between provider and consumer. Much policy debate and experimentation have confronted this conflict in the 1990s, and whether an effective health care system can have a balance between the two is one of the central policy questions of our time and into the future.

This line of reasoning is picked up in both Shortell and Rundall's and Banaszak-Holl, Elms, and Grazman's investigations of the theoretical logic behind the application of network theory and strategic adaptation. By using the realm of physician-organization settings, Shortell and Rundall build on Wholey and Burns's broad discussion of exchange and relational activities. They provide readers with a system of thinking that helps reveal the failure of many of the 1990s' efforts to integrate physician practices into organizations, which were done with the hope of applying the armamentarium of managerial devices to control costs, increase quality, induce efficiencies, and enhance overall performance. Banaszak-Holl and colleagues perform a similar task but in the realm of nonacute care community-based services. By focusing on this sector that is infrequently studied, and in which conventional notions of organizations and markets are difficult to apply, these authors demonstrate through this unique empirical area how notions of networks and exchange can be easily applied.

Taken together, the chapters beginning with Scott's and ending with that of Banaszak-Holl and colleagues provide us with a common thread of theoretical inquiry that emphasizes the intertwining of social factors with market forces. A more catholic view of organizational markets may render a more realistic and faithful representation of what actually happens in health care. The empirical mandate is to devise studies that examine exchanges and their network paths more explicitly, and not merely to measure "market concentration" or "share," while also not being content with the stock measures of organizational attributes such as size, number of beds, ownership category, and the like. And there is the prospect of moving into other realms of the health care sector. For example, the approach of Banaszak-Holl and colleagues could probably be fruitfully applied to alternative organizational settings such as regional health systems or national consortia of health care organizations, for example, the Council of Teaching Hospitals.

Readers will be able to find extensive discussion on issues aside from an exploration of the tension between institutional and market forces. However, in the quest to find a position on the question of whether market forces can or could work were it not for institutional pressures, often reflected in regulatory oversight, both scholars and policymakers must come to terms with the empirical evidence that we have to date, evidence that has produced the chapters in this book. And if one concludes that there is promise in some middle ground between market and institutional forces—a sort of "make markets work approach" to health policy—the quest is to find a workable balance or a dynamic tension between both poles such that enough market discipline can be forged to effect valued objectives while at the same time recognizing that economic markets are social constructions wherein exchange takes place. This means that norms and values, the stuff of institutions, will always exist and will not always conform to pure economic objectives.

The Importance of the Internal Life of Organizations

Much of this volume is devoted to varying arguments about the importance and utility of recasting our image of organizations and markets as a vision of exchange. However, the Kimberly and Minvielle chapter on quality in health care is a forceful reminder that organizations, even as "semipermeable membranes" out of and into which exchanges begin and terminate, have internal dynamics in and of themselves. The force of bureaucratic forms, whether of the machine or professional variety, cannot be ignored in understanding an organization's relations with its constituent environments and markets.

For instance, relational networks among professionals that exist inside a health system are extensively connected and extend well beyond the organization's boundaries into professional associations and reference groups that confer normative sense and direction to almost all professional activity. This connection is a major ingredient in the formation and maintenance of professional bureaucracy. In the realm of quality assessment and improvement, the commingling of internal organization and external relations could probably be no more entangled than in any other feature of clinicians' professional lives.

As a starting point for further inquiry, the themes presented in the Kimberly and Minvielle chapter are very relevant to other historic organizational innovations in the health care industry in the

United States, such as reengineering and the shift to and departure from matrix management. In fact, the adoption of almost any innovation as well as the termination of administrative and production experiments within a particular organization setting can be fruitfully examined from the conjoined perspectives of networks, exchange, and internal organization dynamics.

Zazzali demonstrates that a key ingredient in exchange and relational activities is trust. His chapter focuses on the "glue" that binds actors and organizations together and the havoc wreaked in both social and economic exchange patterns when it is not present. In the spirit of the earlier chapters of this volume, his argument is that trust may mitigate the agency and transaction costs for those in exchange relationships in the health sector. If Zazzali is correct that trust may decrease uncertainty in these exchange relationships, then there could be less of a need for increased monitoring, haggling, and enforcement, which constitute the bulk of agency and transaction costs theorizing. But trust is an essential element in any institutional arrangement, including economic institutions, at least according to a good deal of classical sociological theory from Durkheim to Parsons to Merton, among others. It is unclear that when trust is absent markets themselves can perform well, and this is an area in great need of further examination.

The study of trust presents its own set of challenges. In recent years there has been an explosion of research employing multilevel modeling techniques. Such techniques are good ways of assessing the relationships between variables that exist at different levels of analysis. These methods have proven to be quite useful in organizational applications, in which the dependent variable may exist at one level of analysis (such as individual patients) while the explanatory variables may encompass contextual factors, including organizational variables.

Multilevel models are particularly applicable when examining how trust in the health sector, perceived by individuals, may be a function of organizational relationships. In his chapter on trust,

Zazzali proposes that changes at one level of analysis meant to build trust may negatively influence trust at other levels of analysis. Specifically, relatively new organizational relationships and configurations meant to build trust between organizational entities are largely foreign to consumers of health services (and many providers) and may lead consumers to distrust the organizations and providers affiliated with them. This and many other propositions could be empirically assessed using a multilevel model of individual consumer trust in health care organizations as a dependent variable with explanatory variables including various organizational-level variables.

A Different Paradigm

Following chapters that wrestle with the institutional-market question, Begun, Zimmerman, and Dooley offer a completely different view of where theory can be fruitful. By viewing organizations as complex adaptive systems embedded in organizational fields that are also complex and adaptive, these authors believe that the density, complexity, and inherent dynamism of health care organizational life are better understood by application of "complexity science" than through conventional theories.

Juxtaposed against institutional versus market forces questions that have occupied most of this book's authors, the model that Begun and colleagues propose asks completely different questions. There is less interest, for example, in whether market forces and institutional arrangements can be "made" to coexist in some way such that the benefit of market discipline can be captured while also accommodating the inevitable institutional pressures that will arise because of the inherent social nature of organizational arrangements. Rather, the interest lies less in tagging organizational innovations as "successes" or "failures," as happy adaptations to market forces and the like, but in describing and predicting the natural unfolding of dynamic processes with complex and intertwined origins. The effort of conventional theory to reduce complex phenomena to a few factors and to explain such phenomena with a simplified and reduced set of so-called explanatory variables does injustice to the reality of organizational life and its intimate interdependence with its environments. The time-honored dictum of Occam's Razor always to seek the most simplified explanation is turned on its head with complexity science's adaptive systems approach. This is, indeed, a radical departure from conventional organization theory, and the incorporation of "surprise" and the unexpected in organizational life only adds to the novelty of this perspective, given that "normal" theory prefers predictable relationships and patterns in a broadly generalizing fashion.

As if to underscore the fruitful possibilities of this very different paradigm, Luke and Walston argue that no single conventional theory is capable of capturing the unpredictable richness of organizational change and strategic intent of the 1990s. Their effort to combine a host of approaches stands as a sort of testimony that there is room for innovative thinking about organizations, thinking of the sort that Begun and colleagues espouse. Nevertheless, Luke and Walston insist that undergirding any examination of organizational activity in relation to its environment is a strong institutional impulse, harkening back to this volume's main focus on the normative and value-laden content of environmental and market contexts within which health care organizations operate through networks and exchange relations.

In the end, however, it is the reader who may be best able to see the connections from one chapter to the next in this volume and to ferret out fruitful research themes and avenues for further inquiry. Our hope is that this book has helped crystallize convergences of thinking about health care organizations that are based on the foment of the health care sector of the 1990s. Although our intention has been to synthesize and summarize the applications of theory to 1990s events as well as to encourage theory development in its own right, it has also been our objective to challenge ourselves to think in new and unusual ways about the empirical world in which we work, and to explore the prospect that our theories need refinement, improvement, and perhaps even abandonment. We hope this book has helped in this task in some modest way.

References

Abrahamson, E., and Rosenkopf, L. "Institutional and Competitive Bandwagons: Using Mathematical Modeling as a Tool to Explore Innovation
Diffusion." *Academy of Management Review*, 1993, *18*, 487–517.

The Advisory Board. *The Grand Alliance*. Washington, D.C.: The Advisory
Board, 1993.

Ahuja, G. "Collaboration Networks, Structural Holes, and Innovation: A
Longitudinal Study." *Administrative Science Quarterly*, 2000, *45*(3),
425–455.

"AIDS Drugs for Poor Nations." Editorial, *The New York Times*. March 12, 2001.
Late edition, section A, p. 14.

Aldrich, H. *Organizations Evolving*. Thousand Oaks, Calif.: Sage, 1999.

Alexander, J. A., Burns L. R., and others. "An Exploratory Analysis of Market-
Based Physician-Organization Arrangements." *Hospital and Health Services
Administration*, 1996, *413*, 311–329.

Alexander, J. A., Comfort, M. E., and Weiner, B. J. "Governance in Public-
Private Community Health Partnerships: A Survey of the Community
Care Networks Demonstration Sites." *Nonprofit Management and Leader-
ship*, 1997, *8*(4), 311–332.

Alexander, J. A., and D'Aunno, T. A. "Transformation of Institutional Environments: Perspectives on the Corporatization of U.S. Health Care." In
S. S. Mick (ed.), *Innovations in Health Care Delivery: Insights for Organization Theory* (pp. 53–85). San Francisco: Jossey-Bass, 1990.

Alexander, J. A., and Morlock, L. "Power and Politics in Health Services
Organizations." In S. Shortell and A. Kaluzny (eds.), *Health Care Manage-
ment: Organizations, Design and Behavior* (4th edition) (pp. 244–269).
New York: Delmar Publications, 1999.

Alexander, J. A., Morrisey, M., and Shortell, S. "Effects of Competition, Regulation and Corporatization on Hospital Physician Relationships." *Journal of Health and Social Social Behavior,* 1986, *27*(3), 220–235.

Alexander, J. A., and Scott, W. R. "The Effects of Regulation on the Administrative Structure of Hospitals: Toward an Analytic Framework." *Hospital and Health Services Administration,* 1984, *29*(3), 71–85.

Alexander, J. A., and Weiner, B. J. "Determinants of the Adoption of Corporate Models of Governance by Non-Profit Organizations." *Non-Profit Management and Leadership,* 1998, 8(3), 223–242.

Alexander, J. A., Weiner, B. J., and Bogue, R. "Changes in the Structure, Composition and Activity of Hospital Governing Boards, 1989–1997: Evidence from Two National Surveys. *The Milbank Quarterly,* 2001, 79(2), 253–279.

Alexander, J. A., Weiner, B. J., and Succi, M. "Community Accountability Among Hospitals Affiliated with Health Care Systems." *The Milbank Quarterly,* 2000, 78(2), 157–184.

Alexander, J. A., Vaughn, T., and others. "Organizational Approaches to Integrated Healthcare Delivery: A Taxonomic Analysis of Physician-Organizational Arrangements." *Medical Care Research & Review,* 1996, *53*(1), 71–93.

Alexander, J. A., and others. "The Ties that Bind: Inter-Organizational Linkages and Physician System Alignment." *Medical Care,* 2001a, *39*(7), 30–45.

Alexander, J. A., and others. "Risk Assumption and Physician Alignment with Health Care Systems." *Medical Care,* 2001b, *39*(7), 46–61.

Alford, R. R. "The Political Economy of Health Care: Dynamics without Change." *Politics and Society,* 1972, *2*, 27–64.

Alter, C. F., and Hage, J. *Organizations Working Together.* Newbury Park, Calif.: Sage, 1993.

Amburgey, T. L., Dacin, T., and Kelly, D. "Disruptive Selection and Population Segmentation: Interpopulation Competition as a Segregating Process." In J. A. Baum and J. V. Singh (eds.), *Evolutionary Dynamics of Organizations* (pp. 240–256). New York: Oxford University Press, 1994.

American Academy of Pediatrics. "Issues in the Application of the Resource-Based Relative Value Scale System in Pediatrics: A Subject Review." *Pediatrics,* 1998, *102,* 996–998.

American Hospital Association, Section for Health Care Systems. *Renewing the U.S. Health Care System.* Washington, D.C.: The Office of Constituency Sections, 1990.

American Hospital Association. *Overview: AHA's National Reform Strategy.* Chicago: American Hospital Association, 1992.

American Hospital Association. *Healthcare Networks and Systems* (1999 data). Chicago: Health Forum/American Hospital Association, 2000a.

American Hospital Association. *AHA Annual Survey of Hospitals* (1999 data). Chicago: Health Forum/American Hospital Association, 2000b.

American Hospital Association. *Guide to the Health Care Field* (2001 ed.). Chicago: American Hospital Association, 2001.

American Medical Association. "Brazil May Defy the United States and Make More AIDs Drugs." *Journal of American Medical Association,* Feb. 5, 2001. (www.ama-assn.org/special.hiv/newsline/reuters/02068951.html).

Anand, B., and Khanna, T. "Do Firms Learn to Create Value? The Case of Alliances." *Strategic Management Journal,* 2000, *21,* 295–315.

Anderson, O. W., Herold, T. E., Buler, B. W., Kohrman, C., and Morrison, E. M. (1985). *HMO Development: Patterns and Prospects.* Chicago: Pluribus Press, University of Chicago, 1985.

Anderson, P. "Complexity Theory and Organization Science." *Organization Science,* 1999, *10*(3), 216–232.

Andrews, K. R. *The Concept of Corporate Strategy.* Homewood, Ill.: Dow Jones-Irwin, 1971.

Annison, M., and Wilford, D. (eds.). *Trust Matters: New Directions in Health Care Leadership.* San Francisco: Jossey-Bass, 1998.

Anonymous. "Keeping Its CHIN Up: Wisconsin Health Information Network." *CIO,* 1997, *10,* 60–62.

Anonymous. "An Interview with Merlin I. Olson." *Health Care Review,* 1999, *5,* 1–4.

APM/University HealthSystem Consortium. "How Markets Evolve?" *Hospitals and Health Networks,* 1995, *60,* 60.

Argyris, C., and Schön, D. *Organizational Learning: A Theory of Action Perspective.* New York: Addison-Wesley, 1978.

Arndt, M., and Bigelow, B. "Commentary: The Potential of Chaos Theory and Complexity Theory for Health Services Management." *Health Care Management Review,* 2000, *25*(1), 35–38.

Arthur, B. W. "Competing Technologies, Increasing Returns, and Lock-In by Historical Events." *Economic Journal,* 1989, *99,* 6–31.

Atchison, T. A. "Reply." *Frontiers of Health Services Management,* 1999, *16*(1), 49–50.

Atkinson, B. "Wisconsin Cities Win with WHIN (Wisconsin Health Information Network)." *Infocare,* 1995, *36,* 38–40.

Auerbach, J., and Coates, T. "HIV Prevention Research: Accomplishments and Challenges for the Third Decade of AIDS." *American Journal of Public Health*, 2000, 90(7), 1029–1032.

Axelrod, R. *The Evolution of Cooperation*. New York: Basic Books, 1984.

Axelrod, R., and Cohen, M. D. *Harnessing Complexity: Organizational Implications of a Scientific Frontier*. New York: Free Press, 1999.

Badertscher, D. "Practices Retain Control with a Non-Acquisition Model PPMC." *Healthcare Financial Management*, 1998, 52(5), 66–68.

Bain, J. S., and Qualls, D. "Introduction and Economic Theory Concerning Industrial Organization." In S. B. Bacharach (ed.), *Industrial Organization: A Treatise*, Greenwich, Conn.: JAI Press, 1987.

Baker, W. E. "The Social Structure of a National Securities Market." *American Journal of Sociology*, 1984, 89, 775–811.

Baker, W. E., and Faulkner, R. R. "The Social Organization of Conspiracy: Illegal Networks in the Heavy Electrical Equipment Industry." *American Sociological Review*, 1993, 58, 837–860.

Banaszak-Holl, J., Allen, S., Mor, V., and Schott, T. "Organizational Characteristics Associated with Agency Position in Community Care Networks." *Journal of Health and Social Behavior*, 1998, 39, 368–385.

Barley, S. R., Freeman, J., and Hybels, R. "Strategic Alliances in Commercial Biotechnology." In N. Nohria and R. G. Eccles (eds.), *Networks and Organizations: Structure, Form, and Action* (pp. 311–345). Boston: Harvard Business School Press, 1992.

Barr, S. "The 1990 Florida Dental Investigation: Is the Case Really Closed?" *Annals of Internal Medicine*, 1996, 124(2), 250–254.

Batalden, P. B., and Mohr, J. J. "Building Knowledge of Health Care as a System." *Quality Management in Health*, 1997, 5, 1–12.

Baum, J. A. "Organizational Ecology." In S. Clegg, C. Hardy, and W. R. Nord (eds.), *Handbook of Organizational Studies* (pp. 77–114). Thousand Oaks, Calif.: Sage, 1996.

Baum, J. A., and Oliver, C. "Institutional Linkages and Organizational Mortality." *Administrative Sciences Quarterly*, 1991, 36(2), 187–218.

Baum, J. A., Calabrese, T., and Silverman, B. S. "Don't Go It Alone: Alliance Network Composition and Startups' Performance in Canadian Biotechnology." *Strategic Management Journal*, 2000, 21, 267–294.

Bazzoli, G. "Consequences of Hospital Financial Distress." *Hospital and Health Services Administration*, 1995, 40, 472–495.

Bazzoli, G. J., Chan, B., Shortell, S. M., and D'Aunno, T. "The Financial Performance of Hospitals Belonging to Health Networks and Systems." *Inquiry*, 2000, 37(3), 234–252.

Bazzoli, G., Dynan, L., Burns, L., and Lindrooth, R. "Is Provider Capitation Working? Effects on Physician-Hospital Integration and Costs of Care." *Medical Care*, 2000, 38(3), 311–24.

Bazzoli, G. J., Shortell, S. M., Dubbs, N., Chan, B., and Kralovec, P. "A Taxonomy of Health Networks and Systems: Bringing Order Out of Chaos." *Health Services Research*, 1999, 33(6), 1683–1717.

Becker, S. W., and Gordon G. "An Entrepreneurial Theory of Formal Organizations. Part 1: Patterns of Formal Organizations." *Administrative Science Quarterly*, 1966, 11, 315–344.

Begun, J. W. "Chaos and Complexity: Frontiers of Organizational Science." *Journal of Management Inquiry*, 1994, 3(4), 329–335.

Begun, J. W., and Lippincott, R. C. *Strategic Adaptation in the Health Profession: Meeting the Challenges of Change.* San Francisco: Jossey-Bass, 1993.

Begun, J. W., and Luke, R. D. "Factors Underlying Organizational Change in Local Health Care Markets, 1982–1995." *Health Care Management Review*, 2001, 26(2), 62–72.

Begun, J. W., and White, K. R. "The Profession of Nursing as a Complex Adaptive System: Strategies for Change." In J. J. Kronenfeld (ed.), *Research in the Sociology of Health Care* (pp. 189–203). Greenwich, Conn.: JAI Press, 1999.

Bellandi, D. "Events Unfold for Nonprofits." *Modern Healthcare*, 2001, 31(1), 28.

Berwick, D. "Continuous Improvement as an Ideal in Health Care." *New England Journal of Medicine*, 1989, 320(1), 43–46.

Berwick, D., Godfrey, A., and Roessner, J. *Curing Health Care.* San Francisco: Jossey-Bass, 1990.

Berwick D. "Quality of Health Care. Part 5: Payment by Capitation and the Quality of Care." *New England Journal Medicine*, 1996, 335(16), 1227–1231.

Bigley, G. A., and Pearce, J. L. "Straining for Shared Meaning in Organization Science: Problems of Trust and Distrust." *Academy of Management Review*, 1998, 23(3), 405–421.

Blendon, R. J., and Benson, J. M. "Americans' Views on Health Policy: A Fifty-Year Historical Perspective." *Health Affairs*, 2001, 20(2), 33–46.

Blendon, R. J., and others. (1998). "Understanding the Managed Care Backlash." *Health Affairs*, 1998, 17(4), 80–94.

Blumenthal, D., and Edwards, J. N. "Involving Physicians in Total Quality Management: Results of a Study." In A. C. Scheck (ed.), *Improving Clinical Practice: Total Quality Management and the Physician.* San Francisco: Jossey-Bass, 1995.

Blumenthal, D., and Epstein, A. M. "Quality of Health Care. Part 6: The Role of Physicians in the Future of Quality Management." *New England Journal of Medicine*, 1996, *335*, 1328–1331.

Blumenthal, D., and Kilo, C. M. "A Report Card on Continuous Quality Improvement." *The Milbank Quarterly*, 1998, *76*(4), 625–648.

Bohlmann, R. "Organized Practice 2000 and Beyond: Chaos or Opportunity?" *Medical Group Management Journal*, 2000, *47*(3), 40–42, 44–46.

Bolland, J. M., and Wilson, J. V. "Three Faces of Integrative Coordination: A Model of Interorganizational Relations in Community-Based Health and Human Services. *Health Services Research*, 1994, *29*(3), 341–366.

Bonnel, R. "Economic Analysis of HIV/AIDS." *Report from The World Bank.* 2000. At http://www.iaen.org/.

Borys, B., and Jemison, D. B. "Hybrid Organizations as Strategic Alliances: Theoretical Issues in Organizational Combinations." *Academy of Management Review*, 1989, *14*, 234–249.

Boulding, K. E. "The Concept of Need for Health Services." *Milbank Memorial Fund*, 1966, *44*, 202–221.

Brandenburger, A. M., and Nalebuff, B. J. *Co-opetition*. New York: Doubleday, 1996.

Brint, S., and Karabel, J. "Institutional Origins and Transformations: The Case of American Community Colleges." In W. W. Powell and P. J. DiMaggio (eds.), *The New Institutionalism in Organizational Analysis* (pp. 337–360). Chicago: University of Chicago Press, 1991.

Brook, R., McGlynn, E. A., and Cleary, P. D. "Quality of Health Care. Part 2: Measuring Quality of Care." *New England Journal of Medicine*, 1996, *335*(13), 966–970.

Brown, J. S., and Duguid, P. "Organizational Learning and Communities-of-Practice: Toward a Unified View of Working, Learning, and Innovation." *Organization Science*, 1991, *2*, 57.

Brown, M. "Mergers, Networking, and Vertical Integration: Managed Care and Investor-Owned Hospitals." *Health Care Management Review*, 1996, *21*(1), 29–37.

Buckley, P. J., and Casson, M. "A Theory of Cooperation in International Business." In F. Contractor and P. Lorange (eds.), *Cooperative Strategies in International Business*. Lexington, Mass.: Lexington Books, 1988.

Buckley, S. "Brazil Becomes Model in Fight Against AIDS; Government, Activists Team to Defy Epidemic Through Distribution of Drugs." *Washington Post*, Sept. 17, 2000, A22.

Bunderson, J. S., Lofstrom, S. M., and Van de Ven, A. H. (1998). "Allina Medical Group: A Division of Allina Health System." In P. M. Ginter, L. M.

Swayne, and W. J. Duncan (eds.), *Strategic Management of Health Care Organizations* (3rd edition) (pp. 602–619). Malden, Mass.: Blackwell Publishers, 1998.

Bureau of Labor Statistics. *Occupational Outlook Handbook: Physicians.* Washington, D.C.: U.S. Department of Labor, 2000. At http://www. bls.gov/oco/ ocosØ74.htm.

Burke, W. W. "Metaphors to Consult By." *Group and Organizational Management,* 1992, *17*(3), 255–259.

Burns, L. R., and Robinson, J. "Physician Practice Management Companies: Implications for Hospital Based Integrated Delivery Systems." *Frontiers of Health Services Management,* 1997, *14*(2), 3–35.

Burns, L. R., and Thorpe, D. "Trends and Models in Physician-Hospital Organizations." *Health Care Management Review,* 1993, *18*(4), 7–20.

Burns, L. R., and Thorpe, D. P. "Why Provider-Sponsored Health Plans Don't Work." *Healthcare Financial Management Resource Guide,* 2000, *54*(sup.), 12–16.

Burns, L. R., and Wholey, D. "The Diffusion of Matrix Management: Contagion Effects, Structural Effects, and Institutional Effects on Innovation Adoption." *Academy of Management Journal,* 1993, *36,* 106–138.

Burns, L. R., and Wholey, D. "Responding to a Consolidating Healthcare System: Options for Physician Organizations." *The Future of Integrated Delivery Systems,* 2000, *1,* 261–323.

Burns, L. R., Bazzoli, G., Dynan, L., and Wholey, D. "Managed Care, Market Stages, and Integrated Delivery Systems: Is There a Relationship?" *Health Affairs,* 1997, *16*(6), 204–18.

Burns, L. R., Cacciamani, J., Clement, J., and Aquino, W. "The Fall of the House of AHERF: The Allegheny Bankruptcy." *Health Affairs,* 2000, *19*(1), 7–41.

Burns, L. R., Alexander, J.A., and others. "Physician Commitment to Organized Delivery Systems." *Medical Care,* 2001, *39*(7), 9–29.

Burns, L. R., Walston, S. L., and others. "Just How Integrated Are Integrated Delivery Systems? Results from a National Survey." *Health Care Management Review,* 2001, *26*(1), 20–39.

Burrows, S. N., and Moravec, R. C. "Direct Contracting: A Minnesota Case Study." *Healthcare Financial Management,* 1997, *51*(8), 50–55.

Burt, R. S. "Social Contagion and Innovation: Cohesion Versus Structural Equivalence." *American Journal of Sociology,* 1987, *92,* 1287–1335.

Burt, R. S. "The Stability of American Markets." *American Journal of Sociology,* 1988, *94,* 356–395.

Burt, R. S. *Structural Holes: The Social Structure of Competition.* Cambridge, Mass.: Harvard University Press, 1992a.

Burt, R. S. "The Social Structure of Competition." In N. Nohria and R. G. Eccles (eds.), *Networks and Organizations: Structure, Form, and Action* (pp. 57–91). Boston, Mass.: Harvard Business School Press, 1992b.

Burt, R. S., and Carlton, D. S. "Another Look at the Network Boundaries of American Markets." *American Journal of Sociology,* 1989, 95, 723–753.

Butera, P. "A Network Solution Puts Hospitals, Doctors, Medical Labs, Employers, and Insurers in a Win-WHIN Situation." *Signals,* 1992, 5, 6–7.

Campbell, J. L., and Lindberg, L. N. "Property Rights and the Organization of Economic Activity by the State." *American Sociological Review,* 1990, 55, 634–647.

Capron, L., and Mitchell, W. "Bilateral Resource Redeployment and Capabilities Improvement Following Horizontal Acquisitions." *Industrial and Corporate Change,* 1998, 7, 453–484.

Carroll, G. R., and Hannan, M. T. "Density Dependence in the Evolution of Populations of Newspaper Organizations." *American Sociological Review,* 1989, 54, 524–548.

Carroll, G. R., and Swaminathan, A. "Why the Microbrewery Movement? Organizational Dynamics of Resource Partitioning in the American Brewing Industry After Prohibition." *American Journal of Sociology,* 2000, 106, 715–762.

Carroll, G. R., Delacroix, J., and Goodstein, J. "The Political Environments of Organizations: An Ecological View." In B. M. Staw and L. L. Cummings (eds.), *Research in Organizational Behavior* (pp. 359–392). Greenwich, Conn.: JAI Press, 1988.

Cassidy, J. "Catholic Identity Is Based on Flexible, Reasonable Tradition." *Health Progress,* 1994, 75(1), 16–17, 25.

Catholic Health Association. *Setting Relationships Right: A Working Proposal for Systemic Healthcare Reform.* St. Louis: Catholic Health Association, 1992.

Catholic Health Association. "Mission-Driven Market Strategies: Lessons from the Field." *Health Progress,* 1998, 79(4), 50–53.

Center for Studying Health System Change. *Cleveland Community Report—Draft 1.* Washington, D.C.: Center for Studying Health System Change, 2000a.

Center for Studying Health System Change. *Provider Systems Thrive in Robust Economy.* Washington, D.C.: Center for Studying Health System Change, 2000b.

Centers for Disease Control and Prevention. "Trends in Sexual Risk Behaviors Among High School Students—United States, 1991–1997. *Morbidity Mortality Weekly Report*, 1998, *47*, 749–52.

Centers for Disease Control and Prevention. *HIV Prevention Strategic Plan Through 2005*. Atlanta: Centers for Disease Control and Prevention, 2001.

Charns, M. P., Young G. J., Daley J., Khuri, S. F., and Henderson, W. G. "Coordination and Patient Care Outcomes." In J. R. Kimberly and E. Minvielle (eds.), *The Quality Imperative: Measurement and Management of Quality in Health Care*. London: Imperial College Press, 2000.

Chassin, M. R. "Quality of Health Care. Part 3: Improving the Quality of Care." *New England Journal of Medicine*, 1996, *335*(14), 1060–1063.

Chassin, M. R., Galvin, R. W., and the National Roundtable on Health Care Quality. "The Urgent Need to Improve Health Care Quality." *Journal of the American Medical Association*. 1998, *280*, 1000–1005.

Chesney, R. "Privacy and Its Regulation: Too Much Too Soon, or Too Little Too Late? *Pediatrics*, 2001, *107*, 1423–1425.

Choi, T., and Dooley, K. "Conceptualizing Supply Networks as a Complex System: Its Meaning, Its Properties, and Managerial Implications." *Journal of Operations Management*. 2000, *19*, 351–366.

Christianson, J., Feldman, R., Weiner, J. P., and Drury, P. "Early Experience with a New Model of Employer Group Purchasing in Minnesota." *Health Affairs*, 1999, *18*, 100–114.

Christianson, J. B., Moscovice, I. S., Johnson, J., Kralewski, J., and Grogan, C. "Evaluating Rural Hospital Consortia." *Health Affairs*, 1990, *9*, 135–147.

Clement, J. P., and others. "The Financial Performance of Hospitals Affiliated with Strategic Hospital Alliances." *Health Affairs*, 1997, *16*(6) 193–203.

Cochran, C. E. "The Common Good and Healthcare Policy." *Health Progress*, 1999a, *80*(3), 41–44, 47.

Cochran, C. E. "Institutional Identity; Sacramental Potential: Catholic Healthcare at Century's End." *Christian Bioethics*, 1999b, *5*(1), 26–43.

Cochran, C. E. "Keeping Hospitals Catholic." *Commonweal*, Feb. 25, 2000, 12–16.

Cochran, C. E., and White, K. R. "Does Catholic Ownership Matter?" *Health Progress*, 2002, *83*, 14–16, 50.

Cochrane, J. D. "Are Unions the Future of Medicine?" *Integrated Healthcare Report*, Feb. 1999, 1–12.

Coddington, D. C., Moore, K. D., and Fischer, E. A. *Integrated Health Care: Reorganizing the Physician, Hospital, and Health Plan Relationships.* Englewood, Colo.: Center for Research in Ambulatory Health Care Administration, 1994.

Coffey, R. J., Fenner, K. M., and Stogis, S. L. (1997). *Virtually Integrated Health Systems: A Guide to Assessing Organizational Readiness and Strategic Partners.* San Francisco: Jossey-Bass, 1997.

Cohen, W., and Levinthal, D. "Absorptive Capacity: A New Perspective on Learning and Innovation." *Administrative Science Quarterly,* 1990, *35,* 128–152.

Cole, R. E., and Scott, W. R. (eds.). *The Quality Movement and Organization Theory.* Thousand Oaks, Calif.: Sage, 2000.

Coleman, J. S. "Social Capital in the Creation of Human Capital." *American Journal of Sociology,* 1988, *94,* 95–120.

Coleman, J. S., Katz, E., and Menzel, H. *Medical Innovation: A Diffusion Study.* New York: Bobbs-Merrill, 1966.

Commons, J. R. *The Economics of Collective Action.* New York: Macmillan, 1950.

Conrad, D. A., and Dowling, W. L. "Vertical Integration in Health Services: Theory and Managerial Implications." *Health Care Management Review,* 1990, *15*(4), 9–22.

Conrad, D. A., and Shortell, S. M. "Integrated Health Services: Promises and Performance." *Frontiers of Health Services Management,* 1996, *3*(1), 3–40.

Conrad, D. A., Mick, S. S., Watts-Madden, C., and Hoare, G. "Vertical Structures and Control in Health Care Markets: A Conceptual Framework and Empirical Review." *Medical Care Review,* 1988, *45,* 49–100.

Cook, K. S., and Whitmeyer, J. M. "Two Approaches to Social Structure: Exchange Theory and Network Analysis." *Annual Review of Sociology,* 1992, *18,* 109–127.

Cooper, A. C. "Networks, Alliances, and Entrepreneurship." In M. A. Hitt, R. D. Ireland, S. M. Camp, and D. L. Sexton (eds.). *Strategic Entrepreneurship: Creating a New Integrated Mindset.* Oxford, U.K.: Blackwell, 2001.

Corbin, J., and Strauss, A. *Unending Work and Care.* San Francisco: Jossey-Bass, 1988.

Corman, S., Kuhn, T., McPhee, R., and Dooley, K. "Studying Complex Discursive Systems: Centering Resonance Analysis of Organizational Communication." *Human Communication Research,* 2002, *23,* 157–206.

Council on Graduate Medical Education. *Managed Health Care: Implications for the Physician Workforce and Medical Education.* Washington, D.C.: U.S. Department of Health and Human Resources, 1995.

Coyle, M. J. "No Toyotas in Health Care: Why Medical Care Has Not Evolved to Meet Patient Needs." *Health Affairs*, 2001, *20*, 44–55.

Crozier, M. *The Bureaucratic Phenomenon*. Chicago: University of Chicago Press, 1964.

Cutler, D. M. *The Changing Hospital Industry: Comparing Not-for-Profit and For-Profit Institutions*. Chicago: University of Chicago Press, 2000.

Dacin, T. M. "Isomorphism in Context: The Power and Prescription of Institutional Norms." *Academy of Management Journal*, 1997, *40*, 46–81.

Damanpour, F. "Bureaucracy and Innovation Revisited: Effects of Contingency Factors, Industrial Sectors, and Innovation Characteristics." *Journal of High Technology Management Research*, 1996, *7*(2), 149–173.

Darlington, S. "Brazil Becomes Model in AIDS Fight." Reuters News Media, 2000. At www.aegis.org/news/re/2000/re001107.html.

D'Aunno, T., and Zuckerman, H. "A Life-Cycle Model of Organizational Federations: The Case of Hospitals." *Academy of Management Review*, 1987, *12*(3), 534–545.

D'Aunno, T., Succi, M., and Alexander, J. A. "The Role of Institutional and Market Forces in Divergent Organizational Change." *Administrative Science Quarterly*, 2000, *45*, 679–703.

D'Aveni, R. A. "Top Managerial Prestige and Organizational Bankruptcy." *Organization Science*, 1990, *1*, 121–142.

David, P. A. "Clio and the Economics of QWERTY." *American Economic Review*, 1985, *75*, 232–237.

Davies, H.T.O., and Rundall, T. G. "Managing Trust in Managed Care." *The Milbank Quarterly*, 2000, *78*(2), 1–29.

Davis, G. F. "Agents Without Principles? The Spread of the Poison Pill Through the Intercorporate Network." *Administrative Science Quarterly*, 1991, *36*, 583–613.

Dawes, R. "Behavioral Decision-Making and Judgment." In D. T. Gilbert, S. T. Fiske, and G. Lindzey (eds.), *The Handbook of Social Psychology* (4th edition). Boston: McGraw-Hill and Oxford, 1998.

Deming, W. E. *Out of the Crisis*. Cambridge, Mass.: Massachusetts Institute of Technology, 1986.

Dent, E. B. "Complexity Science: A Worldview Shift." *Emergence*, 1999, *1*(4), 5–19.

Des Jarlais, D., and others. "HIV Incidence Among Injection Drug Users in New York City, 1992–1997: Evidence for a Declining Epidemic. *American Journal of Public Health*, 2000, *90*, 352–359.

Devers, K. J., Sofaer, S., and Rundall, T. "Qualitative Methods in Health Services Research." *Health Services Research*, 1999, *34*(5), Part II.

DeWitt, C. "Getting Down to Business." *Hospitals*, 1981, 55(19), 76–78.

Dickler, R., and Shaw, G. "The Balanced Budget Act of 1997: Its Impact on U.S. Teaching Hospitals." *Annals of Internal Medicine*, 2000, *132*, 820–824.

Dill, A. E., and Rochefort, D. A. (1989). "Coordination, Continuity, and Centralized Control: A Policy Perspective on Service Strategies for the Chronically Mentally Ill." *Journal of Social Issues*, 1989, 45(3), 145–159.

DiMaggio, P. J., and Powell, W. W. "The Iron Cage Revisited: Institutional Isomorphism and Collective Rationality in Organizational Fields." *American Sociological Review*, 1983, 48, 147–160.

DiMaggio, P., and Powell, W. "The Iron Cage Revisited: Institutional Isomorphism and Collective Rationality in Organizational Fields." In W. Powell and P. DiMaggio (eds.), *The New Institutionalism in Organizational Analysis* (pp. 63–82). Chicago: University of Chicago Press, 1991.

Dobbin, F., and Dowd, D. J. "How Policy Shapes Competition: Early Railroad Foundings in Massachusetts." *Administrative Science Quarterly*, 1997, *42*, 501–529.

Donabedian, A. *Aspects of Medical Care Administration: Specifying Requirements for Health Care*. Cambridge, Mass.: Harvard University Press, 1973.

Donabedian, A. "Social Responsibility for Personal Health Services: An Examination of Basic Values." *Inquiry*, 1980a, 8, 3–19.

Donabedian, A. *Explorations in Quality Assessment and Monitoring, Vol. 1.: The Definition of Quality and Approaches to Its Assessment*. Chicago: Health Administration Press, 1980b.

Dooley, K. "Organizational Complexity." In M. Warner (ed.), *International Encyclopedia of Business and Management*, vol. 6 (pp. 5013–5022). London: Thompson Learning, 2002a.

Dooley, K. "Simulation Research Methods." In J. Baum (ed.), *Companion to Organizations* (pp. 829–848). London: Blackwell, 2002b.

Dooley, K., and Plsek, P. "A Complex Systems Perspective on Medication Errors." Working Paper, Arizona State University, 2001.

Dooley, K., and Van de Ven, A. "Explaining Complex Organizational Dynamics." *Organization Science*, 1999, *10*(3), 358–372.

Downie, A. "Brazil: Showing Others the Way." *San Francisco Chronicle*, 2001. At www.aegis.org/news/sc/(2001)/sc010310.html.

Doz, Y. "Technology Partnerships Between Larger and Smaller Firms: Some Critical Issues." *International Studies of Management and Organization*. 1988, *17*, 31–57.

Doz, Y., Olk, P. M., and Ring, P. "Formation Processes of R&D Consortia: Which Path to Take? Where Does it Lead?" *Strategic Management Journal,* 2000, *21,* 239–266.

Dranove, D., and Shanley, M. "Costs Reductions or Reputation Enhancement as Motives for Mergers: The Logic of Multihospital Systems." *Strategic Management Journal,* 1995, *16,* 55–74.

Dranove, D., Peteraf, M., and Shanley, M. "Do Strategic Groups Exist? An Economic Framework for Analysis." *Strategic Management Journal,* 1998, *19,* 1029–1044.

Dukerich, J. M., Golden, B. R., and Shortell, S. M. "Is Beauty in the Eye of the Beholder? Predicting Physician Cooperative Behaviors and the Impact of Organizational Identification, Identity, and Image." Working paper. Berkeley, Calif., 2002.

Dutton, J. E., Dukerich, J. M., and Harquail, C. V. "Organizational Images and Member Identification." *Administrative Science Quarterly,* 1994, *39,* 239–263.

Dyer, J. H., and Nobeaka, K. "Creating and Managing a High-Performance Knowledge-Sharing Network: The Toyota Case." *Strategic Management Journal,* 2000, *21,* 345–367.

Dyer, J. H., and Singh, H. "The Relational View: Cooperative Strategies and Sources of Interorganizational Competitive Advantage." *Academy of Management Review,* 1998, *23,* 660–679.

Eccles, R. *The Transfer Pricing Problem: A Theory for Practice.* Lexington, Mass.: Lexington Books, 1981.

Eddy, D. M. "Performance Measurement: Problems and Solutions." *Health Affairs,* 1998, *17,* 7–25.

Edelman, L. B., and Suchman, M. C. "The Legal Environments of Organizations." *Annual Review of Sociology,* 1997, *23,* 479–515.

Eisenberg, J. M. *Doctors' Decisions and the Cost of Medical Care.* Ann Arbor: Health Administration Press, 1986.

Eisenhardt, K. "Agency Theory: An Assessment and Review." *Academy of Management Review,* 1989, *14*(1), 57–74.

Ellison, M. S. "Physician Unions Continue to Grow; What Lies Ahead?" *Physicians Financial News,* 2000, *18*(1), 1, 14, 15.

Emanuel, E. J., and Emanuel, L. L. "What Is Accountability in Health Care?" *Annals of Internal Medicine,* 1996, *124*(2), 229–239.

Emerson, R. M. "Power-Dependence Relations." *American Sociological Review,* 1962, *27,* 31–41.

Eoyang, G. H., and Berkas, T. H. "Evaluating Performance in a Complex, Adaptive system (CAS)." In M. R. Lissak and H. P. Gunz (eds.), *Managing Complexity in Organizations: A View in Many Directions* (pp. 313–335). Westport, Conn.: Quorum, 1999.

Ethical and Religious Directives for Catholic Health Care Services. United States Conference of Catholic Bishops. Publication No. 5–454. Washington, D.C.: USCCB Publishing, 2001.

Eve, R. A., Horsfall, S., and Lee, M. E. (eds.). *Chaos, Complexity, and Sociology: Myths, Models, and Theories.* Thousand Oaks, Calif.: Sage, 1997.

Farren, S. *A Call to Care: The Women Who Built Catholic Healthcare in America.* St. Louis: The Catholic Health Care Association, 1996.

Federal Register, 1/6/95. The Family and Medical Leave Act of 1993.

Feldman, R. R., and Wholey, D. R. *Do HMOs Have Monopsony Power?* Minneapolis: Division of Health Services Research, Policy and Administration, School of Public Health, University of Minnesota, 1999.

Feldstein, P. *Health Care Economics.* New York: Wiley, 1988.

Fennell, M. L., and Alexander, J. A. "Organizational Boundary Spanning in Institutionalized Environments." *Academy of Management Journal,* 1987, *30,* 456–476.

Feorene, B. T. "The Grass Wasn't Greener: Hospital-Physician Partnering in the Post-PPMC World." *Medical Network Strategy Report,* 1999, 8(2), 1, 8, 11.

Ferlie, W. B., and Shortell, S. M. "Improving Quality of Health Care in the United Kingdom and the United States: A Framework for Change." *The Milbank Quarterly,* 2001, 79(2), 281–315.

Fiol, C. M. "Squeezing Harder Doesn't Always Work: Continuing the Search for Consistency in Innovation Research." *Academy of Management Review,* 1996, *21*(4), 1012–1021.

Fligstein, N. *The Tranformation of Corporate Control.* Cambridge, Mass.: Harvard University Press, 1990.

Fligstein, N. "Markets as Politics: A Political-Cultural Approach to Market Institutions." *American Sociological Review,* 1996, *61,* 656–673.

Fligstein, N. "Social Skill and Institutional Theory." *American Behavioral Scientist,* 1997, *40,* 397–405.

Fligstein, N., and Brantley, P. "Bank Control, Owner Control, or Organizational Dynamics: Who Controls the Large Modern Corporation?" *American Journal of Sociology,* 1992, *98,* 280–307.

Flood, A. B. "Risk, Trust, and the HMO: An Editorial." *Journal of Health and Social Behavior,* 1998, *39,* 187–188.

Flynn, R., Williams, G., and Pickard, S. *Markets and Networks: Contracting in Community Health Services*. Philadelphia: Open University Press, 1996.

Freeland, E. P. "The Dynamics of Nonprofit and Public Organizational Growth in Health Care and Higher Education: A Study of U.S. States." Doctoral Dissertation, Princeton University. *Dissertation Abstracts International*, 1992.

Friedland, R., and Alford, R. R. "Bringing Society Back In: Symbols, Practices and Institutional Contradictions." In W. W. Powell and P. J. DiMaggio (eds.), *The New Institutionalism in Organizational Analysis* (pp. 232–263). Chicago: University of Chicago Press, 1991.

Friedman, L., and Goes, J. "Why Integrated Health Networks Have Failed." *Frontiers of Health Services Management*, 2001, *17*(4), 3–28.

Freidson, E. *Professional Dominance: The Social Structure of Medical Care*. Chicago: Aldine, 1970a.

Freidson, E. *Profession of Medicine: A Study in the Sociology of Applied Knowledge*. New York: Dodd, Mead, 1970b.

Freidson, E. *Doctoring Together: A Study of Professional Social Control*. New York: Elsevier, 1975.

Freidson, E. *Professional Powers: A Study of the Institutionalization of Formal Knowledge*. Chicago: University of Chicago Press, 1986.

Gabel, J., Ginsburg, P., Pickreign, J., and Reschovsky, J. "Trends in Out-of-Pocket Spending by Insured American Workers, 1990–1997." *Health Affairs*, 2001, *20*(2), 47–57.

Galaskiewicz, J., and Wasserman, S. "Mimetic and Normative Processes Within an Interorganizational Field: An Empirical Test." *Administrative Science Quarterly*, 1989, *34*(3), 454–479.

Gallistel, C. *The Organization of Learning*. Cambridge, Mass.: MIT Press, 1990.

Galloro, V. "Allina Under Fire." *Modern Healthcare*, 2001a (March 26), 4, 14.

Galloro, V. "The Big Breakup." *Modern Healthcare*, 2001b (July 30), 4–5.

Garceau, O. *The Political Life of the American Medical Association*. Cambridge, Mass.: Harvard University Press. 1941.

Gargiulo, M., and Benassi, M. "Trapped in Your Own Net? Network Cohesion, Structural Holes, and the Adaptation of Social Capital." *Organization Science*, 2000, *11*, 183–196.

Gerth, H. H., and Mills, C. W. *From Max Weber: Essays in Sociology*. New York: Oxford University Press, 1958.

Ghemawat, P. *Strategy and the Business Landscape*. Upper Saddle River, N.J.: Prentice-Hall. 2000.

Giddens, A. *The Constitution of Society: Outline of the Theory of Structuration.* Berkeley, Calif.: University of California Press, 1984.

Gilbert, R. J. "Symposium on Compatibility: Incentives and Market Structure." *Journal of Industrial Economics,* 1992, *60,* 1–8.

Gillies, R. R., and others. "Implementing Continuous Quality Improvement." In J. R. Kimberly and E. Minvielle (eds.), *The Quality Imperative: Measurement and Management of Quality in Health Care.* London: Imperial College Press, 2000.

Ginsburg, P. "Analyzing the Changing Health System: The Path Taken and the Road Beyond." Annual Report. Washington, D.C.:Center for Studying Health System Change, 2000.

Gleick, J. *Chaos: Making a New Science.* New York: Viking, 1987.

Glouberman, S., and Mintzberg, H. "Managing the Care of Health and the Cure of Disease. Part I: Differentiation." *Health Care Management Review,* 2001a, *26*(1), 56–69.

Glouberman, S., and Mintzberg, H. "Managing the Care of Health and the Cure of Disease. Part II: Integration." *Health Care Management Review,* 2001b, *26*(1), 70–87.

Goldstein, J. *The Unshackled Organization: Facing the Challenge of Unpredictability Through Spontaneous Reorganization.* Portland, Oreg.: Productivity Press, 1994.

Goldstein, J. "Emergence: A Construct Amid a Thicket of Conceptual Snares." *Emergence,* 2000, *2*(1), 5–22.

Goodrick, E., and Salancik, G. R. "Organizational Discretion in Responding to Institutional Practices: Hospitals and Cesarean Births." *Administrative Science Quarterly,* 1996, *41,* 1–29.

Goodwin, B. *How the Leopard Changed Its Spots: The Evolution of Complexity.* New York: Charles Scribner's Sons, 1994.

Granovetter, M. "The Strength of Weak Ties." *American Journal of Sociology,* 1973, *78,* 1360–1380.

Granovetter, M. "Economic Action and Social Structure: The Problem of Embeddedness." *American Journal of Sociology,* 1985, *91*(3), 481–510.

Gray, B. H. "Trust and Trustworthy Care in the Managed Care Era. *Health Affairs,* 1997, *16*(1), 34–49.

Grazman, D., and Van de Ven, A. (1996). "The History of Allina Health System." Working Paper. Minneapolis: Strategic Management Research Center, University of Minnesota, 1996.

Greco, P., and Eisenberg, J. "Changing Physicians' Practices." *New England Journal of Medicine,* 1993, *329,* 1271–1274.

Greening, D. W. "Testing a Model of Organizational Response to Social and Political Issues." *Academy of Management Journal*, 1994, *37*(3), 467–498.

Greenwood, R., and Hinings, C. R. "Understanding Radical Organizational Change: Bringing Together the Old and New Institutionalism." *Academy of Management Review*, 1996, *21*, 1022–1054.

Grenier-Sennelier, C., Maillet-Gouret, M. C., Ribet-Reinhart, N., Jeny-Loeper, C., and Minvielle, E. Une Expérience Concrète du Programme Assurance Qualité: Le Cas de la Prévention des Chutes dans un Hôpital de Soins de Suite et de Réadaptation. *La Revue Française de Gériatrie*, 1998, *23*, 303–315.

Griffith, J. R., and White, K. R. *The Well-Managed Healthcare Organization* (5th edition). Chicago: AUPHA Press/Health Administration Press, 2002.

Grossman, J. M. "Health Plan Competition in Local Markets" (Comment). *Health Services Research*, 2000, *35*, 17–35.

Gulati, R. "Does Familiarity Breed Trust? The Implications of Repeated Ties for Contractual Choice in Alliances." *Academy of Management Journal*, 1995a, *38*, 85–112.

Gulati, R. "Social Structure and Alliance Formation Patterns: A Longitudinal Analysis." *Administrative Science Quarterly*, 1995b, *40*, 619–652.

Gulati, R. "Alliances and Networks." *Strategic Management Journal*, 1998, *19*, 293–317.

Haas-Wilson, D., and Gaynor, M. (1998). "Increasing Consolidation in Healthcare Markets: What Are the Antitrust Policy Implications?" *Health Services Research*, 1998, *33*, 1403–1419.

Hagg, I., and Johanson, J. *Firms in Networks: A New View of Competitive Power.* Stockholm: Business and Social Research Institute, 1983.

Hallyn, F. *The Poetic Structure of the World: Copernicus and Kepler.* New York: Zone Books, 1990.

Hannan, M. T., and Carroll, G. R. *Dynamics of Organizational Populations: Density, Legitimation, and Competition.* New York: Oxford University Press, 1992.

Hannan, M. T., and Freeman, J. "The Population Ecology of Organizations." *American Journal of Sociology*, 1977, *82*, 929–964.

Hannan, M. T., and Freeman, J. "Structural Inertia and Organizational Change." *American Sociological Review*, 1984, *49*, 149–164.

Hannan, M. T., and Freeman, J. *Organizational Ecology.* Cambridge, Mass.: Harvard University Press, 1989.

Hansmann, H. "The Effect of Tax Exemption and Other Factors on the Market Share of Nonprofit Versus For-Profit Firms." *National Tax Journal*, 1987, *40*(1), 71–82.

Harrigan, K. *Strategic Flexibility: A Management Guide for Changing Times*. Lexington, Mass.: Lexington Books, 1985.

Harris-Shapiro, J., and Greenstein, M. S. "RBRVS—1999 Update." *Journal of Health Care Finance*, 1999, 26(2), 48–52.

Hatchuel, A. and Weil, L. B. *L'Expert et le Systeme*. Paris: Economica, 1992.

Haunschild, P. R., and Miner, A. S. "Modes of Imitation: The Effects of Outcome Salience and Uncertainty." *Administrative Science Quarterly*, 1997, 42, 472–500.

Haveman, H., and Rao, H. "Hybrid Forms and Institution/Organization Co-Evolution in the Early California Thrift Industry." In W. W. Powell and D. L. Jones (eds.), *How Institutions Change*. Chicago: University of Chicago Press, forthcoming.

Havlicek, P. L. *Medical Group Practices in the U.S.: A Survey of Practice Characteristics*. Chicago: American Medical Association, 1999.

HCIA. "A Comprehensive Review of Hospital Finances in the Aftermath of the Balanced Budget Act of 1997." 2001. At http://www.hcia.com/ studies/fahs/8total.htm.

Hechter, M. *The Principles of Group Solidarity*. Berkeley, Calif.: University of California Press, 1987.

Heffler, S., and others. "Health Spending Growth Up in 1999: Faster Growth Expected in the Future." *Health Affairs*, 2001, 20(2), 193–203.

Hehir, J. B. "Identity and Institutions." *Health Progress*, 1995, 76, 17–23.

Henny, J. "Speech to the Association of American Medical Colleges, Council of Teaching Hospitals." Washington, D.C. May 11, 2000. At www.aau.edu/research/Henney5.11.00.html

Herzlinger, R. E. *Market-Driven Health Care: Who Wins, Who Loses in the Transformation of America's Largest Service Industry?* Reading, Mass.: Addison-Wesley, 1997.

Heydebrand, W. V. "Autonomy, Complexity, and Non-Bureaucratic Coordination in Professionnal Organizations." In W. V. Heydebrand (ed.), *Comparative Organizations* (pp. 158–189). Englewood Cliffs, N.J.: Prentice-Hall, 1973.

Hibbard, J. H., Slovic, P., and Jewett, J. J. "Informing Consumer Decisions in Health Care: Implications from Decision-Making Research." *The Milbank Quarterly*, 1997, 75, 395–414.

Hill, R. "PPMCs: What Happens when Doctors Flock Together?" *Business and Health*, 1998, 16(9), 43–48.

Hirsch, P. M., and Lounsbury, M. "Ending the Family Quarrel: Toward a Reconciliation of Old and New Institutionalisms." *American Behavioral Scientist*, 1997, 40, 406–418.

Hofer, T. P., and others. "The Unreliability of Individual Physician Report Cards for Assessing the Costs and Quality of Care of a Chronic Disease." *Journal of the American Medical Association*, 1999, *281*, 2098–2105.

Hoff, T. J. "Professional Commitment Among U.S. Physician Executives in Managed Care." *Social Science and Medicine*, 2000, *50*, 1433–1444.

Hoffman, A. J. "Institutional Evolution and Change: Environmentalism and the U.S. Chemical Industry." *Academy of Management Journal*, 1999, *42*, 351–371.

Holahan, J., Zuckerman, S., Evans, A., and Rangarajan, S. "Medicaid Managed Care in Thirteen States: As More States Make Managed Care Mandatory for their Medicaid Populations, Questions Persist about the Quality of Care and the Effect on Safety Net Providers." *Health Affairs*, 1998, *17*(3), 43–63.

Howatt, G. "Medica Lays Off 20 Percent of Its Staff." *Minneapolis Star Tribune*, November 6, 2001, D1, D2.

Huber, G. P. "Organizational Learning: The Contributing Processes and the Literatures." *Organizational Science*, 1991, *2*, 88–115.

Hurtado, M. P., Swift, E. K., and Corrigan, J. M. *Envisioning the National Health Care Quality Report*. Washington, D.C.: Institute of Medicine, National Academy Press, 2001.

Ibarra, H. "Network Centrality, Power, and Innovation Involvement: Determinants of Technical and Administrative Roles." *Academy of Management Journal*, 1993, *36*, 471–501.

Ingram, P. L., and Roberts, P. W. "Friendships Among Competitors in the Sydney Hotel Industry." *American Journal of Sociology*, 2000, *106*(2), 387–423.

Ingram, P. L., and Simons, T. "Institutional Resource Dependence Determinants of Responsiveness to Work-Family Issues." *Academy of Management Journal*, 1995, *38*, 1466–1482.

Institute of Medicine. *To Err Is Human*. Washington, D.C.: National Academy Press, 1999.

Institute of Medicine. *Crossing the Quality Chasm: A New Health System for the Twenty-First Century*. Washington, D.C.: National Academy Press, 2001.

Interstudy. *The Competitive Edge: The HMO Industry Report. 11*(2). St. Paul, Minn.: InterStudy Publications, 2001.

Jencks, S. F., and Wilensky, G. R. "The Health Care Quality Improvement Initiative: A New Approach to Quality Assurance in Medicare." *Journal of the American Medical Association*, 1992, *268*(7), 900–903.

Jensen, M., and Meckling, W. "Theory of the Firm: Managerial Behavior, Agency Costs and Ownership Structure." *Journal of Financial Economics*, 1976, *3*, 305–360.

Jenson, G., Morrisey, M., Gaffney, S., and Liston, D. "The New Dominance of Managed Care Insurance Trends in the 1990s." *Health Affairs*, 1997, *16*, 125–136.

Jepperson, R. "Institutions, Institutional Effects, and Institutionalism." In W. Powell and P. DiMaggio (eds.), *The New Institutionalism in Organizational Analysis*. Chicago: University of Chicago Press, 1991.

Johnson, J. A. "Interview: Thomas C. Dolan, Ph.D., FACHE, CAE, President and Chief Executive Officer of the American College of Healthcare Executives." *Journal of Healthcare Management*, 2000, *45*, 3–7.

Jones, G. R. *Organizational Theory: Text and Cases*. Reading, Mass.: Addison-Wesley, 1995.

Kanter, R. M. "Becoming Pals: Pooling, Aligning, and Linking Across Companies." *Academy of Management Executive*, 1989, *3*, 183–193.

Kanter, R. M. "Collaborative Advantage: The Art of Alliances." *Harvard Business Review*, 1994, *72*, 96–103.

Kao, A. C., Green, D. C., Davis, N. A., Koplan, J. P., and Cleary, P. D. "Patients' Trust in their Physicians: Effects of Choice, Continuity, and Payment Method." *Journal of General Internal Medicine*, 1998, *13*, 681–686.

Kao, A. C., Green, D. C., Zaslavsky, A. M., Koplan, J. P., and Cleary, P. D. "The Relationship Between Method of Physician Payment and Patient Trust." *Journal of the American Medical Association*, 1998, *280*, 1708–1714.

Katz, M. L., and Shapiro, C. "Network Externalities, Competition, and Compatibility." *American Economic Review Papers and Proceedings*, 1985, *75*, 424–440.

Katz, M. L., and Shapiro, C. "Systems Competition and Network Effects." *Journal of Economic Perspectives*, 1994, *8*, 93–115.

Kauffman, C. J. "The Modern Association: Preserving a Catholic Presence in the U.S. Healthcare System." *Health Progress*, 1990, *71*(6), 35–46.

Kauffman, S. A. *The Origins of Order: Self-Organization and Selection in Evolution*. New York: Oxford University Press, 1993.

Kauffman, S. A. *At Home in the Universe: The Search for Laws of Self-Organization and Complexity*. New York: Oxford University Press, 1995.

Kelly, D., and Amburgey, T. L. "Organizational Inertia and Momentum: A Dynamic Model of Strategic Change." *Academy of Management Journal*, 1991, *34*, 591–612.

Kelly, S., and Allison, M. A. *The Complexity Advantage: How the Science of Complexity Can Help Your Business Achieve Peak Performance*. New York: McGraw-Hill, 1999.

Kennedy, D. V., and Jennings, M. C. "Beyond HMOs: Trends in Employer Direct Contracting." *Healthcare Financial Management*, 1998, *52*, 45–48.

Kerr, E. A., and others. "Managed Care and Capitation in California: How Do Physicians at Financial Risk Control Their Own Utilization?" *Annals of Internal Medicine*, 1995, *123*, 500–504.

Kiel, L. D., and Elliott, E. (eds.). *Chaos Theory in the Social Sciences: Foundations and Applications*. Ann Arbor, Mich.: University of Michigan Press, 1997.

Kimberly, J. R., and Minvielle, E. (eds.). *The Quality Imperative: Measurement and Management of Quality in Health Care*. London: Imperial College Press, 2000.

Klemperer, P. "Competition When Consumers Have Switching Costs: An Overview with Applications to Industrial Organization, Macroeconomics, and International Trade." *Review of Economic Studies*, 1995, *62*, 515–539.

Kletke, P. R., Emmons, D. W., and Gillis, K. D. "Current Trends in Physicians' Practice Arrangements." *Journal of the American Medical Association*, 1996, *276*(7), 55–60.

Knoke, D. *Political Networks: The Structural Perspective*. Cambridge, U.K.: Cambridge University Press, 1990.

Knutson, D. "Case Study: The Minneapolis Buyers Health Care Action Group." *Inquiry*, 1998, *35*, 171–177.

Kohn, L. T. "Organizing and Managing Care in a Changing Health System." *Health Services Research*, 2000, *35*, 37–52.

Kohn, L. T., Corrigan, J., and Donaldson, M. S. (eds.). *To Err Is Human: Building a Safer Health System*. Washington, D.C.: National Academy Press, 2000.

Kraatz, M. "The Role of Interorganizational Networks in Shaping Strategic Adaptation: Evidence from Liberal Arts Colleges." *Academy of Management Meeting Best Papers Proceedings*, 1995, 246–250.

Kraatz, M., and Zajac, E. J. "Exploring the Limits of the New Institutionalism: The Causes and Consequences of Illegitimate Organizational Change." *American Sociological Review*, 1996, *61*, 812–836.

Krackhardt, D. "The Strength of Strong Ties: The Importance of Philos." In N. Nohria and R. C. Eccles (eds.), *Networks and Organizations: Structure, Form and Action* (pp. 216–239). Boston: Harvard Business School Press, 1992.

Krackhardt, D., and Porter, L. W. "The Snowball Effect: Turnover Embedded in Communications Networks." *Journal of Applied Psychology*, 1986, *71*, 50–55.

Kramer, R., and Tyler, T. (eds.). *Trust in Organizations: Frontiers of Theory and Research*. Thousand Oaks, Calif.: Sage, 1996.

Kranton, R. E., and Minehart, D. F. "Networks Versus Vertical Integration." *RAND Journal of Economics*, 2000, *31*, 570–601.

Kuhn, T. S. *The Structure of Scientific Revolutions*. Chicago: University of Chicago Press, 1962.

Laffel, G., and Blumenthal, D. "The Case for Using Industrial Quality Management Sciences in Health Care." *Journal of the American Medical Association*, 1989, *262*(20), 2869–2873.

Lakoff, G., and Johnson, M. *Metaphors We Live By*. Chicago: University of Chicago Press, 1980.

Langlais, R. J., and Cutler, J. C. "Case Study of a Successful Hospital-Physician Partnership: The Virtual Merger Between Chesire Medicine Center and Dartmouth Hitchcock-Keene Clinic." *The Governance Institute*, Spring, 2001, 1–20.

Larson, A. "Network Dyads in Entrepreneurial Settings: A Study of the Governance of Exchange Processes." *Administrative Science Quarterly*, 1992, *37*, 76–104.

Latkin, C. A., Madell, W., Vlahov, D., Oziemkowska, M., and Celentano, D. "The Long-Term Outcome of Personal Network-Oriented HIV Prevention Intervention for Injection Drug Users: The SAFE Study. *American Journal of Community Psychiatry*, 1996, *24*, 341–364.

Lawrence, D. M., Mattingly, P. H., and Ludden, J. M. "Trusting in the Future: The Distinct Advantage of Nonprofit HMOs." *The Milbank Quarterly*, 1997, *75*(1), 5–10.

Leape, L. L. "Practice Guidelines and Standards: An Overview." *Quality Review Bulletin*, 1990, *12*, 42–49.

Leblebici, H., Salancik, G. R., Copay, A., and King, T. "Institutional Change and the Transformation of Interorganizational Fields: An Organizational History of the U.S. Radio Broadcasting Industry." *Administrative Science Quarterly*, 1991, *35*, 333–363.

LeBlanc, A. J. "Undercompensated, Unpopular Services in Hospitals: The Case of HIV/AIDS." Doctoral dissertation, Pennsylvania State University. *Dissertation Abstracts International*, 1991.

LeBlanc, A. J., and Hurley, R. E. "Adoption of HIV-Related Services Among Urban U.S. Hospitals: 1988 and 1991." *Medical Care*, 1995, *33*, 881–891.

Leicht, K. T., and Fennell, M. L. *Professional Work: A Sociological Approach*. Malden, Mass.: Blackwell, 2001.

Lesser, C., and Ginsburg, P. "Update on the Nation's Health Care System: 1997–1999." *Health Affairs*, 2000, *19*, 206–216.

Levin, D. Z. "Institutionalism, Learning, and Patterns of Selective Decoupling: The Case of Total Quality Management." Working paper. New Brunswick, N.J.: Rutgers University, 2001.

Levine, S., and White, P. E. "Exchange as a Conceptual Framework for the Study of Interorganizational Relationships." *Administrative Science Quarterly*, 1961, 5, 583–601.

Levine, S., White, P. E., and Paul, B. D. "Community Interorganizational Problems in Providing Medical Care and Social Services." *American Journal of Public Health*, 1963, 53, 1183–1195.

Levinthal, D. A., and March, J. G. "The Myopia of Learning." *Strategic Management Journal*, 1993, 14, 95–112.

Lewin, R. *Complexity: Life at the Edge of Chaos*. New York: Macmillan, 1992.

Lewin, R., and Regine, B. *The Soul at Work: Listen . . . Respond . . . Let Go: Embracing Complexity Science for Business Success*. New York: Simon and Shuster, 2000.

Lewin, R., Parker, T., and Regine, B. (1998). "Complexity Theory and the Organization: Beyond the Metaphor." *Complexity*, 1998, 3(4), 36–40.

Lichtenstein, B. B. "Self-Organized Transitions: A Pattern Amid the Chaos of Transformative Change." *Academy of Management Executive*, 2000, 14(4), 128–141.

Light, D. W. "The Restructuring of American Health Care." In T. Litman and L. Robins (eds.), *Health Politics and Policy*. Albany, N.Y.: Delmar Publishers, 1991.

Light, D. W. "Countervailing Power: The Changing Character of the Medical Profession in the United States." In F. Hafferty and J. McKinley (eds.), *The Changing Character of the Medical Profession: An International Perspective*. New York: Oxford University Press, 1993.

Lin, B., and Wan, T. H. "Analysis of Integrated Healthcare Networks' Performance: A Contingency-Strategy Management Perspective." *Journal of Medical Systems*, 1999, 23(6), 467–485.

Linenkugel, N. *Lessons from Mergers*. Chicago: Health Administration Press, 2001.

Lipson, D. "Medicaid Managed Care and Community Providers: New Partnerships." *Health Affairs*, 1997, 16(4), 91–107.

Lissak, M. R. "Complexity and Management: It Is More than Jargon." In M. R. Lissak and H. P. Gunz (eds.), *Managing Complexity in Organizations: A View in Many Directions* (pp. 11–28). Westport, Conn.: Quorum, 1999.

Loizeau, D. "L'effondrement Tranquille de la Gestion de la Qualité: Résultats d'une Enquête Réalisée dans Douze Hôpitaux Publics au Québec." *Ruptures*, 1996, 3, 187–208.

Lomas, J. "Editorial: Quality Assurance and Effectiveness in Health Care: An Overview." *Quality Assurance in Health Care*, 1990, *2*, 12–15.

Long, J. S. *Social Network Analysis: A Handbook*. London: Sage Publications, 1991.

Lorrain, F., and White, H. C. "Structural Equivalence of Individuals in Social Networks." *Journal of Mathematical Sociology*, 1971, *1*, 49–80.

Luke, R. D., and Begun, J. W. "Industry Distinctiveness and the Teaching of Strategic Management in Health Administration Programs." *Journal of Health Administration Education*, 1987, *5*, 387–405.

Luke, R. D., and Begun, J. W. "Have IDNs Failed in Healthcare?" *Frontiers of Health Services Management*, 2001, *17*, 47–52.

Luke, R. D., Begun, J. W., and Pointer, D. D. "Quasi-Firms: Strategic Interorganizational Forms in the Health Care Industry." *The Academy of Management Review*, 1989, *14*, 1–14.

Luke, R. D., Begun, J. W., and Walston, S. "Strategy in Health Care Organizations and Markets." In S. Shortell and A. Kaluzny (eds.), *Health Care Management: Organizational Design and Behavior*. New York: Delmar, 2000.

Lumpkin, J. "E-Health, HIPAA, and Beyond." *Health Affairs*, 2000, *19*(6), 149–151.

Lumsdon, K., and Hagland, M. "For-Profits: The Right Medicine for Some Markets?" *Hospitals and Health Networks*, 1994, *12*, 34.

Maguire, S., and McKelvey, B. (eds.). "Special Issue on Complexity and Management: Where Are We?" *Emergence*, 1999, *1*, 2.

Manning, W., and others. "Health Insurance and the Demand for Medical Care: Evidence from a Randomized Experiment." *The American Economic Review*, 1987, *77*(3), 251–277.

March, J. G. *A Primer on Decision Making: How Decisions Happen*. New York: Free Press, 1994.

Marcotty, J., and Burcum, J. "Allina Leader Agrees Perks Were Wrong." *Minneapolis Star Tribune*, September 7, 2001, A1, A9.

Marion, R. *The Edge of Organization: Chaos and Complexity Theories of Formal Social Systems*. Thousand Oaks, Calif.: Sage, 1999.

Marion, R., and Bacon, J. "Organizational Extinction and Complex Systems." *Emergence*, 2000, *1*(4), 71–96.

Marquis, S., and Long, S. "Trends in Managed Care and Managed Competition: 1993–1997." *Health Affairs*, 1999, *18*(6), 75–88.

Marsh, L. C., and Feinstein, A. *Of Minds and Men: Changing Behavior in the New Physician Enterprise*. New York: Salomon Brothers, 1997.

Marsteller, J., and Shortell, S. M. "Social Network Theory and Quality Improvement Collaborations." Paper presented at International Meeting of Quality Improvement Evaluation Research Group, Center for Health Research, University of California, Berkeley, California, October 23, 2001.

Marszalek-Gaucher, E., and Coffey, R. J. *Total Quality in Healthcare: From Theory to Practice*. San Francisco: Jossey-Bass, 1993.

Marty, M. E. "Can We Still Hear the Call?" *Health Progress*, 1995, 76(1), 18–21.

Maude-Griffin, R., Feldman, R., and Wholey, D. R. *A Nash Bargaining Model of the HMO Premium Cycle*. Minneapolis: Division of Health Services Research and Policy, University of Minnesota, 2001.

Mauss, M. *The Gift: Forms and Functions of Exchange in Archaic Societies*. New York: Norton, 1967.

Mays, G., Hurley, R., and Grossman, J. "Consumers Face Higher Costs as Health Plans Seek to Control Drug Spending." *Center for Studying Health System Change, Issue Brief*, 2001, 45.

McCall, N., Komisar, H. L., Petersons, A., and Moose, S. "Medicare Home Health Before and After the BBA." *Health Affairs*, 2001, 20(3), 189–198.

McCormick, R. A. *Corrective Vision: Explorations in Moral Theology*. Kansas City, Mo.: Sheed & Ward, 1994.

McCormick, R. A. "The Catholic Hospital Today: Mission Impossible?" *Origins*, March 16, 1995, 648–653.

McCue, M. J., Clement, J. P., and Luke, R. D. "Strategic Hospital Alliances: Do the Type and Market Structure of Strategic Hospital Alliances Matter?" *Medical Care*, 1999, 37, 1013–1022.

McDaniel, R. R. Jr. "Strategic Leadership: A View from Quantum and Chaos Theories." *Health Care Management Review*, 1997, 22(1), 21–37.

McDaniel, R. R. Jr., and Driebe, D. J. "Complexity Science and Health Care Management." In M. D. Fottler, G. T. Savage, and J. D. Blair (eds.), *Advances in Health Care Management*. (pp. 11–36). Oxford, United Kingdom: Elsevier, 2001.

McLaughlin, C. "Employers as Agents for Their Employees." *Health Services Research*, 2001, 36(5), 827–830.

Mead, G. H. *Mind, Self, and Society*. C. W. Morris (ed.). Chicago: University of Chicago Press, 1934.

Mechanic, D. "Managed Care: Rhetoric and Realities." *Inquiry*, 1994, 31, 124–128.

Mechanic, D. "Medical Organization and the Erosion of Trust." *The Milbank Quarterly*, 1996, 74(2), 171–189.

Mechanic, D. "Managed Care as a Target of Distrust." *The Journal of the American Medical Association*, 1997, *277*(22), 1810–1811.

Mechanic, D. "The Functions and Limitations of Trust in the Provision of Medical Care." *Journal of Health Politics, Policy and Law*, 1998a, *23*(4), 661–686.

Mechanic, D. "Managed Care, Rationing, and Trust in Medical Care." *Journal of Urban Health*, 1998b, *75*(1), 118–122.

Mechanic, D. "Public Trust and Initiatives for New Health Care Partnerships." *The Milbank Quarterly*, 1998c, *76*(2), 281–302.

Mechanic, D., and Rosenthal, M. "Responses of HMO Medical Directors to Trust Building in Managed Care." *The Milbank Quarterly*, 1999, *77*, 283–303.

Mechanic, D., and Schlesinger, M. "The Impact of Managed Care on Patients' Trust in Medical Care and their Physicians." *The Journal of the American Medical Association*, 1996, *275*(21), 1693–1697.

Melhado, E. M. "Competition Versus Regulation in American Health Policy." In E. M. Melhado, W. Feinberg, and H. M. Swartz (eds.), *Money, Power, and Health Care* (pp. 15–102). Ann Arbor, Mich: Health Administration Press, 1988.

Meyer, J. W., and Rowan, B. "Institutionalized Organizations: Formal Structure as Myth and Ceremony." *American Journal of Sociology*, 1977, *83*, 340–363.

Meyer, J. W., and Scott, W. R. "Centralization and Legitimacy Problems of Local Governments." In J. W. Meyer and W. Richard Scott (eds.), *Organizational Environments: Ritual and Rationality* (pp. 199–216). Thousand Oaks, Calif.: Sage, 1983.

Meyer, J. W., and Scott, W. R. *Organizational Environments: Ritual and Rationality*. Thousand Oaks, Calif.: Sage, 1993.

Meyer, J. W., Scott, W. R., and Strang, D. "Centralization, Fragmentation, and School District Complexity." *Administrative Science Quarterly*, 1987, *32*, 186–201.

Mick, S. S. (ed.). *Innovations in Health Care Delivery: Insights for Organization Theory*. San Francisco: Jossey-Bass, 1990.

Mick, S. S., and Conrad, D. A. "The Decision to Integrate Vertically in Health Care Organizations." *Hospital and Health Services Administration*, 1988, *33*(3), 345–360.

Millenson, M. *Demanding Medical Excellence: Doctors and Accountability in the Information Age*. Chicago: University of Chicago Press, 1997.

Miller, R. H., and Luft, H. S. "Managed Care: Past Evidence and Potential Trends." *Frontiers of Health Services Management*, 1993, *9*(3), 3–37.

Milward, H. B., and Provan, K. G. "Governing the Hollow State." *Journal of Public Administration Research and Theory*, 2000, *10*(2), 359–379.

Miner, A. S., and Anderson, P. C. "Population Level Learning and Industry Change." *Advances in Strategic Management*, 1999, *16*, 1–32.

Miner, A. S., and Haunschild, P. R. "Population-Level Learning." In L. L. Cummings and B. M. Staw (eds.), *Research in Organizational Behavior* (pp. 115–166). Greenwich, Conn.: JAI Press, 1995.

Mintzberg, H. *The Structuring of Organizations*. Englewood Cliffs, N.J.: Prentice-Hall, 1978.

Mintzberg, H. *Power In and Around Organizations*. Englewood Cliffs, N.J.: Prentice-Hall, 1983.

Mintzberg, H. "Strategy Formulation: Schools of Thought." In J. Frederickson (ed.), *Perspectives on Strategic Management*. Boston: Ballinger, 1990.

Mintzberg, H. *The Rise and Fall of Strategic Planning: Reconceiving Roles for Planning, Plans, Planners*. New York: Free Press, 1994.

Mintzberg, H. *The Positioning School: A Guided Tour Through the Wilds of Strategic Management*. New York: Free Press, 1998.

Minvielle, E. "Gérer la Singularité à Grande Echelle." *Revue Francaise de Gestion*, 1996, *109*, 119–124.

Mitchell, S. M., and Shortell, S. M. "The Governance and Management of Effective Community Health Partnerships: A Typology for Research, Policy and Practice." *The Milbank Quarterly*, 2000, *78*(2), 241–289.

Mitchell, W., Baum, J., Banaszak-Holl, J., Berta, W., and Bowman, D. "Opportunity and Constraint: Chain-to-Component Transfer Learning in Multiunit Chains." In N. Bontis and C. W. Choo (eds.), *Strategic Management of Intellectual Capital and Organizational Knowledge: A Collection of Readings*. New York: Oxford University Press, 2000.

Mohr, R. A. "An Institutional Perspective on Rational Myths and Organizational Change in Health Care." *Medical Care Review*, 1992, *49*, 233–255.

Moisdon, J. C. *Du Mode D'existence des Outils de Gestion*. Paris: Sedi Arslan, 1997.

Montgomery, C. A., and Porter, M. E. *Strategy: Seeking and Securing Competitive Advantage*. Boston, Harvard Business School Press, 1991.

Mor, V., Fleishman, J. A., Allen, S. M., and Piette, J. D. *Networking AIDS Services*. Ann Arbor, Mich.: Health Administration Press, 1994.

Morgan, G. *Images of Organization* (2nd edition). Thousand Oaks, Calif.: Sage, 1997.

Morrisey, M. A., Sloan, F. A., and Valvona, J. "Defining Geographic Markets for Hospital Care." *Law and Contemporary Problems*, 1988, *51*, 165–194.

Morrisey, M. A., Alexander, J. A., Burns, L., and Johnson, V. "The Effects of Managed Care on Physicians and Clinical Integration in Hospitals." *Medical Care*, 1999, *37*(4), 350–361.

Morrissey, J. "Study Shows Value of Wisconsin CHIN." *Modern Healthcare*, 1995, *25*, 50.

Morrison, I. *Health Care in the New Millennium: Vision, Values, and Leadership.* San Francisco: Jossey-Bass, 2000.

Moscovice, I., Johnson, J., Finch, M., Grogan, C., and Kralewski, J. "The Structure and Characteristics of Rural Hospital Consortia." *Journal of Rural Health*, 1991, *7*, 575–588.

Moscovice, I., and others. "Understanding Integrated Rural Health Networks." *The Milbank Quarterly*, 1997, *75*, 563–588.

Nath, D., and Gruca, T. S. "Convergence Across Alternative Methods for Forming Strategic Groups." *Strategic Management Journal*, 1997, *18*, 745–760.

Newman, K. "Organizational Transformation During Institutional Upheaval." *Academy of Management Review*, 2000, *25*, 602–619.

Nielsen, R. "Cooperative Strategies." *Planning Review*, 1986, *14*, 16–20.

Nohria, N., and Berkley, J. D. "The Virtual Organization: Bureaucracy, Technology and the Imposition of Control." In C. Heckscher and A. Donnellon (eds.), *The Post-Bureaucratic Organization: New Perspectives on Organizational Change* (pp. 32–47). Thousand Oaks, Calif.: Sage, 1992.

Nonaka, I. "A Dynamic Theory of Organizational Knowledge Creation." *Organization Science*, 1994, *5*, 102–113.

Ocasio, W. "The Enactment of Economic Adversity: A Reconciliation of Theories of Failure-Induced Change and Threat-Rigidity." In L. L. Cummings and B. M. Staw (eds.), *Research in Organizational Behavior* (pp. 287–331). Greenwich, Conn.: JAI Press, 1995.

Ogrod, E. "Compensation and Quality: A Physician's View." *Health Affairs*, 1997, *16*(3), 82–86.

Okun, A. *Equality and Efficiency: The Big Tradeoff.* Washington D.C.: Brookings, 1975.

Oliver, C. "Strategic Responses to Institutional Processes." *Academy of Management Review*, 1991, *16*, 145–179.

Oliver, C. "The Antecedents of Deinstitutionalism." *Organization Studies*, 1992, *13*, 563–588.

Oliver, A. L., and Montgomery, K. "A Network Approach to Outpatient Service Delivery Systems: Resource Flows and System Influence." *Health Services Research*, 1996, *30*(6), 771–789.

Olson, E., and Eoyang, G. *Facilitating Organizational Change: Lessons from Complexity Science.* San Francisco: Jossey-Bass, 2001.

Ouchi, W. G. "Review of Markets and Hierarchies." *Administrative Science Quarterly*, 1977, 22, 541–544.

Ouchi, W. G. "Markets, Bureaucracies, and Clans." *Administrative Science Quarterly*, 1980, 25, 129–142.

Palmer, R. H. "Considerations in Defining Quality of Health Care." In R. H.Palmer, A. Donabedian, and G. J. Povar (eds.), *Striving for Quality in Health Care: An Inquiry into Policy and Practice* (pp. 1–53). Ann Arbor, Mich.: Health Administration Press, 1991.

Parsons, T., and Smelser, N. J. *Economy and Society*. New York: The Free Press, 1956.

Pauly, M. V. *Doctors and Their Workshops: Economic Models of Physician Behavior*. Chicago: University of Chicago Press, 1980.

Pemble, K. R. "Regional Health Information Networks: The Wisconsin Health Information Network, A Case Study." *Proceedings of the Annual Symposium in Computer Applications in Medical Care*, 1994, 401–405.

Perrow, C. "Hospitals: Technology, Structure and Goals." In J. G. March (ed.), *Handbook of Organizations* (Chapter 22). New York: Rand McNally, 1965.

Perrow, C. "A Framework for the Comparative Analysis of Organizations." *American Sociological Review*, 1967, 32, 194–208.

Pfeffer, J. *New Directions for Organization Theory: Problems and Prospects*. New York: Oxford University Press, 1997.

Pfeffer, J., and Salancik, G. *The External Control of Organizations: A Resource Dependence Perspective*. New York: Harper and Row, 1978.

Place, M. D. "Catholic Identity: A Unifying Force." *Health Progress*, 1999, 80(2), 10, 14.

Podolny, J. M. "A Status-Based Model of Market Competition." *American Journal of Sociology*, 1993, 98, 829–872.

Podolny, J. M., and Page, K. L. "Network Forms of Organization." *Annual Review of Sociology*, 1998, 24, 57–76.

Podolny, J. M., Stuart, T., and Hannan, M. T. "Networks, Knowledge, and Niches: Competition in the Worldwide Semiconductor Industry, 1984–1991." *American Journal of Sociology*, 1996, 102, 659–689.

Poole, K., and Van de Ven, A. H. "Using Paradox to Build Management and Organization Theory." *Academy of Management Review*, 1989, 14(4), 562–578.

Popper, K. *The Logic of Scientific Discovery*. London: Routledge, 1959.

Porter, M. E. *Competitive Strategy: Techniques for Analyzing Industries and Competitors*. New York: Free Press, 1980.

Porter, M. E. "What Is Strategy?" *Harvard Business Review*, 1996, Nov.-Dec., 61–78.

Powell, W. W. "Neither Market nor Hierarchy: Network Forms of Organization." In B. M. Straw and L. L. Cummings (eds.), *Research in Organizational Behavior* (pp. 295–336). Greenwich, Conn.: Jai Press, 1990.

Powell, W., and DiMaggio, P. (eds.). *The New Institutionalism in Organizational Analysis*. Chicago: University of Chicago Press, 1991.

Powell, W. W., Koput, K., and Smith-Doerr, L. "Interorganizational Collaboration and the Locus of Innovation: Networks of learning in Biotechnology." *Administrative Science Quarterly*, 1996, *41*, 116–145.

Powell, W. W., Koput, K. W., Smith-Doerr, L., and Owen-Smith, J. "Network Position and Firm Performance: Organizational Returns to Collaboration in the Biotechnology Industry." *Research in the Sociology of Organizations*, 1999, *16*, 129–159.

Priesmeyer, H. R. *Organizations and Chaos: Defining the Methods of Nonlinear Management*. Westport, Conn.: Quorum, 1992.

Priesmeyer, H. R., and Sharp, L. F. "Phase Plane Analysis: Applying Chaos Theory in Health Care." *Quality Management in Health Care*, 1995, *4*(1), 62–70.

Priesmeyer, H. R., Sharp, L. F., Wammack, L., and Mabrey, J. D. (1996). "Chaos Theory and Clinical Pathways: A Practical Application." *Quality Management in Health Care*, 1996, *4*(4), 63–72.

Prigogine, I., and Stengers, I. *Order Out of Chaos: Man's New Dialogue with Nature*. New York: Bantam, 1984.

Prince, T. R. "Assessing Catholic Community Hospitals Versus Nonprofit Community Hospitals, 1989–1992." *Health Care Management Review*, 1994, *19*(4), 25–37.

Prince, T. R., and Ramanan, R. "Operating Performance and Financial Constraints of Catholic Community Hospitals, 1986–1989." *Health Care Management Review*, 1994, *19*(4), 38–48.

Proenca, E. J. "Community Orientation in Health Services Organizations: The Concept and Its Implementation." *Health Care Management Review*, 2000, *23*(2), 28–38.

ProPac. *An Evaluation of Winners and Losers under Medicare's Prospective Payment System*. Washington, D. C.: Prospective Payment Assessment Commission, 1992.

Provan, K. "The Federation as an Interorganizational Linkage Network." *Academy of Management Review*, 1983, *8*, 79–89.

Provan, K., and Milward, H. B. "Integration of Community-Based Services for the Severely Mentally Ill and the Structure of Public Funding: A Comparison of Four Systems." *Journal of Health Politics, Policy and Law*, 1994, *19*(4), 865–894.

Provan, K., and Milward, H. B. "A Preliminary Theory of Interorganizational Network Effectiveness: A Comparative Study of Four Community Mental Health Systems." *Administrative Science Quarterly*, 1995, *40*, 1–33.

Provan, K., and Sebastian, J. "Networks Within Networks: Service Link Overlap, Organizational Cliques, and Network Effectiveness." *Academy of Management Journal*, 1998, *31*, 453–463.

Randel, L., Pearson, S. D., Sabin, J. E., Hyams, T., and Emanuel, E. J. "How Managed Care Can Be Ethical." *Health Affairs*, 2001, *20*, 43–56.

Raube, K., and Merrell, K. "Maternal Minimum-Stay Legislation: Cost and Policy Implications." *American Journal of Public Health*, 1999, *89*(6), 922–923.

Reinhardt, U. E. "The Rise and Fall of the Physician Practice Management Industry." *Health Affairs*, 2000, *19*(1), 42–55.

Rettig, R., and Levinsky, N. (eds.). *Kidney Failure and the Federal Government*. Washington, D.C.: National Academy Press, 1991.

Rice, T. H. *The Economics of Health Reconsidered*. Chicago: Health Administration Press, 2000.

Robinow, A. "Ensuring Health Care Quality: A Purchaser's Perspective—A Health Care Coalition." *Clinical Therapeutics*, 1997a, *19*, 1545–1554.

Robinow, A. "The Buyers Health Care Action Group: Creating a Competitive Care System Model." *Managed Care Quarterly*, 1997b, *5*, 61–64.

Robinson, J. C. "Health Care Purchasing and Market Changes in California." *Health Affairs*, 1995, *14*, 117–130.

Robinson, J. C. "Consolidation of Medical Groups into Physician Practice Management Organizations." *Journal of the American Medical Association*, 1998a, *279*, 144–149.

Robinson, J. C. "Financial Capital and Intellectual Capital in Physician Practice Management." *Health Affairs*, 1998b, *17*, 53–74.

Robinson, J. C. *The Corporate Practice of Medicine: Competition and Innovation in Health Care*. Berkeley, Calif.: University of California Press, 1999.

Robinson, J. C. "Theory and Practice in the Design of Physician Payment Incentives." *The Milbank Quarterly*, 2001, *79*(2), 149–177.

Robinson, J. C., and Casalino, L. P. "Vertical Integration and Organizational Networks in Health Care." *Health Affairs*, 1996, *15*(1), 7–22.

Rogers, E. M. *Diffusion of Innovations* (4th edition). New York: Free Press, 1995.

Roggenkamp, S. D., and White, K. R. "Is Hospital Case Management a Rationalized Myth?" *Social Science & Medicine*, 2001, *53*(8), 1057–1066.

Roper, W., and Cutler, C. "Health Plan Accountability and Reporting: Issues and Challenges." *Health Affairs*, 1998, *17*(2), 152–155.

Rosenberg, T. "Look at Brazil." *New York Times Magazine*. January 28th, 2001, 26–54.

Rousseau, D. M., Sitkin, S. B., Burt, R. S., and Camerer, C. "Not So Different After All: A Cross-Discipline View of Trust." *Academy of Management Review*, 1998, *23*(3), 393–404.

Roussos, S. T., and Fawcett, S. B. "A Review of Collaborative Partnerships as a Strategy for Improving Community Health." *Annual Review of Public Health*, 2000, *21*, 369–402.

Rowley, T., Behrens, D., and Krackhardt, D. "Redundant Governance Structures: An Analysis of Structural and Relational Embeddedness in the Steel and Semiconductor Industries." *Strategic Management Journal*, 2000, *21*, 369–386.

Ruef, M., and Scott, W. R. "A Multidimensional Model of Organizational Legitimacy: Hospital Survival in Changing Institutional Environments." *Administrative Science Quarterly*, 1998, *43*, 877–904.

Ruggie, M. "Why the United States Does Not Have a National Health Program." *Contemporary Sociology*, 1994, *23*, 138–141.

Rumelt, R. P. *Strategy, Structure, and Economic Performance*. Boston: Harvard Business School Press, 1974.

Rundall, T. G., Starkweather, D. B., and Norrish, B. R. *After Restructuring: Empowerment Strategies at Work in America's Hospitals*. San Francisco: Jossey-Bass, 1998.

Safran, D. G., and others. "Linking Primary Care Performance to Outcomes of Care." *Journal of Family Practice*, 1998, *47*, 213–220.

Savage, G. T., and Roboski, A. M. "Integration as Networks and Systems: A Strategic Stakeholder Analysis." *Advances in Health Care Management*, 2001, *2*, 37–62.

Schein, E. H. *Organizational Culture and Leadership* (2nd edition). San Francisco: Jossey-Bass, 1992.

Scherer, F. M., and Ross, D. *Industrial Market Structure and Economic Performance*. Boston: Houghton Mifflin, 1990.

Schmidt, L. A. "The Corporate Transformation of American Health Care: A Study in Institution Building." Doctoral Dissertation, University of California at Berkeley, 1999.

Schonfeld, E. "Doctors Unite: Physician Practice Management Companies Offer Healthy Returns." *Fortune*, March 3, 1997, 200.

Schumacher, D. N. *Cornerstones of Health Care in the Nineties: Forcing a Framework of Excellence*. Ann Arbor, Mich.: Commission of Professionals of Hospital Activities, 1991.

Schuster, M. E., McGlynn, E., and Brook, R. H. "How Good Is the Quality of Health Care in the United States?" *The Milbank Quarterly*, 1998, *76*, 517–563.

Scott, J. *Social Network Analysis: A Handbook*. Thousand Oaks, Calif.: Sage, 2000.

Scott, W. R. "Managing Professional Work: Three Models of Control for Health Organizations." *Health Services Research*, 1982, *17*, 213–240.

Scott, W. R. "Health Care Organizations." In J. W. Meyer and W. R. Scott (eds.), *Organizational Environments: Ritual and Rationality*. Thousand Oaks, Calif.: Sage, 1983.

Scott, W. R. "Innovation in Medical Care Organization, A Synthetic Review." *Medical Care Review*, 1990, *47*, 165–192.

Scott, W. R. *Goals, Power, and Control in Organizations: Rational, Natural, and Open Systems* (3rd edition). Englewood Cliffs, N.J.: Prentice-Hall, 1992.

Scott, W. R. "Conceptualizing Organizational Fields: Linking Organizations and Societal Systems." In H.-U. Derlien, U. Gerhardt, and F. W. Scharpf (eds.), *Systemrationalitat und Partialinteresse* (pp. 203–221). Baden Baden, Germany: Nomos Verlagsgesellschaft, 1994.

Scott, W. R. *Institutions and Organizations*. Thousand Oaks, Calif.: Sage, 1995.

Scott, W. R. *Organizations: Rational, Natural, and Open Systems* (4th edition). Upper Saddle, N.J.: Prentice-Hall, 1998.

Scott, W. R. *Institutions and Organizations* (2nd edition). Thousand Oaks, Calif.: Sage, 2001.

Scott, W. R., and Lammers, J. C. "Trends in Occupations and Organization in the Medical Care and Mental Health Sectors." *Medical Care Review*, 1985, *42*, 37–76.

Scott, W. R., and Meyer, J. W. "The Organization of Societal Sectors." In J. W. Meyer and W. R. Scott (eds.), *Organizational Environments: Ritual and Rationality* (pp. 129–153). Thousand Oaks, Calif.: Sage, 1983.

Scott, W. R., and Meyer, J. W. (eds.). *Institutional Environments and Organizations: Structural Complexity and Individualism*. Thousand Oaks, Calif.: Sage, 1994.

Scott, W. R., Mendel, P. J., and Pollack, S. "Environments and Fields: Studying the Evolution of a Field of Medical Care Organizations." In W. W. Powell and D. L. Jones (eds.), *Bending the Bars of the Iron Cage: Institutional Dynamics and Processes*. Chicago: University of Chicago Press, forthcoming.

Scott, W. R., Ruef, M., Mendel, P. J., and Caronna, C. A. *Institutional Change and Healthcare Organizations: From Professional Dominance to Managed Care*. Chicago: University of Chicago Press, 2000.

Selznick, P. "Foundations of the Theory of Organization." *American Sociological Review*, 1948, *13*, 25–35.

Selznick, P. *TVA and the Grass Roots*. Berkeley, Calif.: University of California Press, 1949.

Selznick, P. "Institutionalism Old and New." *Administrative Science Quarterly*, 1996, *41*, 270–277.

Senge, P. *The Fifth Discipline: The Art and Practice of the Learning Organization*. (New York: Doubleday/Currency, 1990.

Senge, P., and Carstedt, G. "Innovating Our Way to the Next Industrial Revolution." *Sloan Management Review*, 2001, *42*, 24–38.

Sewell, W. H. Jr. "A Theory of Structure: Duality, Agency, and Transformation." *American Journal of Sociology*, 1992, *98*, 1–29.

Shan, W., Walker, G., and Kogut, B. "Interfirm Cooperation and Startup Innovation in the Biotechnology Industry." *Strategic Management Journal*, June 1994, *15*(5), 387–394.

Shapiro, S. P. "The Social Control of Impersonal Trust." *American Journal of Sociology*, 1987, *93*(3), 623–658.

Sharp, L. F., and Priesmeyer, H. R. "Tutorial: Chaos Theory—A Primer for Health Care." *Quality Management in Health Care*, 1995, *3*(4), 71–86.

Shelanski, H. A., and Klein, P. G. "Empirical Research in Transaction Cost Economics: A Review and Assessment." *Journal of Law, Economics, and Organization*, 1995, *11*, 335–361.

Sheppard, B. H., and Sherman, D. M. "The Grammars of Trust: A Model and General Implications." *Academy of Management Review*, 1998, *23*(3), 422–437.

Shortell, S. M. "The Medical Staff of the Future: Replanting the Garden." *Frontiers of Health Services Management*, 1985, *1*, 3–48.

Shortell, S. M. *Effective Hospital-Physician Relationships*. Ann Arbor, Mich.: Health Administration Press, 1991.

Shortell, S. M. "Community Health Improvement Approaches: Accounting for the Relative Lack of Impact." *Health Services Research*, 2000, *35*(3), 555–560.

Shortell, S. M., and Zajac, E. J. "Healthcare Organizations and the Development of the Strategic Management Perspective." In S. S. Mick (ed.), *Innovations in Health Care Delivery* (pp. 144–180). San Francisco, Jossey-Bass, 1990.

Shortell, S. M., O'Brien, J. L., and Carman, J. M. "Assessing the Impact of Continuous Quality Improvement/Total Quality Management: Concept Versus Implementation." *Health Services Research*, 1995, *30*, 377–401.

Shortell, S. M., Gillies, R. R., Anderson, D. A., and Erickson, K. M.. *Remaking Health Care in America: Building Organized Delivery Systems*. San Francisco: Jossey-Bass, 1996.

Shortell, S. M., Waters, T. M., Clarke, K. W., and Budetti, P. P. "Physicians as Double Agents: Maintaining Trust in An Era of Multiple Accountabilities." *The Journal of the American Medical Association*, 1998, *280*(12), 1102–1108.

Shortell, S. M., Gillies, R. R., Anderson, D. A., Erickson, K. M., and Mitchell, J. B. *Remaking Health Care in America* (2nd edition). San Francisco: Jossey-Bass, 2000.

Shortell, S. M., Gillies, R. R., Anderson, D. A., Mitchell, J. B., and Morgan, K. L. "Creating Organized Delivery Systems: The Barriers and Facilitators." *Hospital and Health Services Administration*, 1993, 38(4), 447–466.

Shortell, S. M., and others. "Implementing Evidence-Based Medicine: The Role of Market Pressures, Compensation Incentives and Culture Physician Organizations." *Medical Care*, 2001, 39(7), 79–91.

Singh, J. V., and Lumsden, C. J. "Theory and Research in Organizational Ecology." *Annual Review of Sociology*, 1990, 16, 161–195.

Skocpol, T. "The Rise and Resounding Demise of the Clinton Plan." *Health Affairs*, 1995, 14(1), 66–85.

Skocpol, T. *Social Policy in the United States: Future Possibilities in Historical Perspective*. Princeton, N.J.: Princeton University Press, 1995.

Sleeper, S., Wholey, D. R., Hamer, R., Schwartz, S., and Inoferio, V. "Trust Me: Technical and Institutional Determinants of Health Maintenance Organization Shifting Risk to Physicians." *Journal of Health and Social Behavior*, 1998, 39(3), 189–200.

Smith, H. H. "Two Lines of Authority Are One Too Many." *Modern Hospital*, 1955, 84, 59–64.

Snail, T. S., and Robinson, J. C. "Organizational Diversification in the American Hospital." *Annual Review of Public Health*, 1998, 19, 417–453.

Snyder, J. "Valley Hospitals Use Computer Alerts to Foil Errors." *Arizona Republic*, Dec. 10th, 2001.

Somers, A. *Hospital Regulation: The Dilemma of Public Policy*. Princeton, N.J.: Princeton University Press, 1969.

Souder, W., and Moenhart, R. "Integrating Marketing and R&D Personnel Within Innovation Projects: An Information Uncertainty Model." *Journal of Management Studies*, 1992, 29, 485–512.

Stacey, R. D. *Managing the Unknowable: Strategic Boundaries Between Order and Chaos in Organizations*. San Francisco: Jossey-Bass, 1992.

Stacey, R. D. *Strategic Management and Organizational Dynamics: The Challenge of Complexity* (3rd edition). London: Trans-Atlantic, 1999.

Stacey, R. D., Griffin, D., and Shaw, P. *Complexity and Management: Fad or Radical Challenge to Systems Thinking?* New York: Routledge, 2000.

Starfield, B. *Primary Care: Concept, Evaluation, and Policy*. New York: Oxford University Press, 1992.

Starfield, B., Cassady, C., Nanda, J., Forrest, C. B., and Berk, R. "Consumer Experiences and Provider Perceptions of the Quality of Primary Care:

Implications for Managed Care." *Journal of Family Practice*, 1998, *46*, 216–226.

Starkey, K., Barnatt, C., and Tempest, S. "Beyond Networks and Hierarchies: Latent Organizations in the U.K. Television Industry." *Organization Science*, 2000, *11*, 299–305.

Starkweather, D. "Hospital Board Power." *Health Services Management Research*, 1988, *1*(27), 74–86.

Starr, P. M. *The Social Transformation of American Medicine*. New York: Basic Books, 1982.

Starr, P. M. "Health Care Reform and the New Economy." *Health Affairs*, 2000, *19*(6), 23–32.

Stepsis, U., and Liptak, D. (eds.). *Pioneer Healers: The History of Religious Women in American Health Care*. New York: Crossroad, 1989.

Stevens, R. *American Medicine and the Public Interest*. New Haven, Conn.: Yale University Press, 1971.

Stevens, R. *In Sickness and in Wealth: American Hospitals in the Twentieth Century*. New York: Basic Books, 1989.

Stiles, R. A., Mick, S. S., and Wise, C. G. "The Logic of Transaction Cost Economics in Health Care Organization Theory." *Health Care Management Review*, 2001, *26*(2), 85–92.

Strang, D., and Soule, S. A. "Diffusion in Organizations and Social Movements: From Hybrid Corn to Poison Pills." *Annual Review of Sociology*, 1998, *24*, 265–290.

Strang, D., and Tuma, N. B. "Spatial and Temporal Heterogeneity in Diffusion." *American Journal of Sociology*, 1993, *99*, 614–639.

Stuart, T. E., and Podolny, J. M. "Local Search and the Evolution of Technological Capabilities." *Strategic Management Journal*, 1996, *17*, 21–38.

Sturm, R. "Cost and Quality Trends Under Managed Care: Is There a Learning Curve in Behavioral Health Carve-Out Plans?" *Journal of Health Economics*, 1999, *18*, 593–604.

Suchman, M. "Managing Legitimacy: Strategic and Institutional Approaches." *Academy of Management Review*, 1995, *20*, 571–610.

Sullivan, J. M. "An Opportunity for Positive Change: We Have the History, Experience, and Will to Preserve a Catholic Presence in Healthcare." *Health Progress*, 1993, *74*(7), 56–65.

Tang, B. "The Impact of Competition on the Financial Performance of Catholic Hospitals." Doctoral dissertation, Saint Louis University, 1995.

Taylor, F. W. *Scientific Management*. New York: W.W. Norton, 1911.

Taylor, M. "The Dust Finally Clears." *Modern Healthcare*, December 18, 2000, 3, 14.

Theodorson, G. A., and Theodorson, A. G. *A Modern Dictionary of Sociology.* New York: Thomas Y. Crowell, 1969.

Thompson, J. *Organizations in Action.* New York: McGraw-Hill, 1967.

Thornton, P. H. "Accounting for Acquisition Waves: Evidence from the U.S. College Publishing Industry." In W. R. Scott and S. Christensen (eds.), *The Institutional Construction of Organizations* (pp. 199–225). Thousand Oaks, Calif.: Sage, 1995.

Thorpe, K. E. "The Health System in Transition: Care, Cost, and Coverage." *Journal of Health Politics, Policy and Law,* 1997, *22*(2), 339–361.

Tucker, D. J., Baum, J.A.C., and Singh, J. V. "The Institutional Ecology of Human Service Organizations." In Y. Hasenfeld (ed.), *Human Service Organizations* (pp. 47–72). Thousand Oaks, Calif.: Sage, 1992.

Turbayne, C. M. *The Myth of Metaphor.* Columbia, S.C.: University of South Carolina Press, 1962.

Turner, J. H. *Sociology: Concepts and Uses.* New York: McGraw-Hill, 1994.

UNAIDS/WHO. "UNAIDS/WHO Epidemiological Fact Sheets on HIV/AIDS and Sexually Transmitted Infections, 2000 update." Geneva: WHO, 2000a.

UNAIDS/WHO. *AIDS Epidemic Update.* Geneva: WHO, 2000b.

U.S. Census Bureau. *The 65 Years and Over Population: 2000.* Washington, D.C.: U.S. Census Bureau, 2000.

U.S. Health Care Financing Administration. *Children's Health Insurance Program.* 2001a. At http://www.hcfa.gov/init/kidssum.htm.

U.S. Health Care Financing Administration. *Medicare Managed Care.* 2001b. At http://www.hcfa.gov/medicare/mgdcar1.htm.

Uzzi, B. "The Sources of Consequences of Embeddedness for the Economic Performance of Organizations: The Network Effect." *American Sociological Review,* 1996, *61,* 674–698.

Uzzi, B. "Social Structure and Competition in Interfirm Networks: The Paradox of Embeddedness." *Administrative Science Quarterly,* 1997, *42,* 35–67.

Uzzi, B. "Embeddedness in the Making of Financial Capital: How Social Relations and Networks Benefit Firms Seeking Financing." *American Sociological Review,* 1999, *64,* 481–505.

Van de Ven, A., Polley, D. E., Garud, R., and Venkataraman, S. *The Innovation Journey.* New York: Oxford University Press, 1999.

Van Etten, P. "Camelot or Common Sense? The Logic Behind the UCSF/ Stanford Merger." *Health Affairs,* 1999, *18*(2), 143–151.

Von Hippel, E. "Cooperation Between Rivals: Informal Know-How Trading." *Research Policy,* 1987, *16,* 291–302.

Vowell, T. H. "Preserving Catholic Identity In Mergers: An Ethical and Canon Law Perspective." *Health Progress*, 1992, *73*(2), 28–33.

Wade, J. B., Swaminathan, A., and Saxon, M. S. "Normative and Resource Flow Consequences of Local Regulations in the American Brewing Industry, 1845–1918." *Administrative Science Quarterly*, 1998, *43*, 905–935.

Wagner, E. H., and others. "The Kaiser Family Foundation Community Health Promotion Grants Program: Findings from an Outcome Evaluation." *Health Services Research*, 2000, *35*(3), 561–589.

Wakefield, J. "Complexity's Business Model." *Scientific American*, January 2001, 31, 34.

Waldrop, M. M. *Complexity: The Emerging Science at the Edge of Order and Chaos.* New York: Simon & Schuster, 1992.

Walker, G., Kogut, B., and Shan, W. "Social Capital, Structural Holes and the Formation of an Industry Network." *Organization Science*, 1997, *8*, 109–125.

Walston, S. L., Kimberly, J. R., and Burns, L. R. "Owned Vertical Integration and Health Care Promise and Performance." *Health Care Management Review*, 1996, *21*, 83–92.

Wasserman, S., and Faust, K. *Social Network Analysis: Methods and Applications.* Cambridge, U.K.: Cambridge University Press, 1994.

Waters, T., and others. "Factors Associated with Physician Involvement in Care Management." *Medical Care*, 2001, *39*(7), 79–91.

Weick, K. E. *The Social Psychology of Organizing*. Reading, Mass.: Addison-Wesley, 1969.

Weick, K. E. "Educational Organizations as Loosely Coupled Systems." *Administrative Science Quarterly*, 1976, *21*, 1–19.

Weick, K. E. *Sensemaking in Organizations*. Thousand Oaks, Calif.: Sage, 1995.

Weiner, B. J., and Alexander, J. A. "Corporate and Philanthropic Models of Hospital Governance: A Taxonomic Evaluation." *Health Services Research*, 1993, *28*(3), 325–355.

Weiner, B. J., and Alexander, J. A. "The Challenges of Governing Public-Private Community Health Partnerships." *Health Care Management Review*, 1998, *23*, 39–55.

Weiner, B. J., and Alexander, J. A. "The Dynamics of Governing Community Health Partnerships: An Empirical Study." *Association for Health Services Research*, 1999, *16*(2), 64.

Weisman, C. S., Khoury, A. J., Cassirer, C., Sharpe, V. A., and Morlock, L. "The Implications of Affiliations Between Catholic and Non-Catholic Health Care Organizations for Availability of Reproductive Health Services." *Women's Health Issues*, 1999, 9(3), 121–134.

Wells, R. "How Institutional Theory Speaks to Change in Organizational Populations." *Health Care Management Review*, 2001, *26*(2), 80–84.

Wennberg, J., and Guttenshon, A. "Variations in Medical Care Among Small Areas." *Science*, 1973, *182*, 1102–1108.

Westney, D. E. "Domestic and Foreign Learning Curves in Managing International Cooperative Strategies." In F. J. Contractor and P. Lorange (eds.), *Cooperative Studies in International Business* (pp. 349–346). Lexington, Mass.: Lexington Books, 1988.

Westphal, J., Gulati, R., and Shortell, S. M. "Customization or Conformity: An Institutional and Network Perspective on the Content and Consequences of TQM Adoption." *Administrative Science Quarterly*, 1997, *39*, 367–390.

Wheatley, M. J. *Leadership and the New Science*. San Francisco: Berrett-Koehler, 1992.

White, K. R. "Catholic Healthcare: Isomorphism or Differentiation?" Doctoral dissertation, Virginia Commonwealth University. Dissertation Abstracts International, 1996.

White, K. R. "Hospitals Sponsored by the Roman Catholic Church: Separate, Equal, and Distinct?" *The Milbank Quarterly*, 2000, *78*(2), 213–239.

White, K. R., and Begun, J. W. "How Does Catholic Hospital Sponsorship Affect Services Provided?" *Inquiry*, 1998/99, *35*, 398–407.

White, K. R., and Ozcan, Y. A. "Church Ownership and Hospital Efficiency." *Hospital & Health Services Administration*, 1996, *41*, 297–310.

White, K. R., Cochran, C. E., and Patel, U. B. "Hospital Provision of End-of-Life Services: Who, What, and Where?" *Medical Care*, 2002, *40*(1), 17–25.

Wholey, D. R., and Burns, L. R. "Tides of Change: The Evolution of Managed Care in the United States." In C. Bird, P. Conrad, and A. Fremont (eds.), *Handbook of Medical Sociology*. Englewood Cliffs, N.J.: Prentice-Hall, 2000.

Wholey, D. R., and Christianson, J. B. "Product Differentiation Among Health Maintenance Organizations: Causes and Consequences of Offering Open-Ended Products." *Inquiry*, 1994, *31*, 25–39.

Wholey, D. R., and Huonker, J. W. "Effects of Generalism and Niche Overlap on Network Linkages Among Youth Service Agencies." *Academy of Management Journal*, 1993, *36*(2), 349–371.

Wholey, D. R., Christianson, J. B., and Sanchez, S. "Organizational Size and Failure Among Health Maintenance Organizations." *American Sociological Review*, 1992, *57*, 829–842.

Wholey, D. R., Christianson, J. B., and Sanchez, S. "Professional Reorganization: The Effect of Physician and Corporate Interests on the Formation of Health Maintenance Organizations." *American Journal of Sociology*, 1993, *99*(1), 175–211.

Wholey, D. R., Engberg, J., and Bryce, C. *The Evolution of Productivity Among Health Maintenance Organizations: 1985 to 1995*. Minneapolis: Division of Health Services Research and Policy, School of Public Health, University of Minnesota, 1999.

Wholey, D. R., Feldman, R., and Christianson, J. B. "The Effect of Market Structure on HMO Premiums." *Journal of Health Economics*, 1995, *14*, 81–105.

Wholey, D. R., Feldman, R., Christianson, J. B., and Engberg, J. "Scale and Scope Economies Among Health Maintenance Organizations." *Journal of Health Economics*, 1996, *15*, 657–684.

Williamson, O. E. *Markets and Hierarchies, Analysis and Antitrust Implications: A Study in the Economics of Internal Organization*. New York: Free Press, 1975.

Williamson, O. E. "Transaction Cost Economics: The Governance of Contractual Relations." *Journal of Law and Economics*, 1979, *22*, 3–61.

Williamson, O. E. "The Economics of Organization: The Transaction Cost Approach." *American Journal of Sociology*, 1981, *87*(3), 548–577.

Williamson, O. E. "Credible Commitments: Using Hostages to Support Exchange." *The American Economic Review*, 1983, *73*(4), 519–540.

Williamson, O. E. "Credible Commitments: Further Remarks." *The American Economic Review*, 1984, *74*(3), 488–490.

Williamson, O. E. *The Economic Institutions of Capitalism*. New York: Free Press, 1985.

Williamson, O. E. *Economic Organizations: Firms, Markets and Policy Control*. New York: University Press, 1986.

Williamson, O. E. *The Mechanisms of Governance*. New York: Oxford University Press, 1996.

Williamson Institute. *Database on Markets and Systems*. Richmond, Va.: Virginia Commonwealth University, 2001.

Wilson, R., and Schindler, T. F. "Tradition in Transition: What It Means to Be a Catholic Healthcare Facility Today." *Health Progress*, 1990, *71*(8), 26–31.

Womak, J. P., Jones, D. T., and Roos, D. *The Machine that Changes the World: The Story of Lean Production*. New York: Rawson Associations, 1990.

Woolf, S. H. "Practice Guidelines: A New Reality on Medicine: Impact on Patient Care." *Annals of Internal Medicine*, 1993, *153*, 2646–2655.

World Bank. *Confronting AIDS: Public Priorities in a Global Epidemic*. Oxford: Oxford University Press, 1997.

Yamagishi, T., Gillmore, M. R., and Cook, K. S. "Network Connections and the Distribution of Power." *Exchange Networks*, 1988, *93*, 4.

Young, D. W., and McCarthy, S. M. *Managing Integrated Delivery Systems*. Chicago: Health Administration Press, 1999.

Young, G. J., Parker, V. A., and Charns, M. P. "Provider Integration and Local Market Conditions: A Contingency Theory Perspective." *Health Care Management Review*, 2001, 26(2), 73–79.

Zajac, E. J., D'Aunno, T. A., and Burns, L. R. "Managing Strategic Alliances." In S. M. Shortell and A. D. Kaluzny (eds.), *Health Care Management: Organization Design and Behavior* (4th edition). Albany, N.Y.: Delmar, 2000.

Zald, M. N., and Denton, P. "From Evangelism to General Service: The Transformation of the YMCA." *Administrative Science Quarterly*, 1963, 8, 214–234.

Zelman, W. A. *Changing Health Care Marketplace: Private Ventures, Public Interests*. San Francisco: Jossey-Bass, 1996.

Ziegenfuss, J. T. "Organizational Barriers to Quality Improvement in Medical and Health Care Organizations." *American College of Medical Quality*, 1991, 6(4), 115–122.

Zimmerman, B. "Strategy, Chaos and Equilibrium: A Case Study of Federal Metals *Inc.*" Unpublished doctoral dissertation, York University, Toronto, Canada, 1991.

Zimmerman, B. "The Inherent Drive Towards Chaos." In P. Lorange, B. Chakravarthy, J. Roos, and A. Van de Ven (eds.), *Implementing Strategic Processes: Change, Learning and Cooperation* (pp. 373–393). London: Blackwell Business, 1993.

Zimmerman, B., and Dooley, K. "Mergers Versus Emergers: Rethinking Structural Change in Health Care Systems." *Emergence*, 2002, 3, 65–82.

Zimmerman, B., Lindberg, C., and Plsek, P. *Edgeware: Insights from Complexity Science for Health Care Leaders*. Irving, Tx: Voluntary Hospital Association, 1998.

Zinn, J. S., Aaronson, W. E., and Rosko, M. D. "Strategic Groups, Performance, and Strategic Response in the Nursing Home Industry." *Health Services Research*, 1994, 29, 187–205.

Zucker, L. G. "The Role of Institutionalization in Cultural Persistence." *American Sociological Review*, 1977, 42, 726–743.

Zucker, L. G. "Production of Trust: Institutional Sources of Economic Structure." *Research in Organizational Behavior*, 1986, 8, 53–111.

Zucker, L. G. "Institutional Theories of Organization." *Annual Review of Sociology*, 1987, 13, 443–464.

Zuckerman, H. S., and Kaluzny, A. "Strategic Alliances in Health Care: The Challenges of Cooperation." *Frontiers of Health Services Management*, 1991, 7(5), 3–23.

Zuckerman, H. S., and others. "Physicians and Organizations: Strange Bedfellows or a Marriage Made in Heaven?" *Frontiers of Health Services Management*, 1998, *14*, 3–34.

Zuckerman, S., Bazzoli, G., Davidoff, A., and LoSasso, A. "How Did Safety-Net Providers Cope in the 1990s?" *Health Affairs*, 2001, *20*(4), 159–168.

Name Index

• •

Subject Index